TREATING PARENT–INFANT RELATIONSHIP PROBLEMS

Treating Parent–Infant Relationship Problems

STRATEGIES FOR INTERVENTION

Edited by

Arnold J. Sameroff
Susan C. McDonough
Katherine L. Rosenblum

THE GUILFORD PRESS
New York   London

© 2004 The Guilford Press
A Division of Guilford Publications, Inc.
72 Spring Street, New York, NY 10012
www.guilford.com

Printed in the United States of America

This book is printed on acid-free paper.

Last digit is print number: 9   8   7   6   5   4   3   2   1

Library of Congress Cataloging-in-Publication Data

Treating parent–infant relationship problems: strategies for intervention / edited
by Arnold J. Sameroff, Susan C. McDonough, Katherine L. Rosenblum.
    p. cm.
Includes bibliographical references and index.
    ISBN 1-57230-957-1 (Hardcover: alk. paper)
    1. Infants—Mental health.   2. Family psychotherapy.   3. Parent and
infant.   4. Infants—Development.   I. Sameroff, Arnold J.   II. McDonough,
Susan C.   III. Rosenblum, Katherine L.
    RJ502.5.T77 2004
    616.89′ 156—dc22

                                                          2003020437

*To the families who moved us to find
ways to understand and help*

ABOUT THE EDITORS

Arnold J. Sameroff, PhD, is a developmental psychologist who specializes in infant mental health. He is a professor in the Department of Psychology at the University of Michigan and Director of the Center for Development and Mental Health at the Center for Human Growth and Development, Ann Arbor, Michigan. Dr. Sameroff's theoretical and empirical writings have been a foundation for the field of developmental psychopathology. He is currently President of the International Society on Infant Studies.

Susan C. McDonough, PhD, MSW, is a social worker who specializes in treating relationship problems of parents and infants with special needs. She is an associate research scientist in the School of Social Work and the Center for Human Growth and Development at the University of Michigan. Dr. McDonough directs the University of Michigan Post-Graduate Certificate Training Program in Clinical Work with Infants, Toddlers and Their Families and is an international consultant for infant and family mental health programs.

Katherine L. Rosenblum, PhD, is a clinical and developmental psychologist who specializes in research on parents' representations of their infants and on infant emotional development. She is a research investigator at the Center for Human Growth and Development at the University of Michigan. Dr. Rosenblum has taught the clinical applications of attachment research to multidisciplinary groups at the University of Michigan and the University of Vienna.

CONTRIBUTORS

Nadia Bruschweiler-Stern, MD, Centre Brazelton Suisse, Clinique des Grangettes, Geneva, Switzerland

Antoinette Corboz-Warnery, MD, Centre d'Etude de la Famille, Université de Lausanne, Prilly, Switzerland

Winnie Dunn, PhD, OTR, FAOTA, Department of Occupational Therapy Education, University of Kansas Medical Center, Kansas City, Kansas

Byron Egeland, PhD, Institute of Child Development, University of Minnesota, Minneapolis, Minnesota

Robert N. Emde, MD, Department of Psychiatry, University of Colorado Health Sciences Center, Denver, Colorado

Martha Farrell Erickson, PhD, Children, Youth and Family Consortium, University of Minnesota, Minneapolis, Minesota

Kevin D. Everhart, PhD, Department of Psychiatry, University of Colorado Health Sciences Center, Denver, Colorado

Elisabeth Fivaz-Depeursinge, PhD, Centre d'Etude de la Famille, Université de Lausanne, Prilly, Switzerland

Miri Keren, MD, Infant Mental Health Unit, Geha Mental Health Center, Petach-Tikvah, Israel; Sackler Medical School, Tel Aviv University, Tel Aviv, Israel

Julie A. Larrieu, PhD, Department of Psychiatry and Neurology, Institute of Infant and Early Childhood Mental Health, Tulane University Health Sciences Center, New Orleans, Louisiana

Alicia F. Lieberman, PhD, Department of Psychiatry, University of California–San Francisco; Child Trauma Research Project, San Francisco General Hospital, San Francisco, California

Susan C. McDonough, PhD, MSW, Center for Human Growth and Development, University of Michigan, Ann Arbor, Michigan

Katherine L. Rosenblum, PhD, Center for Human Growth and Development, University of Michigan, Ann Arbor, Michigan

Arnold J. Sameroff, PhD, Center for Human Growth and Development and Department of Psychology, University of Michigan, Ann Arbor, Michigan

Daniel N. Stern, MD, Department of Psychology, University of Geneva, Geneva, Switzerland; Department of Psychiatry, Cornell Medical School, New York, New York

Brian K. Wise, MD, Department of Psychiatry, University of Colorado Health Sciences Center, Denver, Colorado

Charles H. Zeanah, MD, Department of Psychiatry and Neurology, Institute of Infant and Early Childhood Mental Health, Tulane University Health Sciences Center, New Orleans, Louisiana

ACKNOWLEDGMENTS

To produce a book on therapies for infants and their parents requires a collaboration between editors, contributors, and funders. We wish to acknowledge the generosity of the chapter authors in this volume with both their time and creative energies. The roots of this book are in a research group convened by Robert Emde in 1984 at the Center for Advanced Study in the Behavioral Sciences in Stanford, California. That group produced a book in 1989 that took the position that, during infancy, understanding relationships was a primary requirement for understanding infant mental health. It seemed a logical extension to believe that improving relationships was the primary route to improving infant mental health. To examine this assumption, the editors of the current volume convened a group of experts in therapy with infants and families in Ann Arbor, Michigan, in the spring of 2001. The group included many of the participants from the earlier Stanford effort—Robert Emde, Thomas Anders, Daniel Stern, and Arnold Sameroff—who provided continuity with the original conceptualization of early relationship issues. The resulting integration of theory and practice is the core of this book. All this would not have happened, however, without financial support for convening the meeting and creating a product. For this, we owe gratitude to the Center for Human Growth and Development at the University of Michigan, the National Institute of Mental Health, and especially Irving Harris. Through his foundation and personal efforts, Irving Harris has been a constant supporter of and stimulus to the field of early mental health, helping us in both our Stanford and Ann Arbor efforts.

ARNOLD J. SAMEROFF
SUSAN C. MCDONOUGH
KATHERINE L. ROSENBLUM

CONTENTS

PART III

CODA

PART I

THEMES

CHAPTER 1

PORTS OF ENTRY AND THE DYNAMICS OF MOTHER–INFANT INTERVENTIONS

Arnold J. Sameroff

This book is about relationship problems, but more broadly it is about infant mental health. There are still many for whom the topic of infant mental health seems ridiculous. What would lead someone to believe that a baby could have a mental health problem? Infants are seen as too young to have such troubles or, if early problems do exist, they are believed to be physical ones that can be dealt with by physicians. This view is being replaced as modern understanding of human development has discovered much greater capacities for feeling and knowing in babies than were thought possible only a generation ago when not only parents but also pediatricians believed that newborns could not see and hear. But more importantly, these infant abilities are expressed in a context. Early social and emotional problems are inextricably connected to the relationship between babies and their caregivers. This topic was fully explored in a pioneering book edited by Sameroff and Emde (1989) where early relationships were given clinical, empirical, and theoretical reality.

Treating early relationship problems is important from two aspects, the relief of current suffering and the prevention of long-term consequences. But both of these aspects raise complex questions. In the current situation, who is suffering? And with respect to the future, who will be carrying the seeds of later happiness or unrest, the child or the care-givers? Among adult clients the sufferer is generally clear; it is the pa-tient who self-refers for the alleviation of some psychological distress. Treatment is generally directed, for better or worse, at the self-identified patient. Increasingly the importance of treating relationships is being recognized even for adult psychotherapies. In the case of children, espe-cially young ones, the referral comes from others, most often the par-ents. It is others who are concerned that a child is too sad, too active, or too oppositional. It is others who are suffering and need relief. In this light infant mental health problems are always relational, they are always caregiver–child mental health problems. Stern (see Chapter 2, this vol-ume) has identified this as the new "prototypic patient" for clinical atten-tion.

Even when parents may not be sufficiently concerned or knowl-edgeable about their infant's psychological health to seek help, others in the child's world may be. For example, during the newborn period a nurse may become concerned with the effects of a mother's depression and make a psychiatric referral (see Bruschweiler-Stern, Chapter 8, this volume). In cases of abuse or neglect, neither the child nor the parent self-refers. It is the legal system that makes that determination and has the additional task of getting the parent to see that there is a problem in the caregiver–child relationship. The complicated nesting of infant and maltreating caregivers in a therapeutic milieu is described by Larrieu and Zeanah (see Chapter 10, this volume), with protective services, the judicial system, lawyers, biological parents, and foster parents all consid-ered as significant influences on the child's welfare.

More commonly, infant mental health concerns are raised in the context of pediatric appointments in which parents express anxiety about an infant's behavior. Their worries typically relate to functional regulation problems around issues of excessive crying, sleeping, or feed-ing. If the problem has a physiological basis, it is typically treated in the medical context. If not, the pediatrician or nurse practitioner makes ac-tive or passive recommendations, and often this is sufficient. Active rec-ommendations would be suggestions that the parents' change their behavior, such as letting infants go to sleep in their crib instead of in a parent's arms. Passive recommendations would be reassurances that the child's behavior was in the normal range and that the situation would improve over time with no change in parents' behavior. These three in-terventions—physiological, active, and passive—fit into categories of remediation, redefinition, and reeducation (Sameroff, 1987; Sameroff & Fiese, 2000) that will be more fully explored below.

However, there are parents for whom these strategies are not enough, either because of special problems in the child, in the parents' personality, or in the resources available to support their caregiving efforts. In these cases further referrals become necessary either by the primary care physician or the parents themselves. The variety of treatments available for such referrals is the topic of this book. The range of services available can be delivered by psychologists, psychiatrists, social workers, occupational therapists, physical therapists, or other infant mental health specialists, each with a different slant on how best to help the patient. With these different professional orientations come different perspectives on who the "real" patient is and what is the best way of affecting the system.

THE REAL PATIENT

The title of our book makes it clear who—or rather *what*—we believe the real patient is. It is the parent–infant relationship. As Sameroff and Emde (1989, p. 221) remind us, "Human existence is social existence." Infants' physical existence is tied to the care provided by other human beings. The same can be said for their psychological existence. In the first book to have the words "infant psychiatry" in its title, Rexford, Sander, and Shapiro (1976) observed that infants and their caregivers are part of an interactive and regulative system, mutually influencing and regulating each other. Sameroff and Emde (1989) focused on the issue of diagnosis. They acknowledged that infants are individuals and make contributions to the behavior of their caregivers, but argued further that that individuality must be considered in context and that diagnosis must include those around the infant as well. From this initial focus on diagnosis of infants in relationships, it follows that the treatment of infants must also be relationship oriented.

A text on the treatment of relationship problems in early childhood must be situated in an understanding of infant development. At one extreme are those who believe that a child's future is determined by early behavior. Consequently making sure that the infant has positive mental health is important for everything that will follow. At the other extreme are those who believe that infancy is a passing period that will have little relation to what follows (Lewis, 1997). In this view the foundation of later mental health will be found in later stages of development, with each period's good and bad experiences determining concurrent mental health. In the first view infancy is the most crucial period of development, and in the second view it is only of transient interest. A third view takes elements from both perspectives and sees each developmental stage as laying a foundation for the next. If the foundation is one of competence, the following stage will proceed more easily than if the foundation is problematic, but the outcome of each following stage will be a product of not only what the child brings to the situation or only what is experienced from caregivers but of the interplay between these two domains (Sameroff & Chandler, 1975).

Identification of the real patient will depend on what is believed to be the source of current problems. If one cannot separate the infant from the caregiving context, then the patient must be the relationship. But, as we shall see, repairing a relationship can be accomplished in many different ways. Because relationships are dynamically interacting systems, changing parts of the relationship should affect the totality of the relationship and, most importantly for our interests, the current and future mental health of the child.

THE TRANSACTIONAL MODEL

Planning effective interventions requires a sophisticated view of environmental action that includes attention to many factors. A developmental frame that has been useful for understanding and prescribing treatment options is the transactional model (Sameroff & Chandler, 1975). In this approach how a child turns out is neither a function of the infant alone nor of experience alone. Successful development is a product of the combination of an individual and his or her experience. Although we must know the experiences available to the infant, we cannot lose sight of the important role individual differences in the child play in terms of what the child elicits from the environment and what the child is able to take from the environment.

The birth of an infant is a separation that appears to produce an independent individual who will mature into a psychological adult. This physical independence from other family members gives rise to the idea that there is a psychological independence so that whatever levels of achievement and health the child attains can be attributed to personal resources. Dramatic advances in molecular biology have fostered a view that genes play deterministic roles in the growth process. Such a perception leads to a maturational view of development in which there is an unfolding of intrinsic characteristics. From this perspective individual differences in intelligence or personality or more categorical differences such as retardation or mental disorder can be explained by differences in initial circumstances, the genetic endowment of the individual. But the study of genes has led to the equally dramatic biological advances demonstrating the important role of context in gene expression. Each somatic cell of the body has the same genes, yet each cell is different because of different experiences and even relationships with other cells. Similarly, by analogy, whatever characteristics the infant may have been born with, in different families with different sets of experiences the infant would have developed differently.

Progress within molecular biology has shown the necessity of studying multiple interacting systems if the goal is to understand the processes of development. The path from the fertilized egg to the newborn infant is one of the most complex phenomena in biology. Earlier misconceptions that perinatal brain development reflects rigidly deterministic genetic programs are being replaced by current knowledge that experience has a critical role in the development of the infant's brain. Moreover, neural plasticity can be found even in human adults (Nelson & Bloom, 1997). Positive or negative life experiences can alter both the structure and the function of the brain. This intimate relation between the developing organism and experience is extended into the behavioral domain where a transactional model is used to understand cognitive and social–emotional functioning during infancy. Fox, Calkins, and Bell (1994) compared three models of development: an insult model, where early brain deviations lead to later problems; an environmental model, where the brain is seen as completely plastic; and a transactional model, where genetic programs for developmental processes interact with environmental modifiers. They found much evidence for brain plasticity in response to new experiences but constrained by the developmental status of the nervous system, fitting the transactional model. These studies of neurobiology and behavior support a view of mutual influence between the child and the caregiving context.

Within this transactional model the development of the child is seen as a product of the continuous dynamic interactions of the child and the experience provided by his or her family and social context (see Figure 1.1). There is an equal emphasis placed on the effects of the child and of the environment. The experiences provided by the environment are not

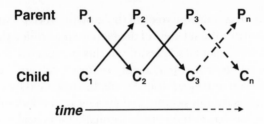

FIGURE 1.1. Transactional process with reciprocal effects between the child and the parent across time.

viewed as independent of the child. The child may have been a strong determinant of current experiences, but developmental outcomes cannot be systematically described without an analysis of the effects of the environment on the child.

Before the recent ascendance of genetic explanations, there were many retrospective studies reporting that children's cognitive and social–emotional difficulties were the result of birth complications. But when later researchers prospectively followed the development of infants with perinatal problems they found that most of them had perfectly normal developmental outcomes. This is not to say that some children with birth complications, especially severe anomalies, did not end up with developmental disabilities but so did some children without birth complications. The research seemed to support the idea that children with birth complications ended up with later developmental problems, not because of changes in the brain but because of the negative impact such children had on their caregivers. An example of such a process can be seen in Figure 1.2.

A complicated childbirth may have made an otherwise calm mother somewhat anxious. Her anxiety during the first months of the child's life may have caused her to be uncertain and less appropriate in her interactions with the child. In response to such inconsistency the infant may have developed some irregularities in feeding and sleeping patterns that give the appearance of a difficult temperament. This difficult temperament decreases parenting pleasure so the mother spends less time with her child. If she or other caregivers are not actively interacting with the child, and especially not talking to the infant, the child may score poorly on later preschool language tests and be less socially mature.

What determined the poor outcome in this example? Was the poor verbal performance caused by the complicated childbirth, the mother's anxiety, the child's difficult temperament, or the mother's avoidance of verbal and social interaction? If one were to design an intervention program for this family, where would it be directed? The most proximal cause is the mother's avoidance of the child, yet one can see that such a view would oversimplify a complex developmental sequence. Would treatment be directed at eliminating the child's difficult temperament or at changing the mother's reaction, or at providing alternative sources of verbal stimulation for the child? Each of these would eliminate a potential dysfunction at some point in the developmental system.

This series of transactions is an example of how developmental achievements are rarely sole consequences of immediate causes and even more rarely sole consequences of earlier events. Not only is the causal chain between perinatal problems and early childhood problems extended over time, but it is also embedded in an interpretive framework. The mother's anxiety is based on an interpretation of the meaning of a complicated childbirth, and her avoidance is based on an interpretation of the meaning of the child's irregular feeding and sleeping patterns. To understand the effects of interventions on the way parents behave toward their infants, there is a need to understand this interpretive framework.

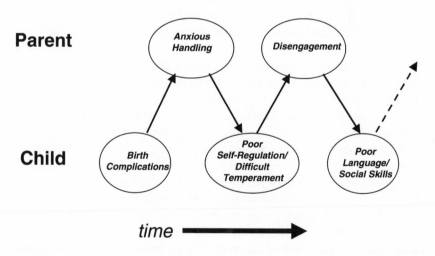

FIGURE 1.2. Transactional process linking perinatal complications and preschool language delays.

THE REPRESENTED AND PRACTICING FAMILY

In addition to the developmental significance of the behavior of the infant and the caregivers clinicians must attend to the meaning system which parents use to understand their children. The influence of families may be understood through the two ways in which they organize experiences: first, through the beliefs that they hold, their family representations; second, through the ways in which they behave toward each other, their family practices (Reiss, 1989; Sameroff & Fiese, 2000).

The *represented family* highlights the internal representation of relationships and how working memories provide a sense of stability. Working models of relationships develop within the context of the family are retained in memory and guide the individual's behavior over time. To study this represented family, we must explore how families impart values and make sense of personal experiences. One dimension of these representations are family narratives that deal with how the family makes sense of its world, its relationships, and its rules of interaction. Fiese et al. (1999) document how such family meaning making is associated with adaptation to illness, alcoholism, and the identity formation of adolescent offspring.

The *practicing family*, in contrast, stabilizes and regulates family members through observable interaction. The interaction patterns are repetitive and serve to provide a sense of family coherence and identity. Family life resides not only in the minds of individuals but is evident in the observed coordinated practices of the group (Grych & Fincham, 1990; Reiss, 1981).

From a transactional perspective, the practicing and represented family both organize behavior across time and both affect each other. Family practices come to have meaning and are translated into the symbolic aspect of the represented family. The represented family, in turn, may affect how the family members regulate and interpret their practices. As an example, consider negative emotion at the dinner table for a parent who experienced abuse and neglect as a child. Because of his or her history the parent does not expect relationships to be rewarding and has created a representation of family as unfulfilling and disappointing (Cicchetti & Toth, 1995). Negative affect at the dinner table confirms the parent's expectation for unrewarding family interactions in the present. Exposure to negative affect may then lead to acting-out behaviors by the children (Katz & Gottman, 1993). This then reinforces the parent in the belief that he or she cannot expect offspring to behave. A family story is created labeling the children as "bad" and uncontrollable. This transactional process results in escalation of problem behavior and an entrench-ment of beliefs that make it more difficult to alter maladaptive patterns of interaction. The storied representation of family behavior becomes tainted with expectations for unfulfilling family relationships confirmed in the directly observable interaction among family members (Fiese & Marjinsky, 1999).

As with other transactional systems there is no direct causal link be-tween parental expectations for unrewarding relationships and child problem behavior. The relation is mediated by a chain of reciprocal events that could lead to many other outcomes with appropriate inter-ventions. Changing parental behavior at dinnertime, negative expecta-tions of the child, or family stories may significantly alter the outcome for the child. A transactional understanding of such processes helps the therapist to identify both problematic developmental processes and po-tential interventions.

SELF-REGULATION AND OTHER-REGULATION

Understanding how infants and their parents influence each other over time is a necessary prologue to the understanding of developmental problems and recommendations for appropriate treatment. Once we have an overview of the complexity of the systems involved, we can turn to the search for nodal points at which intervention strategies can be di-rected. These points will be found in the interfaces among the child, the family, and the cultural systems.

Despite a tendency to see infants as objects existing in a physical world where their talents unfold in some maturational sequence, the re-ality is that from conception the infant is embedded in relationships with others who provide the nutrition for both physical and psychological growth. The developmental changes in this relationship between indi-vidual and context can be represented as an expanding cone (see Figure 1.3). The balance between other-regulation and self-regulation shifts as the child is able to take on more and more responsibility for his or her own well-being.

At birth the infant could not survive without the environment pro-viding nutrition and warmth. To enhance the child's social–emotional self-regulation, the parenting role is to provide a model by helping to quiet the infant when he or she is overaroused and to stimulate the in-fant when he or she is underaroused. Later the child is able to find a blanket when cold and go to the refrigerator when hungry, although

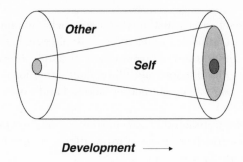

Development ⟶

FIGURE 1.3. Changing balance between other-regulation and self-regulation as a child develops into an adult.

someone else still has to buy the clothing and food for the family. Eventually the child reaches adulthood and can become part of the other-regulation of a new infant, beginning the next generation. Parents too are regulated, at one level by the laws and customs of their society, but also by the relationships in which they are involved. An interesting intervention aspect of this is regulation of the mother during pregnancy and then of the mother and infant after delivery provided by the doula program. A doula is a professional who provides emotional, physical, and informational support to the family just before, during, and just after delivery (Kennell, Klaus, McGrath, Robertson, & Hinkley, 1991).

The importance of parent characteristics relative to child characteristics during early childhood is because of the large asymmetry between self-regulation and other-regulation. As development progresses the asymmetry will become more balanced, and then a new asymmetry will emerge during adolescence with the burgeoning of adult capacities for thought and action. As a consequence intervening with the family rather than the infant alone is the most efficacious therapeutic strategy during infancy and toddlerhood.

TARGETING INTERVENTION EFFORTS

A sensitivity to the complexities of child development has encouraged the implementation of intervention strategies to include multiple members of the child's family (see Fivaz-Depeursinge, Corboz-Warnery, & Keren, Chapter 6, this volume), as well as multiple disciplines concerned with early childhood (see Larrieu & Zeanah, Chapter 10, this volume). Increasingly, early intervention programs designed today are based on a team approach that addresses the many facets of childhood problems (see Egeland & Erickson, Chapter 9, this volume). As it becomes less acceptable to focus on isolated aspects of developmental disorders, the total environmental context of the child needs to be considered (Sameroff, 1995). Once the multiple determinants associated with childhood problems are recognized, a more targeted approach to implementing intervention is in order, based on the specific determinants identified in a specific situation.

A frequent problem in planning treatment is deciding where to concentrate therapeutic efforts—what has been called the "port of entry" (Stern, 1995). Problem areas may include individual, family, community, and cultural factors, but economic and personnel limitations preclude global interventions across all these systems. A careful analysis of the involved systems for a particular family is necessary to define what may be the most effective avenue and form of therapy. A basic point that emerges from this perspective is that there will never be a single intervention strategy that will solve all developmental problems. Cost-effectiveness will be found in the individuation of programs that are targeted at the relevant nodal points for a specific child in a specific family in a specific social context.

PORTS OF ENTRY I: THE THREE R'S OF INTERVENTION

The transactional model has implications for the treatment of relationship problems, particularly for identifying targets and strategies of intervention. The nonlinear premise that continuity in individual behavior is a systems property rather than a characteristic of individuals provides a rationale for an expanded focus of intervention efforts. In the model there is an emphasis on the multidirectionality of change while pinpointing regulatory sources that mediate change. By examining the strengths and weaknesses of the childrearing system, categories of targets can be identified that minimize the necessary scope of the intervention while maximizing cost-effectiveness. In some cases small alterations in child behavior may be all that is necessary to reestablish a well-regulated developmental system. In other cases, changes in the parents' perception of the child may be the most strategic intervention. In a third category are cases that require improvements in the parents' ability to take care of the child. These intervention categories have been labeled *remediation*, *redefinition*, and *reeducation*, respectively, or the "three R's" of intervention (Sameroff, 1987; Sameroff & Fiese, 1990).

An abstraction of the transactional model that focuses on the three R's of early treatment can be seen in Figure 1.4. In the model, development is an iterative process between child and parent. The baby by its activity or appearance stimulates the parent, who makes an interpretation and then responds in turn. For example, a baby's smile elicits a good feeling in the parent, who then reciprocates by smiling back, speaking warmly to the infant or cuddling. Problems arise when one of these links produces a maladaptive or negative response. In our earlier transactional example a crying baby leads to anxiety in the parent, who avoids the infant. The three R's are directed at creating a happier parental reaction and an improved developmental outcome.

Remediation changes the way the child behaves toward the parent. For example, in cases where children present with known organic disorders, intervention may be directed primarily toward remediating biological dysregulations. Such an improvement in the child's physical status will better enable him or her to elicit caregiving from the parents. *Redefinition* changes the way the parent interprets the child's behavior. Attributions to the child of difficulty or willfulness may deter a parent from positive interactions. As the parent is refocused on other, more acceptable attributes of the child, positive engagement may be facilitated. *Reeducation* changes the way the parent behaves toward the child. Providing training in positioning or stimulating techniques for parents of developmentally delayed children is an example of this form of intervention. Examples of these strategies will be found in the ensuing chapters.

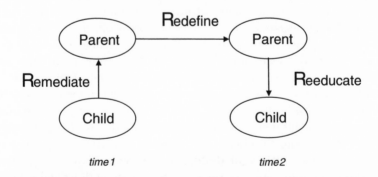

FIGURE 1.4. The three R's of treatment within a transactional model.

Remediation

The strategy of remediation is the class of intervention techniques designed to change the child, with eventual changes occurring in the parent, depicted by the upward arrow in Figure 1.4. Remediation is not aimed at changing the childrearing capacity of the family. The intervention goal is to fit the child to preexisting caregiving competencies that are already adequate if the child behaves as expected. Remediation is typically implemented outside the family system by a professional whose goal is to change an identifiable condition in the child. Once the child's condition has been altered, intervention is complete.

The most clear-cut examples of remediation are those in which there are possibilities for structural repair of a biological condition, for example, short-term medical interventions such as nasogastric feedings for underweight infants. The child is presented to the parents as cured, and they proceed to engage in the normative childrearing appropriate to a healthy infant. Such direct solutions are excellent interventions for a number of early problems, but they occasionally involve controversial applications. The surgical alteration of the appearance of children with Down syndrome would be such a questionable procedure (Pueschel, 1984). In this example, the transactional hypothesis is the basis for the surgeon's belief that if the child looked more like a nonhandicapped child, he or she would be treated more like a nonhandicapped child and consequently would have a developmental outcome more like a nonhandicapped child. Another questionable practice is the medication of infants with diphenhydramine (Benadryl) or young children with fluoxetine (Prozac) equivalents for temperament problems. More accepted is the large number of children given drugs for hyperactivity where, rather than have parents or teachers adapt to the individuality of the child, the child is changed to fit in with existing parent and teacher expectations and behavior.

According to the principles of the transactional model being presented here, there are circumstances where interventions directed toward the child alone may result in changes in the parent. In cases where the child's dysfunction is easily identified and successful intervention techniques are available, remediation of the child may lead to adaptive changes in the parent's representations and responses.

The case of treating malnutrition in infancy highlights how remediation with the child may influence the parents' behavior. Craviotto and DeLicardie (1979) found that the behavioral effects of malnutrition were most prevalent in families where mothers were more traditionally passive in their child care and provided little stimulation to their children. Malnourished infants, on their part, have less energy to smile and vocalize, behaviors that serve to elicit positive parental responses. Moreover, where malnutrition is a social problem, the parents themselves have less energy. In an effort to change this dynamic Barrett, Radke-Yarrow, and Klein (1982) gave a caloric supplementation to malnourished children. The infants who received the nutritional supplements demonstrated greater social responsiveness, more expression of affect, greater interest in the environment, and higher activity at school age. Nutritional supplements increased the infants' energy level, which led to increases in their school-age social, emotional, and intellectual competence. Owing to this increase in their energy level, the nourished infants were better able to participate in the family and were better able to elicit a wide range of behaviors from their parents, including feeding. Their parents, by providing more socially responsive stimulation, facilitated their children's interpersonal behavior. Pollitt et al. (1993) enlarged this developmental model to posit that the effects of malnutrition, especially for low socioeconomic groups, contribute to the formation of styles of social-emotional and behavioral interactions between the malnourished infant and the environment that slow cognitive development.

Remediation is an intervention aimed at changing the child, with the expectation that the child will become a more responsive interaction partner. In this regard, remediation allows the child to be more acceptable to the family. Remediation is indicated when there is a reasonable expectation that the child's condition can be altered and the family and cultural code do not prevent implementation of the intervention. Remediation is most effective when there is a time-limited intervention aimed at the child with the support and assurance that the family can take over routine caregiving activities once the intervention is complete. There are instances, however, where the infant's appearance or behavior cannot be changed or the parents have other problems and a second strategy might be appropriate—the strategy of redefinition.

Redefinition

Redefinition as an intervention strategy is indicated when existing family representations do not fit with the child's behavior (Sameroff & Fiese, 1990). Redefinition is represented by the horizontal arrow in Figure 1.4, linking the infant's input with the parents' output. Redefinition strategies are directed primarily toward the facilitation of more optimal parenting through an alteration in parents' beliefs and expectations. These are warranted when the parents have defined the child as abnormal and are unable or unwilling to provide normal caregiving. Difficulties in caregiving may arise from a variety of sources including a failure of parents to adapt to a disabling condition in the child, failure of the parents to distinguish between their emotional reactions to the child and the child's actual behavior, and maladaptive patterns of care that extend across generations (Sameroff & Fiese, 2000). Examples of the first kind of problem are parents who disqualify themselves as adequate caregivers by automatically translating a child's physical or mental handicap into a condition that can only be treated by professionals, as in the case of physical anomalies or very-low-birthweight (VLBW) babies. Examples of the second kind are parents who become disenchanted with child-rearing because they find a poor fit between their expectations of child behavior and the child's actual performance as in the case of excessive crying. The third situation is marked by caregiving that is constrained by childhood experiences of the parents that prevent them from distinguishing current caregiving demands from their past experiences.

In the case of an atypical condition in the child, redefinition interventions are directed toward normalizing the parents' reactions to their child. An infant born with Down syndrome, for example, may be defined as abnormal because of differences in appearance or developmental pace or merely the label itself, leading the parents to believe that they are incapable of rearing such a child. Redefinition would be directed toward emphasizing to the parents the normal aspects of the child's behavior in order to facilitate caregiving behaviors that are in the parents' repertoire. Such normal child behaviors would include communication efforts like eye contact and emotional responsivity like smiling and laughing.

When a deviant condition in the child is not identified, redefinition interventions directed toward parents focus on the their misperceptions of the child. Redefinition is directed toward changing interactions in the context of immediate experience rather than past events. Low-birthweight (LBW) infants are often sent home in a biologically vulnerable state. Parents may be called upon to continue massage techniques provided in the neonatal intensive care unit, monitor the child's sleep patterns, and adjust feeding practices to meet the needs of their small infant. Whereas parents may feel competent to care for a healthy infant, they may feel overwhelmed by the demands of caring for a vulnerable LBW infant. In this instance the parents define caregiving as an extraor-

dinary experience that they are unable to manage. Redefinition interventions may be aimed at normalizing the care of the infant and decreasing the emphasis on "special care" the child demands. Highlighting the
normal developmental tasks of sleeping, eating, and play would redefine
the parents' role as one that is familiar and consistent with the parents'
image of caregiving. Once the parent considers the normative aspect of
raising an LBW infant, they may be able to proceed with their intuitive
parenting (Barnard, Morisset, & Spieker, 1993; Papousek & Papousek,
1987).

Occasionally, parents are unresponsive to programs aimed at redefining the child's behavior because of beliefs that are entrenched across
generations. The recent work of attachment researchers has demonstrated that current caregiving activities are framed in light of the
parent's relationship with their caregivers (Main & Goldwyn, 1984).
Mothers whose working models of attachment are tempered by inconsistent, unreliable, and/or abusive relationships are more likely to form insecure attachments with their children. The current relationship between the mother and the child is proposed to be a partial reenactment
of the mother's relationship with her mother and current behavior is
guided by generational patterns of relating. Attachment relationships are
malleable, however, and interventions aimed at redefining the attachment relationship have been found to be effective in a sample of high-
risk infants and their mothers. Lieberman, Weston, and Pawl (1991) conducted infant–parent psychotherapy sessions with mothers and infants
who had been classified as anxiously attached. Anxious attachments are
overrepresented in LBW infants and characterized by inconsistent parental response to infant distress and a resistance on the part of the infant to be soothed by familiar caregivers (Easterbrooks, 1989; Wille,
1991). Infant–parent psychotherapy aimed at redefining the current
caregiving relationship improved mother's responsiveness to her child's
signals and increased active engagement between mother and child. Redefinition interventions are aimed at distinguishing the current relationship between the mother and the child from the mother's own upbringing.

Fraiberg, Adelson, and Shapiro (1975) were pioneers in describing
how past experiences of being parented influence current caretaking behaviors. As parents engage in routine caretaking activities with their
children, past experiences of their own childhoods are recalled. Individuals who experienced nurturant parenting recall these positive experiences as they parent their own children. However, individuals who have
experienced inadequate parenting often repeat the same nonoptimal in-

teractions. Mothers of "failure-to-thrive" infants often recount their own upbringing as inadequate in nurturance (Altemeir, O'Connor, Sherrod, & Vietze, 1985). In such cases, interventions may be directed to the parents' memories of past experiences. Redefining the baby as the mother's own, rather than as a symbol of past parenting experiences, has been effective in the treatment of infants failing to thrive (Chatoor, Dickson, Schaeffer, & Egan, 1985).

The mother, the father, or the entire family may be the source of inappropriate attributions concerning the infant. In fact, recognizing how a family may contribute to dysfunctions in the child is central to adapting the family's representations to fit the child's behavior. It is possible to redefine the current relationship in order that more sensitive forms of interaction may be maintained. Mothers who feel that their current caregiving interactions will be appreciated are more likely to engage in positive and reciprocal interactions than mothers who believe that their child is unlikely to be a source of reward and positive esteem.

Redefinition interventions are aimed at altering parents' beliefs and expectations about their child. If beliefs that the child is deviant are changed, then normative caregiving can begin or resume. The parents are freed to use the skills that are already in their repertoire. There are cases, however, where the parents do not have requisite skills or knowledge base for effective parenting. In this case reeducation is indicated.

Reeducation

Reeducation refers to teaching parents how to raise their children and is represented by the downward arrow in Figure 1.4. It is directed toward parents who do not have the knowledge or experience to positively regulate their child's development. Reeducation is typically aimed at families and individuals who are considered at risk due to environmental conditions or characteristics of the parents, for example, teenage mothers or alcoholic parents. Public health initiatives have been used on occasion to reeducate large segments of society to change their caregiving behaviors. Instructional materials such as *Keys to Caregiving* (Spietz, Johnson-Crowley, Sumner, & Barnard, 1990) are aimed at instructing parents as to what to expect from infants at different ages in terms of their behaviors, cues, state modulation, and feeding interactions.

The majority of reeducation efforts are directed toward the family or individual parent and serve to provide information about specific caregiving skills. The Infant Health and Development Program (IHDP; 1990) was one such reeducation intervention aimed at enhancing the development of LBW and VLBW infants. This multisite clinical trial combined family and home-based educational interventions with child-focused center interventions, but for the purposes of illustrating reeducation we will limit our discussion to the home-based educational component. Home visits over a 3-year period provided parents with information on child development, instruction in the use of age-appropriate games, and family support for identified problems. Intervention effects improved the quality of maternal assistance, the child's persistence and enthusiasm, and dyadic mutuality in a laboratory setting (Spiker, Ferguson, & Brooks-Gunn, 1993). Such parent support components are characteristics of the STEEP program (i.e., Steps Toward Effective, Enjoyable Parenting; see Egeland & Erickson, Chapter 9, this volume) among whose goals are to encourage sensitive, predictable parental responses to the baby's cues and signals and to facilitate the parent in efforts to create a home environment that is safe, predictable, and conducive to optimal child development.

In contrast to community-centered reeducation interventions are interventions tailored to meet the needs of individual families. McDonough (2000; see also Chapter 4, this volume) describes the use of feedback to parents while viewing videotapes of family interactions to guide positive family interactions in an Interaction Guidance (IG) program. The feedback portion of the IG session serves to facilitate the parents' understanding of child development and to identify interactive behaviors that are reinforcing to the parents as well as patterns of interaction that lead to less enjoyable exchanges. The IG treatment approach focuses on enhancing existing adaptive patterns of interaction and builds on the family's strengths.

Such reeducation therapies are typically aimed at the practices of the family. These interventions focus on the immediate and momentary exchanges between the parent and the child that are associated with optimal development. It is assumed that once parents have the requisite knowledge about their child's behavior, caregiving will proceed to facilitate development in accord with the cultural code.

Specificity of Interventions

Remediation, redefinition, and reeducation have been described as ports of entry for targeting specific aspects of the transactional process. However, development is part of a system that includes influences from multiple aspects of the cultural, family, and parental context. An examination of instances where interventions do not work or are more or less effective points to how choosing a form of intervention needs to be aligned with resources and characteristics of individual families and children. Educational interventions may be more effective for some mothers than for others. Spiker et al. (1993) propose that there are likely to be at least two types of mothers involved in early intervention programs: those who provide inadequate affective and instructional support to their children, and those who lack instructional skills but possess positive affective qualities. In the first case reeducation would not be sufficient and would warrant redefinition interventions to alter the parents' affective response to their children. In the same regard, redefinition efforts aimed at reframing current interactions between the parent and the child may stimulate childhood experiences and require a more historical consideration of caregiving (Lieberman & Pawl, 1993).

Spillover effects from one area of functioning to another, such as between family practices and family representations, have been documented in therapeutic interventions with families (Zuckerman, Kaplan-Sanoff, Parker, & Young, 1997). For example, it would be difficult to imagine that increasing the satisfaction of parents in their interactions with their infant through reeducation would not also redefine their attitudes and beliefs about the child. Stern (see Chapter 2, this volume) argues that intervention through any port of entry affects the whole system, emphasizing that infants and parenting figures are inextricably connected.

When one is faced with limited resources for early intervention programs it is beneficial to consider the most cost-effective form of intervention that would affect multiple domains of adaptation. If education efforts aimed at parents also influence how they interact with their children and the beliefs they hold about development, then focused education programs may be offered to large groups of parents. However, if the parents are unable to make use of the educational efforts because of a past history of poor caregiving or lack of social support, more intensive redefinition programs might well be warranted. The three forms of intervention can be placed in a transactional diagnosis scheme.

Transactional Diagnosis

We have argued that it may be helpful to focus intervention efforts according to problem identification. Such categorization would not only lead to better program design but to better evaluation models and research designs as well. In the case of remediation, the child is defined as developmentally atypical and interventions would be necessary with any parent. The focus of remediation is to change the child, and there is little alteration directed at the parents. Redefinition interventions are pre-scribed when the parents' relationship with the child inhibits the child's normal growth and development. Treatment is necessary because of the particular maladapted relationship between the parent and the child and does require changes in the parents (most notably their representations). In the case of reeducation, the parent has been identified as being defi-cient in certain skills or knowledge and the child's condition may not need changing. Here the purpose of intervention is to change parents' knowledge and skills.

A decision tree can be described for choosing the appropriate form of transactional early intervention (Sameroff & Fiese, 1990). The first de-cision to be made is whether remediation is appropriate or viable (see Figure 1.5). Remediation cannot be achieved in at least two instances: a case where there is no procedure to modify the condition of the child, or a situation where nothing can be found in the child that needs changing. In such cases, the parents' knowledge of the developmental agenda and their reactions to the child must be examined. When parents show evi-dence of caregiving skills but are not using them with their child, redefi-nition is necessary. When the child's problems can be identified as a re-sult of the parents' lack of knowledge about adaptive childrearing, reeducation is indicated.

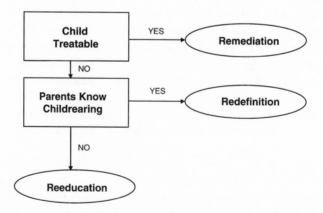

FIGURE 1.5. Transactional diagnosis decision flowchart based on the three R's in-tervention model.

PORTS OF ENTRY II:
THE MOTHERHOOD CONSTELLATION

Where the transactional model is a description of the processes by which individuals are transformed over time through their mutual involvement, with infants changing parents and then the changed parents reciprocally changing infants from birth onward, a model that focuses on the structure of the interacting systems is also necessary. Such a model for relationship therapy has been proposed by Stern-Bruschweiler and Stern (1989) and elaborated by Stern (1995) and labeled the *motherhood constellation*. In the constellation model the practicing family is depicted as the mother and infant's behaviors and the represented family or working models is depicted as the mother and infant's representations (see Figure 2.1, Chapter 2, this volume). What Stern adds is to place the parent–infant relationship into a clinical context where the therapist's behavior and representations are also depicted. Representations of the infant, parent, and therapist have in common that they are the repositories of the subjective experiences of each. What is different is that the infant is not yet able to reflect on his or her experience, whereas the parent and therapist have the capacity to reflect on both the infant's and mother's experience and behavior. The parent and therapist differ in that the parent may not use the reflective capacity, where such reflection is the therapist's profession.

The three R's described earlier centered on the transactional developmental process between the parents and the child with an implicit but not explicit place for the therapist within the model. Stern makes the therapist's role explicit and then moves to what this role might encompass specifically in terms of answering the question, "Who is the patient?" There are three answers in this model: the infant, the parent, or their interaction. Determining which is the patient is to be guided by two considerations, the target of the therapy and the port of entry into the system. These may be the same or different. The target would be homologous to the three R's, the child's behavior as in remediation, the parent's representation as in redefinition, or the parent's behavior as in reeducation. The port of entry could be quite different. If the goal is redefinition, that is, changing the parent's meaning system, the port of entry may be the behavioral interaction, with the expectation of spillover effects into changing the representational target. The three R's conceptualization allows for spillover from one intervention to the other two, but the motherhood constellation conceptualization reframes spillover effects into an optimal port of entry for some relationship problems. In addition, ports of entry are possible through therapists' representations and behavior as they gain knowledge through experience with a specific family.

Stern also adds a different twist to remediation and redefinition as targets. One can change the way babies affect their parents in less drastic ways than making physical changes through surgery or medication. One can demonstrate the variety of behavior in the child's repertoire to the parents to alter (redefine) their perceptions of the child's normality. Such an approach is at the core of the neonatal interventions described by Bruschweiler-Stern (see Chapter 8, this volume). When parents are shown that their child is less fragile than they imagined or that the child has the capacity for alert attention to their faces, redefinitions can occur.

TREATING RELATIONSHIP PROBLEMS

This book is devoted both to enlarging the scope and reducing the focus of therapists' reflections and representations with the goal of improving the treatment of relationship problems. The enlargement of scope is carried out by placing the infant and parent in a transactional *process* model for understanding how developmental influences move through time and a parent constellation *structural* model to appreciate the multiple behavioral and representational levels that have to be considered at any specific point in time. Both the three R's and the motherhood constellation models are devoted to embedding parent–infant problems in a broader context. An appreciation of the breadth of influences on healthy child development does not mean that the therapist must intervene with each influence. Rather, these models provide a diagnostic basis for choosing a therapeutic target and point of entry that would be the most effective for each family at a specific point in time.

There are multiple perspectives for identifying the real patient, but the two of most salience for our purposes are the diagnostic and clinical. The clinical perspective is the focus of most of this book and is captured by the three R's and motherhood constellations as ports of entry. The diagnostic perspective is the focus of Chapter 3, where Rosenblum critically evaluates existing diagnostic schemes for their overemphasis on disorders in the individual and lack of emphasis on disorders in relationships, our specific area of clinical concern.

Each therapy chapter in this book expands on one or more specific port of entry. In Chapter 4 on Interaction Guidance McDonough focuses

primarily on strategies for changing parent–infant interactions, whereas in Chapter 5 on child–parent psychotherapy Lieberman focuses
primarily on changing parent representations. In Chapter 6 Fivaz-
Depeursinge, Corboz-Warnery, and Keren expand a dyadic mother–
infant approach into a triadic one where the behavior and representations of both mother and father are taken into account. The infant's
behavior becomes the port of entry for the next two chapters, but all
three R's come into play. In Chapter 7 Dunn brings the skills of an occupational therapist to helping parents deal with challenging individual
differences in infant sensitivities. By showing parents how to be appropriately responsive to hyper- or hyposensitive and over- and underaroused infants, their interactions are modified to be more satisfying to
both the parent and the child. Similarly, in Chapter 8 Bruschweiler-
Stern uses a neonatal behavioral assessment scale to show parents the
range of normal responses to be found in any infant. This enlarged perspective of their newborn allows the parents to be more accepting of
their roles as mothers and fathers.

The last two therapy chapters expand the domain of clinical concern
from the healthy development of the infant to include the healthy development of the parents and place them in their community and legal contexts. As Harris (1996) documented, concentrating on mothers' mental
health and parenting behavior may be appropriate and essential for most
clinical situations, but such delimited interventions are inadequate for
multiproblem families. In Chapter 9 Egeland and Erikson describe an
intervention model that adds a focus on support networks, life management skills, and parent empowerment to traditional concerns' about the
family interactions with each other. In Chapter 10 Larrieu and Zeanah
use an integrated systems approach that in the special case of child maltreatment involves foster parents, state protective services agencies, and
the legal system as additional ports of entry for resolving parent–infant
relationship problems.

How does one summarize these multiple models and multiple ports
of entry? In Chapter 11 Emde, Everhart, and Wise focus on a theme that
is a common thread throughout the book—the effect of relationships on
relationships. From a developmental perspective they implicate not only
the dyadic and triadic relationships between the mother, the father, and
the infant, but also the relationships between each of these and other
siblings or primary caregivers. More important from a clinical perspective is the influence of the therapist–parent relationship on the relationship between the parent and the child.

Although the therapies presented in this book do not constitute a complete compendium of what therapists do with parents and infants, they not only are all exemplary in their quality but also exemplify the process and structural model we are using to help understand early relationships. They provide a guide that should enable a clinical and developmental audience to judge how best to improve the lives of infants, toddlers, and their families.

REFERENCES

Altemeir, W. A., O'Connor, S. M., Sherrod, K. B., & Vietze, P. M. (1985). Prospective study of antecedents for nonorganic failure to thrive. *The Journal of Pediatrics, 106,* 360–365.

Barnard, K. E., Morisset, C. E., & Spieker, S. (1993). Preventive interventions: Enhancing parent–infant relationships. In C. H. Zeanah (Ed.), *Handbook of infant mental health* (pp. 386–401). New York: Guilford Press.

Barrett, D. E., Radke-Yarrow, M., & Klein, R. E. (1982). Chronic malnutrition and child behavior: Effects of early caloric supplementation on social and emotional functioning at school age. *Child Development, 18,* 541–556.

Chatoor, I., Dickson, S., Schaeffer, S., & Egan, J. (1985). A developmental classification of feeding disorders associated with failure to thrive: Diagnosis and treatment. In D. Drotar (Ed.), *New directions in failure to thrive: Implications for research and practice* (pp. 235–258). New York: Plenum Press.

Cicchetti, D., & Toth, S. L. (1995). Developmental psychopathology and disorders of affect. In D. Cicchetti & D. J. Cohen (Eds.), *Developmental psychopathology: Vol. 2. Risk disorder and adaptation* (pp. 369–420). New York: Wiley.

Craviotto, J., & DeLicardie, E. R. (1979). Nutrition, mental development and learning. In F. Falhner & J. M. Turner (Eds.), *Human growth* (Vol. 3, pp. 481–508). New York: Plenum Press.

Easterbrooks, M. A. (1989). Quality of attachment to mother and father: Effects of perinatal risk status. *Child Development, 60,* 825–830.

Fiese, B. H., & Marjinksy, K. A. T. (1999). Dinnertime stories: Connecting family practices with relationship beliefs and child adjustment. In B. H. Fiese, A. J. Sameroff, H. D. Grotevant, F. S. Wamboldt, S. Dickstein, & D. L. Fravel (Eds.), The stories that families tell: Narrative coherence, narrative interaction, and relationship beliefs. *Monographs of the Society for Research in Child Development* (2, Serial No. 257, pp. 52–68). Malden, MA: Blackwell.

Fiese, B. H., Sameroff, A. J., Grotevant, H. D., Wamboldt, F. S., Dickstein, S., & Fravel, D. L. (1999). The stories that families tell: Narrative coherence, narrative interaction, and relationship beliefs. *Monographs of the Society for Research in Child Development* (64, Serial No. 257). Malden, MA: Blackwell.

Fox, N. A., Calkins, S. D., & Bell, M. (1994). Neural plasticity and development in the first two years of life: Evidence from cognitive and socioemotional domains of research. *Development and Psychopathology, 6*, 677–696.

Fraiberg, S., Adelson, E., & Shapiro, V. (1975). Ghosts in the nursery: A psychoanalytic approach to the problem of impaired mother–infant relationships. *Journal of the American Academy of Child Psychiatry, 14*, 387–421.

Grych, J. H., & Fincham, F. D. (1990). Marital conflict and children's adjustment: A cognitive-contextual framework. *Psychological Bulletin, 108*, 267–290.

Harris, I. B. (1996). *Children in jeopardy: Can we break the cycle of poverty?* New Haven, CT: Yale Child Study Center.

Infant Health and Development Program. (1990). Enhancing the outcomes of low-birthweight, premature infants. *Journal of the American Medical Association, 263*(22), 3035–3042.

Katz, L. F., & Gottman, J. M. (1993). Patterns of marital conflict predict children's internalizing and externalizing behaviors. *Developmental Psychology, 29*, 940–950.

Kennel, J., Klaus, M., McGrath, S., Robertson, S., & Hinkley, C. (1991). Continuous emotional support during labor in a U.S. hospital. *Journal of the American Medical Association, 265*, 2197–2201.

Lewis, M. (1997). *Altering fate: Why the past does not predict the future.* New York: Guilford Press.

Lieberman, A. F., & Pawl, J. H. (1993). Infant–parent psychotherapy. In C. H. Zeanah (Ed.), *Handbook of infant mental health* (pp. 427–442). New York: Guilford Press.

Lieberman, A. F., Weston, D. R., & Pawl, J. H. (1991). Preventive intervention and outcome with anxiously attached dyads. *Child Development, 62*, 199–209.

Main, M., & Goldwyn, R. (1984). Predicting rejection of their infant from mother's representation of her own experience: Implications for the abused and abusing intergenerational cycle. *Child Abuse and Neglect, 8*, 203–217.

McDonough, S. C. (2000). Interaction guidance: An approach for difficult to engage families. In C. H. Zeanah (Ed.), *Handbook of infant mental health* (2nd ed., pp. 485–493). New York: Guilford Press.

Nelson, C. A., & Bloom, F. E. (1997). Child development and neuroscience. *Child Development, 68*, 970–987.

Papousek, H., & Papousek, M. (1987). Intuitive parenting: A dialectic counterpart to the infant's integrative competence. In J. D. Osofsky (Ed.), *Handbook of infant development* (2nd ed., pp. 669–720). New York: Wiley.

Pollitt, E., Gorman, K. S., Engle, P. L., Mattorell, R., & Rivera, J. (1993). Early supplementary feeding and cognition: Effects over two decades. *Monographs of the Society for Research in Child Development, 58*(7, Serial no. 235).

Pueschel, S. M. (1984). *The young child with Down syndrome*. New York: Human Sciences Press.

Reiss, D. (1981). *The family's construction of reality*. Cambridge, MA: Harvard University Press.

Reiss, D. (1989). The represented and practicing family: Contrasting visions of family continuity. In A. J. Sameroff & R. N. Emde (Eds.), *Relationship disturbances in early childhood: A developmental approach* (pp. 191–220). New York: Basic Books.

Rexford, E. N., Sander, L., & Shapiro, L. W. (1976). *Infant psychiatry: A new synthesis*. New Haven, CT: Yale University Press.

Sameroff, A. J. (1987). The social context of development. In N. Eisenberg (Ed.), *Contemporary topics in developmental psychology* (pp. 273–291). New York: Wiley.

Sameroff, A. J. (1995). General systems theories and developmental psychopathology. In D. Cicchetti & D. Cohen (Eds.), *Manual of developmental psychopathology: Vol. 1. Theory and methods* (pp. 659–695). New York: Wiley.

Sameroff, A. J., & Chandler, M. J. (1975). Reproductive risk and the continuum of caretaking casualty. In F. D. Horowitz, M. Hetherington, S. Scarr-Salapatek, & G. Siegel (Eds.), *Review of child development research* (Vol. 4, pp. 187–244). Chicago: University of Chicago Press.

Sameroff, A. J., & Emde, R. N. (Eds.). (1989). *Relationship disturbances in early childhood: A developmental approach*. New York: Basic Books.

Sameroff, A. J., & Fiese, B. H. (1990). Transactional regulation and early intervention. In S. J. Meisels & J. P. Shonkoff (Eds.), *Handbook of early childhood intervention* (pp. 119–149). New York: Cambridge University Press.

Sameroff, A. J., & Fiese, B. H. (2000). Transactional regulation: The developmental ecology of early intervention. In J. P. Shonkoff & S. J. Meisels (Eds.), *Early intervention: A handbook of theory, practice, and analysis* (2nd ed., pp. 135–159). New York: Cambridge University Press.

Spietz, A., Johnson-Crowley, N., Sumner, G., & Barnard, K. E. (1990). *Keys to caregiving: Study guide*. Seattle, WA: NCAST (Nursing Child Assessment Satellite Training), University of Washington School of Nursing.

Spiker, D., Ferguson, J., & Brooks-Gunn, J. (1993). Enhancing maternal interactive behavior and child social competence in low birthweight premature infants. *Child Development, 64*, 754–768.

Stern, D. N. (1995). *The motherhood constellation: A unified view of parent–infant psychotherapy*. New York: Basic Books.

Stern-Bruschweiler, N., Stern, D. N. (1989). A model for conceptualizing the role of the mother's representational world in various mother–infant therapies. *Infant Mental Health Journal, 10*, 16–25.

Wille, D., E. (1991). Relation of preterm birth with quality of infant–mother attachment at one year. *Infant Behavior and Development, 14*, 227–240.

Zuckerman, B., Kaplan-Sanoff, M., Parker, S., & Young, K. T. (1997). The healthy steps for young children program. *Zero to Three, 17*(6), 20–25.

CHAPTER 2

THE MOTHERHOOD CONSTELLATION

Therapeutic Approaches to Early Relational Problems

Daniel N. Stern

PARENT–INFANT RELATIONAL PROBLEMS: A NEW CLINICAL CATEGORY

Historically, parents and infants with problems represent a new clinical population. The problems are not new, of course, but the identification and classification of them is. And with that, new therapeutic or preventive approaches specific to this population have been developed.

The nature of the clinical population determines in very large part the theories and practices applied to them. Consider the following. The "prototypic patient" that Sigmund Freud had in mind when he first created psychoanalysis was a young, intelligent woman with a conversion hysteria psychoneurosis who invariably "fell in love" with her older male therapist. This led to a theoretical and technical construct shaped to the realities encountered, such as the need for neutrality, abstinence, and emotional distance on the part of the therapist. Although there have been important developments in the theory as new psychoneuroses were seen, the prototype still retains considerable influence.

In the 1950s a completely new prototypic patient was encountered, a schizophrenic adolescent who lived with his family. From this encounter, family therapies and systemic therapy (as applied to the clinic) arose that differed widely from the existing psychoanalytic approaches. In the 1960s therapists met a third prototypic patient, one with a personality disorder, especially borderline or narcissistic disorders. And again new theoretical notions were needed that spawned new therapeutic approaches, such as self psychology.

And now, in the last few decades, we are faced with yet another prototypic patient population, namely, parents and infants with relational problems. These relational problems are largely new as main presenting complaints, especially as they appear within the parent–infant relationship. They include most frequently—but are not confined to—developmental delays and their impact on the infant and family, excessive uncontrollable crying, a range of sleeping and eating difficulties, and a sense of nonattachment to the parents.

Once again, various new ideas and practices are evolving. We will look at these. But first a crucial question: Why is this new prototypic patient population different from the preceding ones?

IN WHAT WAYS DO RELATIONAL PROBLEMS BETWEEN PARENTS AND INFANTS REPRESENT A TRULY NEW PROTOTYPIC CLINICAL CATEGORY?

There are many widely accepted observations about mothers in particular that set them apart from other clinical populations.

1. *Giving birth, having a baby, and having problems with the baby are normal life events.* They should not be pathologized. Problems (sometimes even when severe) are usually not illnesses. This is not to deny that true psychiatric disorders can play a significant role in relational problems, but labeling the therapeutic/preventive approaches for mothers and infants under rubrics of "psychiatry" or "clinical psychology" is counterproductive. Most mothers will not want to be thought of as cases or patients. To be successful the intervening teams must carry destigmatized names such as "developmental psychologists" or "guidance counselors" to not scare mothers away. Such destigmatized names are not really deceptive; they are closer to the truth as designations of the new approaches that have been shaped by the needs and realities of this client population.

2. *Parents have a different psychological structure from other clinical populations.* They have a special involvement with their child, which includes a large dose of altruism with psychobiological determinants not

operating to the same extent elsewhere. Because of this, they are often ready to blame themselves rather than find fault with the baby. Also from birth and during the months after it, the mother is in a "normal life crisis" that disorganizes and reorganizes much of her psychological life. And finally, as we shall see, a first-time new mother's mental landscape is different. This includes her preferences, her tendencies for action, and her interests (in men, in women, especially her own mother, and in her career). All of these taken together lead to the far more open psychological system than most other clients present.

3. *The parent–infant relationship has an interpersonal aspect and an intrapsychic aspect.* The interpersonal aspect consists of the overt behaviors that make up the parent–infant interaction. The intrapsychic aspect consists of the representations of how the father and mother see themselves as parents and how they see the baby, taking the form of memories and other past influences. Both sets of influences are unavoidable. During early infancy, powerful societal and cultural influences are certainly there as well, but these act mainly and indirectly through the mother's behavior and mental sets. Socioeconomic class, education, and cultural and family norms and expectations only act on the infant largely by way of how they influence the maternal and paternal behaviors toward the baby. This does not mean that they are any less strong—only more indirect—as far as the infant is concerned.

This situation leads to an approach that takes into account both the objective interpersonal data and the subjective intrapsychic data. This point is important because most approaches fashioned for other client populations can be classified as more interpersonal (e.g., behavioral approaches) or more intrapsychic (e.g., psychodynamic approaches)—and "never the twain shall meet." But with parent–infant relational problems the two must meet, and as equals. The approach must be hybrid even if at some phases of the treatment one or the other is dominant. In a similar vein, the approach must be both nonverbal (since key aspects of the interactions do not involve language) and verbal. Similarly, it must be systemic as well as individual. This multilevel view frees parent–infant interventions from some of the longstanding therapeutic polemics and makes it necessarily an integrated approach.

4. *Mothers rapidly evolve a different psychological organization when they have a baby.* One recent version of this has been called "the motherhood constellation" (Stern, 1995). This new organization is seen as a basic, independent, stable mental organization that emerges in most mothers. It is not viewed as a variation or derivation of some preceding more basic organization. It lasts forever, but remains in an active state

for a variable amount of time, usually from months to years, and then
subsides to remain in a deactivated, latent state, only to be reactivated
again at any life point when the child is in trouble, sick, or unhappy, no
matter whether he or she is 40 weeks old or 40 years old.

THE MOTHERHOOD CONSTELLATION

The nature of the motherhood constellation is discussed in great detail
by Stern (1995), Stern and Bruschweiler-Stern (1998), and Bruschweiler-
Stern (Chapter 8, this volume). In brief, there are seven main features.

1. *Mothers' interest, attention, and curiosity about others shifts with
the advent of pregnancy and/or the birth of the child.* She becomes less
interested in men and far more involved with women. She becomes particularly curious about her own mother, but not as a woman or as the
wife to her father, but rather as her own mother was when the new
mother was a little girl.

2. *Mothers become relatively less attentive to and interested in issues of competition, dominance, and sex and more attuned to issues of cooperation and caring.*

3. *Mothers develop new sensory preferences and sensibilities.* The
priority of their action tendencies shifts. What they notice and act upon
changes. It is as if they have grown another nervous system.

4. *Mothers are centrally preoccupied with issues of loving.* Do they
love their child as they "should?" Are they capable of it? Will they know
if their baby loves them or be able to accept that love? Are they "natural"
mothers, well endowed with all the right instincts?

5. *Mothers fall in love with their new baby.* It does not happen all at
once completely. There is a process, remarkably similar to that seen
when two adults fall in love. I am not talking about loving but about falling in love. The state of falling in love has its own mental organization
consisting of a special repertoire of behaviors, feelings, actions, and
mental preoccupations. Two simple examples suffice. The gaze behavior
of people falling in love is a variant of "normal" gaze behavior. Usually
people do not gaze in each other's eyes for more than 7 seconds without
speaking. The rise in tension is too steep. Mothers and infants, as well as
lovers, can silently gaze into one another's eyes for dozens of seconds.
Similarly, the overvaluation of the baby in the mother's eyes ("She is the
most beautiful baby in the world") is similar to the overevaluation of the
loved one among lovers.

6. *Mothers have a new fear that arises and takes form.* This is one of two additional features of the constellation that underlines the general point of the mother's difference from other clients. When a mother comes home from the hospital with her new baby, she has only one overwhelming preoccupation—to keep the baby alive and thriving. All mothers know this. It is clearly evident. Yet it does not appear in most theories. This preoccupation/fear is manifest in a mother's frequent night visits to the crib when the baby first comes home to reassure herself that the infant is still breathing, in her fearful vigilance in bathing the infant lest the baby slip through the mother's soapy fingers and bang his or her head, in her anxiety that the baby might fall from the changing table, in her worry that the baby might get suffocated in bed with her or be rolled over on by her husband and get crushed, or in her concern that the infant is not eating enough and will have to go back to the hospital. There is a hypervigilance and fearful preoccupation that sweeps all before it.

This hypervigilance should not be viewed as "ambivalence" or a "morbid preoccupation." For the vast majority it is a constructive force attesting to the mother's caring. When nature wants to ensure something—like the survival of the next generation of the species—it builds in great redundancy. Mothers are the victims of nature's conservative plan. They pay dearly with worry, great effort, and fatigue. To label this as pathological would undermine a new mother's vigilance and be simply destructive.

It is telling that most psychological theories have roughly the same list of basic fears (i.e., fears that are attached to the human condition). These include fragmentation, death of self, castration, isolation, falling, thunder, and snakes. Many psychological theories are built around such primary fears. But when we encounter a new mother, a new fundamental fear appears, fear for the survival of another person. In fact, it becomes the dominant fear organizing her behavior. In short, when we are considering mothers, the list of basic fears must be expanded and their priorities altered. This attests to the independence and uniqueness of the mental organization particular to mothers.

7. *New mothers need other, experienced women around them.* This feature will have implications for therapeutic approaches. In most traditional societies new mothers have an entourage of other woman to support them physically and emotionally. This is a central feature of the Doula program that provides an experienced woman to sit with mothers during the labor and birth to provide emotional support (Landry, McGrath, Kennell, Martin, & Steelman, 1998). The importance of this

companionship is not necessarily confined to the immediate perinatal period but extends longer.

The need for and interest in other women is characteristic of this period. During pregnancy, mothers tend to have more thoughts and dreams about their own mother and the caregiving experience they received. The way their own mother or primary caregiver behaved becomes a sort of North Star to help navigate these unfamiliar waters, to be steered either toward or away from certain caregiving behaviors, but a reference point either way. In the same vein, studies of intergenerational attachment show that the mother–baby attachment pattern observed when the baby is a year old is related to the new mother's narrative history of her relationship with her own mother when she was a girl (Main, Kaplan, & Cassidy, 1989). All of this suggests that the new mother becomes actively involved with her own history of being cared for, including her actual caregivers and other models of caregiving, memories of which now become activated and very relevant.

Many mothers create a "benign grandmother fantasy." This is the wish for a benign, experienced, caring older woman around her. (It need not be her own mother.) This benign figure is not needed to help her physically, nor to teach her, but to create a sort of holding environment in which the new mother feels encouraged, validated, appreciated, and psychologically supported so that she, herself, can freely explore her own innately given repertoire of maternal behaviors. Her husband cannot fulfill this role. He has other functions.

In brief, we have a new "prototypic patient" with different fears, wishes, needs, fantasies, and behaviors—a different mental organization. This must be taken into account because it will shape the therapeutic approach, both theoretically and clinically.

APPROACHES TO THE NEW PROTOTYPIC PATIENT

Stern (1995) and Bruschweiler-Stern (1998) have described a model for examining aspects of this new patient. It is shown in Figure 2.1. This figure shows both the observable–interactive–interpersonal influences (within the rectangle) and the intrapsychic influences (outside the rectangle) on these behaviors. This distinction is important because it highlights the necessity that we think interpersonally and intrapsychically at the same time when encountering the parent–infant pair.

Each of the elements of the model represents a potential clinical

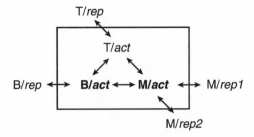

FIGURE 2.1. Model of the elements of a mother–infant therapeutic situation and their interconnections. Everything within the box is overt interpersonal behavior. Everything outside the box is intrapsychic material. M, mother; B, baby; T, therapist; rep, representations; act, actions (i.e., behaviors).

port of entry into the system. And, indeed, each port of entry defines a therapeutic approach. For instance, a more psychodynamic approach targets the mother's representations as the privileged port of entry, emphasizing the mother's past, her conflicts, and current fantasy life as they concern her baby and herself as a mother. The basic idea behind this attention to representations is that the mother's past experience and especially her unresolved conflicts are the major source for determining how she will behave with the baby, shaping the mother–infant interactions, which in turn may produce symptoms in the infant such as sleep or eating or attachment difficulties. Note that the mother's internal problem gets played out in the interaction to which the baby has something to contribute. As a consequence, we still need to consider the interface between the intrapsychic influences (of the mother) and the interpersonal influences (of the interaction). This approach was given its initial impetus by the groundbreaking work of Selma Fraiberg and colleagues in their concept of the "ghosts in the nursery" who reside in the mother's mind but indirectly affects the infant (Fraiberg, Adelson, & Shapiro, 1975). A contemporary variation concept of this is represented by the therapeutic approach (see Lieberman, Chapter 5, this volume).

In these approaches the therapist spends the vast majority of time focused on the mother, her life story and current experiences. The parent–infant interaction is only focused on when it is immediately useful in bringing to light or instantiating some of the mother's representations.

A more behaviorally centered approach considers the overt interaction between parent and infant as the optimal port of entry into the system. Accordingly, the major focus of attention is on the interaction, both sides of it. With this approach, the basic idea is that the interaction itself is the immediate cause of the problems (even though there may be secondary causes) and therefore it is the interaction that must addressed. Translated into technique, such as that practiced by Susan C. McDonough (see Chapter 4, this volume), first the therapist videotapes an interaction between the mother (or both parents) and the child and then observes the recording with the parent(s) immediately afterward. Together they examine what happened, how it felt, and what the parent(s) intended to happen. This is done in a cooperative spirit of curiosity and mutual exploration. The parent(s) and therapist are assumed to have an equal but different expertise about this particular interaction.

Another special feature of this approach is the emphasis on the positive, on what the mother's demonstrated capabilities are and how to build on them. This stands in contradistinction to the more psychodynamic approach that seeks the problems and deficits in the mother that are enacted in the interaction.

The emphasis on building from the positive, from the islands of competence the mother displays, is also determined by the nature of this "new" and special clinical population. Mothers most need a benign regard that encourages them and validates what they can do, rather than a critical eye that identifies their inadequacies.

A third port of entry focuses on the infant's behavior, particularly his or her competencies. This might best be called the "developmental pediatric approach" as it was largely developed by T. Berry Brazelton in a pediatric setting. A variant of this approach is presented in this volume by Nadia Bruschweiler-Stern (Chapter 8, this volume). The basic idea is that parents' representations of their baby that result in undesirable interactive patterns can be rapidly altered by showing the parents who the baby "really is" in terms of his or her capacities to interact, to respond to stimulations especially from the parents, to self-regulate, to be regulated by the parent's behavior, and to express his or her preferences. These demonstrations of who babies are and of what they are capable are addressed, where possible, to the misconceptions that parents have about their babies. While the approach uses the infant's behavior as the port of entry, it always has an eye on the parents' representations and the interaction.

A fourth port of entry consists of the mother's representations that arise in the therapeutic relationship. This might be called a "transference–attachment approach." The basic notion (and this is unique to this "new" clinical population) is that new mothers need an experienced woman who will accompany them on their journey to become the mother they want to become. The experienced woman falls into a category that we have called the "benign grandmother fantasy," (Stern, 1995). Many give her the vital role of an alternate attachment figure for the mother who can "hold," guide, accompany, and validate the mother in her new role (e.g., Lieberman & Pawl, 1993). This need for an experienced woman at this time in the new mother's life is largely recognized around the world today in most cultures, as it was in previous times. The reality of a woman going through this experience alone, as too often happens in our modern Western culture, is to my mind aberrant and makes for trouble.

If the new mother can establish a therapeutic relationship with another woman, she will start to form new representations of who she can be as a mother and who this baby is for her and with her. These representations form under the benign and secure regard of the experienced woman accompanying her. These new representations that are born in the transference act to progressively correct her original representations and interactions with the baby.

A fifth port of entry involves a more systemic family approach. Here the father's presence is essential so that the interactive patterns between the three family members can be examined. The three dyads that make up a family can be observed in the context of the triadic setting. Fivaz-Depeursinge, Corboz-Warnery (1999) have developed and explicated this approach (see also Fivaz-Depeursinge, Corboz-Warnery, & Keren, Chapter 6, this volume). It is focused on the interaction rather than the representations and uses altering the contextualization of the relationships as a way of effectuating interactive change. Many of the classic maneuvers of family systems theory can be adapted to this particular approach.

More distinctions between these ports of entry and their corresponding therapeutic approaches are explored in greater detail elsewhere (Stern, 1995).

EQUIFINALITY OF APPROACHES

Although the advocates of each therapeutic approach or port of entry argue for the efficacy of their technique, comparative studies suggest that the different therapeutic approaches give roughly the same results. They all work more or less equally well, and there is no clear evidence that one is better with this or that subpopulation. There may be practical issues of availability or costs of different programs, but this is a separate issue from effectiveness.

One study addressed the question by comparing two approaches on mother–infant pairs who were randomly assigned to a behavioral approach (McDonough's Interaction Guidance; see Chapter 4, this volume) where the port of entry is the dyadic interaction or to a psychodynamic approach where the port of entry is the mother's representations. The therapeutic results from the two treatments showed no differences (Cramer et al., 1990). What is also notable is that the Interaction Guidance not only changed the interaction as expected but it also changed the mother's representations as much as did the psychodynamic approach; conversely, the psychodynamic approach not only changed the mother's representations as expected but it also changed the interaction as much as did the behavioral approach.

Such findings suggest equifinality of all approaches. However, this relative efficacy is invariably despised and rejected by practitioners (and believers) of a specific approach and its technique. This is understandable in that equifinality suggests that the techniques and theories behind any one approach are less important than factors common to all the approaches. What then are the nonspecific factors, and how do they act?

THE NONSPECIFIC COMMON ASPECTS OF PARENT–INFANT INTERVENTIONS

What is common among all ports of entry is that they are parts of the same system. There is always at least one parent and one child in interaction and with a set of represented relationships. Considering the model in Figure 2.1, it becomes apparent that the chosen port of entry into the system is not determinant of the outcome. Once you have altered one element of the system all the others readjust correspondingly. The dynamic interdependence of the various elements ensures that any effect will get distributed throughout the system. The choice of port of entry is a clinical–theoretical choice but may have less to do with the final outcome than expected. The nature of the system is itself a factor leading to the nonspecificity of approaches.

Another common nonspecific aspect is that the parent–infant system is part of a larger system including the therapist. The therapist or interventionist adds an important extra dimension, the *therapeutic holding environment*. We have stressed the importance of the therapeutic holding environment and in particular the role of women in this holding. All psychotherapies recognize the importance of the therapeutic relationship in terms of a therapeutic alliance or transference/countertransference or a holding environment. In some approaches this recognition is explicit and forms part of the stated approach. In others the importance of this relationship is implicit and clearly given full weight even when it is not part of the stated therapeutic strategy.

Whether explicitly or implicitly, all approaches to parent–infant psychotherapy stress the central role of the therapeutic relationship. They present variations on the same theme of the necessity for a therapeutic holding environment. There is a consensus that the therapeutic holding environment is the major nonspecific factor in all treatments. No treatment can begin, continue, or succeed without this environment in place. It may well account for the majority of all change in all therapeutic approaches. The different forms it takes are but variations depending on the specific technique used. However, the commonalities are greater than the differences.

The Boston Change Process Study Group (2002; Stern et al., 1998; Tronick et al., 1998) has studied the therapeutic process trying to identify the main elements leading to change. We have identified what we call the *intersubjective field* between the patient and therapist. This consists of what each one knows implicitly about the nature of their relationship as it changes from moment to moment. It is a form of sharing and being mutually understood. We find that when the therapist and patient can achieve greater degrees of intersubjective meeting and sharing, a context is created that permits for therapeutic change. This kind of intersubjective meeting and sharing is common to all therapeutic relationships and is one of the more potent common elements promoting change. It is part of the holding environment. In some therapeutic approaches it is explicitly aimed for; in others it is created implicitly.

The particular form of the therapeutic holding environment that evolves in any parent–infant intervention that is treating real parents and infants and not theories is determined by the previously mentioned features special to mothers in this period of their lives: (1) the wish (or fantasy) and need for a benign grandmotherly figure to "hold" her psychologically as she explores her new role; (2) the necessity of a positive atmosphere wherein the mother is supported and validated and not criticized (e.g., where her legitimate fears are construed as evidence of her caring and involvement, not as ambivalence); (3) a relationship that permits the therapist to touch the mother, put an arm around her, and hold her hand as appropriate (note how different this is from the relationship needed in a traditional psychoanalytic setting, where any such action would be deemed a violation of the therapeutic frame); and (4) the need for nonverbal understanding between the mother and therapist that falls into the domain of unverbalized implicit knowledge between them.

The creation of a warm, cooperative accompanying ambience in the treatment setting with a strong emphasis on the capacities the mother shows, even when limited, is essential. The notion of a "transfer cure" is not applicable to this clinical situation, and no effort need be taken to re- solve positive transference. It will dissolve on its own if the therapy is working. Negative transference needs be confronted only if it signifi- cantly impedes the establishment of the therapeutic holding environ- ment.

These then are the alterations in the nonspecific aspects of parent– infant treatment that have evolved and been shaped by the special fea- tures of this new clinical population. All therapeutic approaches have moved closer to this altered framework, even when it is not recognized "officially." Otherwise they would not work.

A recent trend in prevention for families at risk bears out the power of the nonspecific factors of the therapeutic holding environment. Many clinicians have used nonprofessional, older, experienced women as home visitors or therapists. These home visitors receive a short training and regular supervision. Otherwise they use their own experience. They are, of course, well selected (Lyons-Ruth, Connell, Greunbaum, & Botein, 1990; Olds et al., 1998). These reports indicate that the therapeutic hold- ing environment created by the home visitors must be maintained on a once-a-week basis ideally for 18 months to get the best results, which are comparable or better than most traditional approaches. The implications of this approach are enormous, not only practically but for how we con- ceive of the nature of the therapeutic process.

SUMMARY

We have described new mothers as a "new" clinical population requiring different therapeutic approaches both theoretically and technically.

What makes a new mother a different patient or subject is that she evolves a different mental organization than a woman who neither is pregnant nor has recently given birth. We call this mental organization the "motherhood constellation." It differs from other mental organiza- tions in altering the mother's sensibilities, fantasies, action tendencies, preferences, life priorities, mental engagement with her own mother, and basic fears.

One of the more important alterations making up this motherhood constellation is the desire–fantasy–need for the presence of an older, ex- perienced, benign woman or women who can accompany her at this time, encourage her to build on her maternal competencies, discover new ones, and validate her in her new role.

A second major new feature of this new mother is that the relationship between the mother and infant (or the mother, father, and infant) must be understood in terms of both the representations of the parents and the overt interactions between the parent(s) and infant. In other words, the situation calls for equally divided attention between the intrapsychic and the interpersonal. However since the two are so intimately connected and mutually influencing, one can therapeutically enter this interdependent system through any of the main elements that make it up: the parent's representations, the interaction, the infant's competencies, or the family context. Each of these elements has thus been called a "port of entry" to gain access to the entire system. Once the system has been entered using the techniques best adapted to each port of entry, changing one element will result in changing all of them because of the interdependence within the system.

Some immediate implications of the above for all mother–infant therapies including home visitors are the following:

1. It does not matter too much which port of entry is chosen and privileged. The technique to get there will be different, but the end results will be similar since the whole system will be changed.
2. Problems in the parent–infant relationship must be approached with a different therapeutic relationship than those habitual for other patient populations. We have called this the therapeutic holding environment. This environment must be far more positive, validating, and accompanying than traditional therapeutic alliances. It is a feature common to the different approaches.
3. Ideally, the therapists should be experienced women.
4. The emphasis in choosing therapists should be placed on selecting those that have the requisite qualities already, and not on training and "education." Learning can only be a complement to selection. Learning without prior selection is wasteful and productive of poor therapists.

REFERENCES

Boston Change Process Study Group. (2002). Explicating the implicit: The interactive micro-process in the analytic situation (Report No. 3). *International Journal of Psychoanalysis, 79,* 903–921.

Cramer, B., Robert-Tissot, C., Stern, D. N., Serpa-Rusconi, S., DeMuralt, M., Besson, G., Palacio-Espaca, F., Bachmann, J.-P., Knauer, D., Berney, C., &

D'Arcis,U. (1990). Outcome evaluation in brief mother–infant psychotherapy: A preliminary report. *Infant Mental Health Journal, 11,* 278–300.

Fivaz-Depeursinge, E., & Corboz-Warnery, A. (2000). *The primary triangle: A
developmental systems view of fathers, mothers, and infants.* New York: Basic Books.

Fraiberg, S., Adelson, E., & Shapiro, V. (1975). Ghosts in the nursery: A psychoanalytic approach to the problems of impaired infant–mother relationships.
Journal of the American Academy of Child Psychiatry, 14, 338–421.

Landry, A. H., McGrath, S. K., Kennell, J. H., Martin, S., & Steelman, L. (1998).
The effect of doula support during labor on mother–infant interaction at 2
months. *Pediatric Research, 43*(Pt. II), 13.

Lieberman, A. F., & Pawl, J. H. (1993). Infant–parent psychotherapy. In C. H.
Zeanah (Ed.), *Handbook of infant mental health* (pp. 427–442). New York:
Guilford Press.

Lyons-Ruth, K., Connell, D., Greunbaum, H., & Botein, S. (1990). Infants at social risk: Maternal depression and family support services as mediators of
infant development and security of attachment. *Child Development, 61,*
85–98.

Main, M., Kaplan, N., & Cassidy, J. (1989). Security in infancy, childhood and
adulthood: A move to the level of representation. In I. Bretherton & E.
Waters (Eds.), Growing points in attachment theory and research. *Monographs of the Society for Research in Child Development, 50,* 66–106.

Olds, D. L., Pettit, L. M., Robinson J., Henderson, C., Jr., Eckenrode, J.,
Kitzman, H., Cole, B., & Powers, J. (1998). Reducing risks for antisocial
behavior with a program of prenatal and early childhood home visitation.
Journal of Community Psychology, 26, 65–83.

Stern, D. N. (1995). *The motherhood constellation: A unified view of parent–infant psychotherapy.* New York: Basic Books.

Stern, D. N., & Bruschweiler-Stern, N. (1998). *The birth of a mother.* New York:
Basic Books.

Stern, D. N., Sander, L. W., Nahum, J. P., Harrison, A. M., Lyons-Ruth, K., Morgan, A. C., Bruschweiler-Stern, N., & Tronick, E. Z. (1998). Non-interpretive mechanisms in psychoanalytic therapy: The "something more" than interpretation (the Boston Change Process Study Group, Report No. 1).
International Journal of Psycho-Analysis, 79, 903–921.

Tronick, E. Z., Bruschweiler-Stern, N., Harrison, A. M., Lyons-Ruth, K., Morgan, A. C., Nahum, J. P., Sander, L. W., & Stern, D. N. (1998). Dyadically
expanded states of consciousness and the process of therapeutic change.
Infant Mental Health Journal, 19, 290–299.

CHAPTER 3

DEFINING INFANT MENTAL HEALTH

A Developmental Relational Perspective on Assessment and Diagnosis

Katherine L. Rosenblum

Treatment approaches for disturbances in infant mental health are varied, as are the populations served. When parents are the source of referral the concerns that are brought to the attention of an infant mental health specialist are often framed in terms of problems with the *infant's* behavior. For example, parents may be concerned that their infant or toddler "cries too much," "sleeps to little," or acts "too aggressively." Other referrals, often those made by outside professionals, are based on the *caregiver's* behavior, for example, referrals for mothers who experience a postpartum depression or for caregivers whose parenting is believed to place the child at risk. In intervention practice, however, infant mental health specialists have made significant contributions to the field by emphasizing that despite the target of referral the *caregiver–infant relationship* can be the primary target for change.

The focus of this book is the treatment of problems in the caregiver–infant relationship. While most of the chapters address the issue of how to intervene, the present chapter highlights issues related to assessment and diagnosis in an effort to help clarify which interventions may work best for whom and why.

Current research on infant mental health raises a number of important conceptual and practical questions with implications for both diagnosis and intervention. First, who is the client? Is it the infant? The caregiver? Or, rather, is it the relationship? Second, what is the disorder? Does it reside in the infant's behavior, the caregiver's behavior, or in their interaction? And if in the infant, how is it manifest at different ages? For example, does sad or anxious behavior in a 1-year-old manifest itself similarly in a 5-year-old? Answers to these types of questions lead us to different conclusions regarding the best approach to preventing or treating a particular type of disturbance.

Research that aims to address these questions relies heavily upon current conceptualizations of disorder—primarily those reflected in the currently available diagnostic systems, such as the text revision of the fourth edition of the *Diagnostic and Statistical Manual of Mental Disorders* (DSM-IV-TR; American Psychiatric Association, 2000). Diagnostic classification systems can hold great power: they inform our conceptualization of disorder, lead to conclusions about screening and the identification of risk factors, often determine reimbursement for services, and inform approaches to intervention. In the present chapter I argue, however, that the most commonly employed diagnostic system does not fully reflect the state-of-the-art conceptualization of infant disorder, failing to adequately acknowledge important developmental issues as well as the centrality of the caregiver–infant relationship. Current research and clinical practice indicates a need for incorporation of a developmental relational approach to assessment and diagnosis, and recent diagnostic approaches that aim to address these issues are a step in the right direction.

There are surprisingly few studies examining the prevalence of infant mental health problems in the general population. The paucity of data is clearly linked to the limitations of the currently available diagnostic systems. Studies of prevalence require diagnostic systems that adequately identify or define the disorder. Yet the absence of developmentally based prevalence data limits our ability to develop adequate diagnostic systems.

Current advances in the conceptualization of disorder are evident in the establishment of a new approach to studying patterns of disease prevalence, the "developmental epidemiology" approach. The present chapter provides a review of the currently available diagnostic systems for infant mental health assessment. Data from current research on commonly referred infant behavior problems are used to highlight some of the limitations posed by traditional classification systems, and innovative new approaches being taken to the assessment of infant mental health disorder are presented.

DEVELOPMENTAL EPIDEMIOLOGY AND DISORDERS OF INFANT MENTAL HEALTH

Epidemiology is a field of study concerned with the population prevalence of disease. By identifying patterns of distribution of disease across populations, epidemiologists are concerned with identifying individuals and groups vulnerable to the disease and attempt to determine why these groups are vulnerable (Costello & Angold, 2000). An ultimate goal of much epidemiological research is the reduction or eradication of risk for these vulnerable groups of individuals, with a primary focus on disease prevention. Recent advances in the field have led to a new focus on *developmental epidemiology*, which is defined as "being concerned with why vulnerability to, and expression of, different disorders changes over the course of individual development" (Costello & Angold, 2000, p. 59). For example, from a developmental epidemiology perspective it is important to address such issues as why disruptions in attachment relationships during the first 2 years of life, versus during adolescence, hold different consequences for the individual's mental health.

As clinicians we are not always drawn to consider epidemiology. Not surprisingly, the focus is often on how to intervene with the individual child—the particular caregiver and child—or family and social contexts that present for our services. However, in order to develop truly effective interventions we need to understand who our clients are—both who is seen and who is missed. We need to understand the nature of the disorder we treat, and thus our target for change, as well as identify the unmet needs in our communities. Furthermore, in order to assess whether our interventions for targeted individuals or dyads are effective, we need to know something about the origin and course of the disorder—both with and without treatment. Understanding the developmental course of the disorder may lead to different approaches to intervention at different developmental stages. The questions that epidemiological investigations address are central to developmentally sensitive clinical practice: "What works for whom?"; "What is the origin and course of this illness or disorder?"; and, ultimately, "How can we prevent each disorder in other at-risk individuals?"

However, despite the call for a developmental epidemiology, there are limited epidemiological data focused on disorder among infants and toddlers. Studies that report on the prevalence of many infant diagnoses are typically based on limited geographic regions, clinical samples, or special groups, not representative population screening. Much research on infant disorder is done using populations known to be at risk for disorder (e.g., preterm infants) or populations with some manifestation of the disorder under consideration (e.g., excessive crying). There is a notable lack of prospective longitudinal community-based studies of infant mental health disorder. Thus we might know something about whether currently identified individuals are truly at risk for the disorder (e.g., are infants with colic at risk for the development of later problems in self-regulation?), but we know little of the individuals we might have missed at our initial screening (e.g., are some infants without colic also at risk for later problems in self-regulation?).

In order to best identify and describe disorders of infant mental health, we need diagnostic systems that allow for assessment of relevant aspects of infant disorder, including possible developmental and relationship factors. The more evolved the diagnostic systems, the more relevant and helpful are the subsequent epidemiological data. Similarly, the more we know about the specific nature of infant mental health problems, the better able we are to develop meaningful classification systems for the diagnosis of such disorder.

CONCEPTUALIZING DISORDER: ISSUES IN THE CLASSIFICATION OF INFANT MENTAL HEALTH DISORDER

One of the central issues that any taxonomic (or diagnostic classification) system must address is where to place or locate the disease process. Can an infant really be diagnosed with a psychiatric disorder? Are infant conditions psychiatric disorders per se—or rather simply risk factors for later psychopathology? And importantly: Where does a disorder reside? These questions challenge us to determine whether disturbances in the caregiving relationship are simply *associated features* or, rather, an *integral part* of infant mental health disorder. Answers to these questions directly impact the diagnostic criteria used to identify any particular disorder.

There are two basic models for conceptualizing infant mental health disorder: a disease model, which locates the disorder within a person, either the parent or the child, and a relationship model, which locates the disorder in neither individual, but rather in the specific relationship between those two individuals.

Psychiatric diagnostic classification systems have primarily retained a traditional medical approach, where the disease process is located within an individual. Diagnoses are categorical, that is, an individual either meets criteria for a disorder or does not. Traditional psychiatric systems attempt to minimize the assignment of multiple diagnoses by hierarchically organizing disorder categories. In such systems the recommendation is that wide-ranging symptoms should typically best be captured by the one "best fitting" or "most parsimonious" primary diagnosis. This approach is complicated by current research that indicates comorbidity is much more common than previously thought; individuals more often than not meet criteria for more than one diagnosis (Angold, Costello, & Erkanli, 1999). This is true both within and across the internalizing spectrum (e.g., anxiety and depression) and the externalizing spectrum (e.g., oppositional defiant disorder and conduct disorder).

Relationship models for diagnostic classification, on the other hand, emphasize the centrality of the caregiving relationship to infant mental health functioning. These approaches highlight a transactional approach, one that acknowledges the reciprocal, mutual influence of both partners in a relationship (Sameroff & Fiese, 2000). Caregivers and infants are seen as dynamically influencing one another over time, and the relationship is assumed to be more than simply "a sum of its parts" (Sroufe, 1989). The infant's relational context is seen as a critical feature of infant social emotional health as well as infant mental health disorder. While newer diagnostic classification systems have made efforts to incorporate more of a relationship focus, articulating and refining an appropriate "relationship model" classification system remains an ongoing challenge (see First et al., 2002).

It is important to note that a relationship model approach does not inherently deny the existence of problems that may be seen as residing primarily in a parent or infant, but rather emphasizes that such conditions are heavily embedded in and affected by a relational context (Sameroff & Emde, 1989). Clearly, certain relatively persistent infant conditions (e.g., infant colic or Down syndrome) may provide significant challenges for the caregiving system. Similarly, some parental characteristics (e.g., a substance abuse disorder or postpartum depression) may pose constraints for the infant's self-development, for example, by rendering the parent less flexible or responsive to the infant's particular needs or cues. Nonetheless, the emphasis is placed on understanding the dynamic interplay between characteristics of the infant and caregiver in the relationship, as well as the consequences for individual and relational functioning. For example, how does the parent–child relationship support or hinder a child with Down syndrome from fully optimizing his or her developmental potential? In a relationship model, the relationship is seen as an integral part of health or disorder, not simply as an "associated feature."

In the past decade, significant advances have been made in the development of a taxonomy of infant mental health disorder addressing the developmental and relational aspects of the disorder—culminating in an innovative new approach to infant diagnosis, the Zero to Three Diagnostic and Classification system (DC: 0–3; Zero to Three/National Center for Clinical Infant Programs, 1994). While this diagnostic scheme represents a significant advance in being developmentally sensitive as well as relationship sensitive, issues remain. Some clinicians have argued for a more dimensional, rather than categorical, approach to assessment, while another critique raises issues about the assessment of the subjective representational level of psychological functioning. The preceding two chapters in this volume have emphasized the importance of representation in the parent–infant system, both theoretically and as a major port of entry into treating infant mental health problems.

A Standard Approach: The DSM-IV-TR

The most commonly employed diagnostic system in the United States is DSM-IV-TR. Although the DSM-IV-TR is a multiaxial system, certain axes have precedence: "primary" diagnoses are assigned to Axis I; developmental and personality disorders are diagnosed on Axis II; Axis III is used to capture any medical or physical problems; Axis IV is used to designate specific psychosocial risks; a given individual may receive diagnoses on one or several of these axes, and the individual's overall level of functioning is captured on the Global Assessment of Functioning (GAF) scale, which is assigned to Axis V.

All Axis I through Axis V diagnoses are assigned to an individual— in the case of a caregiver and infant, either the infant or the caregiver. With respect to relationship assessment, the DSM-IV-TR also provides for an additional diagnostic possibility, the "V Code." The Parent–Child Relational Problem V code was developed to capture problems in the parent–child relationship, but it is assigned to the individual even when problems in the relationship are seen as being central to the impairment of individual or family functioning or the manifestation of clinically significant problems in the child or parent. The emphasis remains on diagnosing the individual, and V codes are placed in the "Other Conditions" section rather than on an axis. Relational problems are typically considered to be associated features of mental disorder and thus are not included in the primary DSM-IV-TR diagnostic system.

Table 3.1 lists the primary infant-relevant Axis I diagnoses found under "Disorders Usually First Diagnosed in Infancy, Childhood, or Adolescence" in the DSM-IV-TR. These include feeding disorders, motor skills disorder, pervasive developmental disorders, communication disorders, separation anxiety disorder, and reactive attachment disorder. While other diagnoses in the DSM-IV-TR may apply to an infant, child, or adolescent (e.g., mood disorders), diagnostic criteria are not specifically framed in terms of child manifestation of these disorders.

Despite its widespread usage, there are at least three main limitations to the DSM-IV-TR approach. First, the diagnoses for infant disorder are limited in both number and scope. It is a common dilemma for practitioners of infant mental health to fail to identify a DSM-IV-TR diagnosis that adequately or accurately captures the type of problem presented by the clients. Second, as noted previously, the assumption is that the disorder necessarily resides "within" the individual—in other words, in the infant or the caregiver. While the V codes represent an attempt to acknowledge that relationship problems may exacerbate or challenge individual functioning, the focus remains on diagnosing the individual. Keeping V codes in a separate "Other Conditions" section, rather than as part of the primary multiaxial system, inherently implies that the relationship aspect of the disorder is an associated, rather than an integral, feature of the disorder. A direct consequence of giving these types of di-

TABLE 3.1. DSM-IV-TR Diagnoses for Disorders during Infancy and Toddlerhood

Axis I	Axis II	Other conditions (V codes)
Feeding and eating disorders of infancy or early childhood	Mental retardation	Relational problems
Pica		Parent–child relational problem
Rumination disorder		Sibling relational problem
Feeding disorder		Problems related to abuse or neglect
Separation anxiety disorder		Physical abuse of child
Reactive attachment disorder of infancy or early childhood		Sexual abuse of child
Pervasive developmental disorders		Neglect of child
Autistic disorder		
Rett's disorder		
Childhood disintegrative disorder		

agnoses a "secondary" place is seen in the realm of insurance and pay-
ment for services; many insurers do not recognize the V code category of
disorder for reimbursement. Third, the criteria for disorder in the DSM-
IV-TR are not based on developmental norms. Even within the section
on disorders usually assigned during infancy, childhood, or adolescence,
the same criteria typically apply for children under and over 3 years of
age. Diagnoses outside of this section (e.g., the depressive disorders) are
typically framed in terms of adult criteria, and it may be unlikely that infants or children would ever be able to meet certain symptom criteria
(e.g., impaired ability to maintain employment, or duration criteria of 6
or more months for particular symptoms). The DSM-IV-TR approach to
classifying disorder thus is not sufficiently developmentally sensitive,
nor does it adequately capture the centrality of the relationship for infant
mental health functioning.

A "Zero to Three" Approach (The DC: 0–3 System)

The DC: 0–3 system was developed by specialists in the field of infancy
and early childhood development in an effort to address some of the limitations of the DSM-IV-TR, and aims to provide a more accurate and
complete classification of infant mental health disorders. It was not intended to replace but rather to elaborate upon the DSM-IV-TR. The
DC: 0–3 system is also a multiaxial diagnostic system, yet relative to the
DSM-IV-TR use in practice there is a strong emphasis on fully addressing each of the axes, as they are all considered central to clinical case
conceptualization. It provides a broader array of age-relevant diagnoses
and importantly represents a first step at incorporating a relationship
perspective into our diagnostic conceptualization.

As with the DSM-IV-TR, the DC: 0–3 Axis I captures what are to be
considered the "primary infant diagnoses." These include disorders of
relating and communicating, regulatory disorders, adjustment disorder,
eating behavior disorder, sleep behavior disorder, traumatic stress disorder, and a variety of disorders of affect. Note, however, that compared to
the DSM-IV-TR there are a broader range of diagnostic possibilities and
that the behavioral disorders described are more clearly linked to the
types of problems commonly referred to infant mental health practice
(see Table 3.2).

Axis II of the DC: 0–3 is specifically designed to capture the "relationship dimension" of infant mental health; it is a relationship classification system, and a variety of "disordered relationship types" are identified. The types of relationship disorders identified on DC: 0–3 Axis II

TABLE 3.2. DC: 0–3 Diagnoses for Disorders during Infancy and Toddlerhood.

Axis I	Axis II	Axis III	Axis IV	Axis V
Primary Infant Diagnoses	Relationship Disorder Classification	Medical and developmental disorders and conditions	Psychosocial stressors	Functional emotional developmental level
Traumatic stress disorder	Overinvolved			
Disorders of affect	Underinvolved			
Anxiety disorders	Anxious/tense			
Mood disorders: Prolonged bereavement/grief reaction	Angry/hostile			
Mixed disorder of emotional expressiveness	Mixed			
Gender identity disorder	Abusive			
Reactive attachment deprivation/maltreatment disorder	Verbal			
Adjustment disorder	Physical			
Regulatory disorders	Sexual			
Hypersensitive				
Underreactive				
Motor processing—Impulsive, motorically disorganized				
Other regulatory disorder				
Eating behavior disorder				
Sleep behavior disorder				
Disorders of relating and communicating				
Multisystem developmental disorder				

include the overinvolved, underinvolved, anxious/tense, angry/hostile, mixed, and abusive types. The remaining DC: 0–3 axes capture the relevant medical and developmental diagnoses (Axis III), psychosocial stressors (Axis IV), and the functional emotional developmental level of the infant (Axis V).

Note that Axis II represents a significant advance in the incorporation of a relationship focus in diagnostic classification. On Axis II the classification of disorder is applied to a specific relationship, not simply to either individual in the relationship. A given child may have more than one relationship that meets criteria for Axis II disorder (e.g., an infant's relationship with the mother and with the father); the specific relationship is the focus of diagnosis, not the parent or child alone. The diagnostic categories on Axis II are considered to be mutually exclusive; that is, the relationship is either "overinvolved" or one of the other types. If more than one relationship type applies, the "mixed" category is assigned. Although the categorical mixed diagnosis formally allows for the recognition of comorbidity, the broad category does not allow for discernment of which elements of relationship disturbance were observed. For example, a given dyad may be assigned a mixed classification because of both over- and underinvolved relationship patterns, abusive and angry/hostile relationship patterns, or some other unspecified combination. A dimensional approach would avoid such a problem.

In addition, in order for the parent–infant relationship to meet criteria for an Axis II disorder, the clinician must document that the relationship meets a specified level of clinical impairment. When using the DC: 0–3 system, clinicians are required to assess the quality of the parent–infant relationship using the Parent–Infant Relationship Global Assessment Scale (PIR-GAS). Scores on this scale range from 0 (grossly impaired) to 100 (very well adapted), and place specific relationship problems along a dimension from perturbance to disturbance to disorder. In order for the relationship to meet criteria for a "relationship disorder" on Axis II, the PIR-GAS score assigned must be less than 40 (the "disturbed" cut point). Anders (1989) describes the relationship problem spectrum in detail; he notes that each of the three levels—perturbation, disturbance, and disorder—are characterized by differences in terms of the *intensity* of the problem, extent or *frequency* of the disruption, *duration* of the disturbance, and the *malleability* of the problem to change with or without intervention.

A *relationship perturbation* (PIR-GAS scores of 60–79) is a transient disruption in the environment, including, for example, such things as minor physical illnesses. Perturbations reflect disruptions that are often considered normative childhood experiences and typically resolve themselves over time without significant intervention, for example, an ear infection, a parent's return to work, or increased assertiveness on the part of the child. A perturbation may affect the parents' feelings about the child but not their caregiving behavior. A relationship wherein the caregiver is somewhat frustrated by the child's more frequent night waking while she or he is teething may lead to the assignment of a "perturbance" level PIR-GAS score. Typically the individuals in the relationship have satisfactory family and social supports, and the disruption is generally of a short duration (i.e., lasting only several days or weeks).

A *relationship disturbance* (PIR-GAS scores of 40–59) is a pattern of inappropriate or insensitive regulation in interaction, in other words, a "risk condition" that, if continued, would likely lead to subsequent individual or relationship psychopathology. For example, a relationship wherein the caregiver experiences frustration with the child because she or he is persistently difficult to feed, and consequently the caregiver begins to show more intrusive or rejecting behavior toward the child during mealtimes, may meet criteria for a "disturbance" level PIR-GAS score. No other domains of parent–child interaction or functioning reveal disturbance or distress. Relationship disturbances are often of moderate duration (lasting from 1 to 3 months), and the problems are typically evident in only one domain of the relationship.

Finally, a *relationship disorder* (PIR-GAS scores <40) is a more extended pattern of inappropriate or insensitive regulation in interaction; in this case the affected interaction patterns are relatively fixed and not easily altered. Problems at this level are likely to interfere with the successful achievement of developmental milestones by one or both of the partners, the problem is likely to "spill over" into multiple domains, and, particularly if left untreated, tend to be of long duration. These problems may escalate over time and likely reflect a dynamic "transactional" process. For example, consider a relationship wherein a mother and toddler experience significant difficulties in separation such that the mother decides to quit her job. This disruption leads to heightened feelings of isolation and depression for the mother and heightened anxiety and clinginess in the child. The mother's depression reduces her capacity to cope with her child's neediness, and she grows increasingly helpless and overwhelmed in her responses to the toddler's distress. This, in turn, leads to heightened aggressive and oppositional behavior in the child during normal day-to-day interactive routines (e.g., mealtimes or bedtime). It is clear that the disruption in one domain has spilled over into functioning across a range of domains and is interfering with both the in-

fant and the mother's relational and developmental tasks. This type of
relationship problem may meet criteria for a "disorder" level PIR-GAS
score, and problems at this level typically require intervention for improvement in relationship functioning to occur.

Although the DC: 0–3 represents a significant advance with respect
to diagnosing infant mental health disorder, there remain a number of
important challenges. First, there are limited validity data available, with
only a few published articles examining the utility of this diagnostic
scheme and with many of these studies limited by relatively small sample sizes (Emde & Wise, 2003). Second, the DC: 0–3 does not provide
standardized assessment protocols; thus the process of applying this system is likely to be relatively idiosyncratic and not necessarily best informed by state-of-the-art knowledge regarding assessment procedures.
For example, Axis II relationship disorders require clinicians to assess
the behavioral quality of the interaction, the affective tone, and the level
of psychological involvement, yet there is no reference to a currently
available standard procedure for assessing these behavioral and represented levels of the parent–infant relationship.

Assessing Behavior along Multiple Continuums: Dimensional Approaches

Although they differ in a number of significant respects, both the DSM-
IV-TR and the DC: 0–3 system tend to assume at least two of the disease
model tenets: (1) the person or relationship either has ("meets criteria
for") or does not have ("fails to meet criteria for") a disorder, that is, disorders are assumed to be categorical, and (2) disorders are hierarchically
organized, that is, the goal is to assign a single primary diagnosis whenever possible.

There are several potential problems with these assumptions. If an
individual or relationship fails to meet criteria for full-blown disorder,
these diagnostic systems do not provide ways of meaningfully capturing
the presence of a particular symptomatology. This is problematic given
that current research suggests that the distinction between "disorder"
and "nondisorder" is not always categorical; problem severity may be
more continuous in nature, and consequently it is not always possible to
identify a critical threshold (First et al., 2002). In addition, if symptoms
are evident across a variety of domains, the search for a "primary" diagnosis may lead to the occlusion of the particular patterning of all relevant
behavior problems. For example, a child may exhibit both depressed and
aggressive behavior, but these mixed behavioral symptoms may not be

clearly identified in the primary diagnostic assignment. Comorbidity across broad domains of problem behavior is not surprising given that current research also indicates that there may be certain core dimensions of temperament and behavioral functioning that underlie or cut across most Axis I and II pathology. These include dimensions that have been highlighted by infant researchers as central to both normal and atypical infant social–emotional functioning, and include such constructs as affective regulation, impulse control, and anxiety modulation (First et al., 2002).

In response to these limitations, a number of researchers and clinicians have advocated for empirically-based syndrome approaches that are "bottom–up" rather than "top–down" in their derivation. These "dimensional" approaches assume that there are a number of independent child behavior traits and that children all exhibit these behaviors albeit in varying degrees. The emphasis is placed on the reported observed behavior of children rather than imposed adult categories based on clinician reports (Achenbach, 1985; Quay, 1986). Dimensional assessment allows the clinician or observer to rate the presence of a wide range of symptoms across multiple domains of behavior, typically rating the presence of the behavior along a scale that specifies the frequency or intensity of the problem (e.g., "How true is this of your child?" or "How often does this occur?"). Scores are assigned whether the individual meets criteria for a prespecified "disorder level" or not, though with many of these systems, certain scores are identified as norm-based cut points for "clinically relevant" functioning.

There are several clear advantages to this type of approach, including (1) the absence of a hierarchical assumption regarding different diagnostic features, which allows an individual "profile" to emerge that reflects the unique nature and patterning of symptoms for the individual or relationship; (2) many of the most commonly employed dimensional measures include reference group normative data, allowing the clinician to compare the individual's behavior ratings to those of other individuals of the same age and sex; and (3) subclinical threshold problems are still captured.

The most common empirically based measure for child behavior problems is the Child Behavior Checklist (CBCL; Achenbach, 2002a). Either parents (on the CBCL) or teachers (on the Caregiver–Teacher Report Form [C-TRF]; Achenbach, 2002b) rate toddler and young child behavior across a range of domains, with a clear emphasis on problematic behavior. The CBCL and C-TRF yield scores on a number of scales that are summarized into two primary dimensions: internalizing behavior (e.g., sadness/anxiety) and externalizing behavior (e.g., aggression/ oppositionality). Both of these dimensions, as well as the total score, have been extensively studied and validated, and this measure has been used with a wide range of populations. However, the preponderance of the normative data for the CBCL are for older children, and the instrument is only valid for use with children over the age of 1½.

More recently, empirically based measures for use with infants and toddlers have been developed: the Infant–Toddler Social and Emotional Assessment (ITSEA; Carter & Briggs-Gowan, 2000) and a "brief" version of the same instrument (BITSEA; Briggs-Gowan & Carter, 2001). Both provide age-relevant norms for symptomatic behavior across a range of infant-relevant domains. Like the CBCL, these measures are typically completed by parents or primary caregivers. Unlike many other assessment measures the ITSEA includes and emphasizes subscales assessing domains of competence in infant/toddler functioning, rather than focusing solely on age-relevant problem behavior. Thus, more in keeping with a developmental psychopathology framework, the ITSEA captures relevant clinical information regarding sources of both risk and strength in individual infant/toddler functioning (Briggs-Gowan, Carter, Skuban, & Horwitz, 2001).

Research using dimensional approaches for assessment has highlighted several of the limitations of the categorical system approach. First, problem behavior in the externalizing domain (e.g., aggression, oppositionality) is often highly correlated with problem behavior in the internalizing domain (e.g., sadness, anxiety), particularly in high-risk populations (McConaughy & Achenbach, 1994). This is consistent with clinical observations that comorbidity in clinical diagnoses is common, occurring at rates that far exceed chance (Angold et al., 1999; Caron & Rutter, 1991). Assigning a primary disorder may occlude or minimize the role of other important problems in individual or relationship functioning. Second, there is support for the assumption that it may be problematic to use a dichotomous "disorder" versus "nondisorder" approach; variations in subclinical threshold level problems may still be predictive of later problematic adaptation (Achenbach, 1994). In other words, it may be clinically significant that an individual or a relationship demonstrates certain problematic behaviors even if those problems do not yet fully meet criteria for psychiatric disorder.

Although research using dimensional approaches for the assessment of problem behavior shows great promise, current psychiatric diagnostic systems have generally not incorporated this type of approach into standard classification schemes. This is likely due to a bias toward medical models for classification of problems in mental health. From a clinical standpoint, while categorical diagnostic schemes may help provide overarching organization to multiple co-occurring presenting symptoms, they may limit the practitioner's ability to derive a comprehensive diagnostic assessment that fully reflects the range of individual and relationship functioning. Limitations also exist regarding the utility and availability of age-appropriate dimensional systems; for example, the most widely validated and used dimensional approaches tend to focus on the assessment of the child versus the relationship (e.g., the CBCL). Clearly more research is warranted to further develop the empirically based dimensional approaches for the assessment of infant mental health and relationship disturbance problems.

Assessing "Personal Meaning": The Representational Level of Relationships

In addition to the problems with existing schemes related to categorical diagnosis and little allowance for co-occurrence of disorders, there is an additional omission in the lack of attention to personal meaning systems. Many diagnostic systems lack an explicit emphasis on the assessment of the "personal meaning" of the relationship to the individuals involved, even though parents' meaning systems or representations are often the target of infant mental health interventions. These include most of the treatment approaches described in the present volume. Consider the following vignettes; both are responses of mothers of 7-month-old infants to the question, "How would you describe your child's personality?"

> *Parent A:* "She is very demanding. She's spoiled right now, so, like it's her way or no way. She's not real, too much fussy but she knows how to get your attention when she wants something. She just hollers. But, as far as her personality, she's . . . she's, like, pretty quiet. She'll be trying to act like she's innocent when she comes around other people. But when she's just at home, she's bad."

> *Parent B:* "He's very curious, he likes new things, and he's very determined. When he gets his mind set on something he finds a way to get to it. He, um, since he hasn't learned how to crawl yet he gets . . . he gets to where he wants to go by rolling and scooting. And he knows what he wants. He gets upset if you take a toy away from him, but he's—he's got a good personality.

He's pretty mellow, he just wants to have something to do all the time."

These brief responses illustrate how differently parents may experience their infants' needs or demands. Parent A is clearly quite frustrated with her infants' perceived manipulation and demandingness. Parent B describes her infant as needing something "to do all the time," but she sees this in a developmental context and has a generally positive orientation towards her son's personality. This aspect of the relationship requires assessment of the subjective or "represented" level of the relationship. While the DC: 0–3 incorporates subjective psychological-level components in the Axis II criteria, it does not provide guidelines for standard assessment of this aspect of the relationship. Parent meaning systems or representations are implicated in current research in infant mental health, and there is compelling evidence that attachment-based assessment procedures can yield important clinically relevant information regarding the inferred subjective experience of the parent–infant relationship (Zeanah, Larrieu, Heller, & Valliere, 2000).

Attachment-based approaches to assessment include behavioral-, narrative-, and projective-based assessment techniques (George & West, 2001; Zeanah et al., 2000). Narrative, or interview-based, assessment of the parents' representation of their infant holds particular promise for clinical intervention in the parent–infant relationship. These interviews can be used with parents from a wide range of socioeconomic and demographic backgrounds, can be coded reliably, and have been used successfully in clinical settings (Rosenblum, Dayton, & McDonough, in press; Zeanah & Benoit, 1995). Research has demonstrated that parents' representations of their infants, assessed via semistructured interviews, are associated with early infant emotion regulation (Rosenblum et al., 2002), clinical status of the infant (Coolbear & Benoit, 1999), and parental behavior with the infant (Rosenblum et al., in press). Indeed, parents' representations of their infants are associated with subsequent infant attachment security, even when the representations are assessed *prenatally* (Benoit, Parker, & Zeanah, 1997).

The Working Model of the Child Interview (WMCI; Zeanah & Benoit, 1995) is one of the most widely used procedures for assessing parents' representations of their infant for clinical purposes. The interview is approximately 1 hour long, includes open-ended questions regarding the parent's perceptions of the infant's personality and the relationship with the infant, and is coded both categorically and dimensionally. The coding system identifies multiple clinically relevant dimensions, including the caregiver's sensitivity, acceptance of the infant, psychological involvement in the relationship, and the affective tone of the representation. In addition, the representation is designated into one of three categories reflecting the overall organization of the interview: balanced, disengaged, or distorted. These categories incorporate both content (i.e., what is said) and process (e.g., how it is said) features of the parents' interview responses, and yield information regarding how the parent subjectively experiences the relationship with the infant. *Balanced* representations are characterized by a general acceptance of the infant, involvement in the relationship, an ability to tolerate both positive and negative emotions in the self and the infant without being overwhelmed, and an ability to respond sensitively to the infants physical and emotional needs. *Disengaged* representations reflect an emotion-deactivating strategy and are characterized by a tendency to impose a type of emotional distance from the infant. This often manifests either as cool rejecting of the infant or indifference and a lack of psychological investment in parenting. Finally, *distorted* representations reflect an emotion-heightening strategy, which may make the parent appear overwhelmed, confused, self-involved, or distracted by other emotion-laden issues when describing his or her experience of the relationship with the infant.

The subjective meaning level of the relationship is an important part of relationship assessment in infant mental health, and attachment-based measures show promise for the standard assessment of this level of relationship functioning. Extant research suggests that the most effective approaches to intervention may vary according to the nature of the parents' representation of early relationships, and this seems likely to hold true for representations of the current relationship with the child. For example, Bakermans-Kranenburg, Juffer, and van IJzendoorn (1998) found that mothers whose representations of their early attachment relationships to their own parents reflected preoccupation and affect heightening benefited most from parent–infant psychotherapies that included attention to the mothers' early childhood experiences. In contrast, mothers who were dismissive of their early attachment-related experiences benefited most from interventions that focused solely on their current relationship with their infant, with an emphasis on behavioral interaction. Given the data linking relationship representations with infant mental health disorder as well as parent–infant psychotherapy treatment outcomes, it would seem that as part of the process of ongoing refinement of diagnostic systems clinicians should consider more formal incorporation of representational-level criteria for relationship assessment.

REDEFINING INFANT MENTAL HEALTH DISORDER

How can we describe the population served by typical infant mental health programs? The range of problems that may be referred for infant mental health services is indeed quite broad, including such disparate diagnoses as autism and posttraumatic stress disorder. Although nationally representative studies of infant mental health disorder are not available, current research on the prevalence of infant mental health problems in community samples helps to clarify the types of problems that present with relative frequency and some of the diagnostic challenges posed by extant classification systems.

Infant Mental Health Problems: Community Prevalence Studies in the United States and Israel

As part of an infant mental health prevalence study in an urban Israeli setting, Keren, Feldman, and Tyano (2001) trained home-visiting public health nurses to screen all infants in their target community. The nurses were trained to attend to common infant mental health problems, and they referred cases to the local infant mental health clinic whenever there was a possible disorder. Once cases were referred, they were evaluated using the DC: 0–3 system for possible diagnosis.

Reasons for referral included sleep and eating problems, infant anxiety or irritability, language delays, suspected pervasive developmental disorder, aggression/oppositionality, toilet training difficulties, maternal depression, and poor mother–child relationships. There was a developmental dimension to referral, and the primary reasons for referral to the clinical agency varied significantly by age. During the first year of life infant eating problems and maternal depression were the primary reasons for referral. During the second year of life, referrals were primarily for infant sleep and eating problems, and during the third year of life, eating problems and aggression/oppositionality led the charts.

The finding that problems in infant regulatory behavior, that is, problems with sleeping and eating, were among the most common sources of referral is consistent with recent findings from our own research conducted in the United States. We have found that significant numbers of parents report problems or concerns regarding their infants' functioning in the broad regulatory domains of infant sleeping, feeding, and crying. The Michigan Family Study (MFS; McDonough, 1994) focused on the examination of infant regulatory behavior problems and relationship disturbances across the first 3 years of life. As part of a preliminary investigation, over 400 caregivers with 3- to 30-month-old children were interviewed during routine pediatric "well-child" visits regarding their perceptions of their infant's sleeping, crying, and feeding behavior (McDonough, Rosenblum, DeVoe, Gahagan, & Sameroff, 1998). Although these were not clinically identified parents or infants, almost half (45%) of all parents reported that their infant's behavior in one of these domains bothered or concerned them, thus underscoring the normative "perturbation" aspect of problems in these domains. A significant minority appeared to demonstrate more than passing concern with these behaviors; approximately 1 in 10 parents who reported concern also noted that their concerns regarding these problems were so significant as to have affected how they felt about being parents overall. This "spilling over" of problems in the infant domain to problems in parental feelings about parenting is likely to reflect progression along the relationship problem spectrum—from a more transient, limited perturbance to a more pervasive or fixed disturbance or disorder.

There was also a developmental dimension in the MFS data, indicating that the type of infant behavior that gave rise to the most parental concern varied at different ages. For example, the transition to toddlerhood, at about 16–18 months of age, appeared to be a time particularly associated with a number of marked shifts in both infant regulatory functioning and parents' perceptions of their child's behavior. Parental distress regarding their toddlers' crying and feeding increased markedly during this time period. It is possible that these findings reflect either the parents' mismatched developmental expectations or changes in the parent–infant relationships that are triggered by shifts in the infant's growing ability to regulate behaviors (Rosenblum, Devoe, McDonough, Gahagan, & Sameroff, 1998).

These prevalence data converge to suggest that concerns regarding infant regulatory behavior (e.g., sleeping and feeding) are quite common and are often the focus of referral to infant mental health practice. The Keren et al. (2001) study in Israel provides some insight into how these and other types of referrals translate into actual clinical diagnoses using current diagnostic systems. As noted previously, Keren and colleagues conducted comprehensive evaluations and assigned relevant DC: 0–3 diagnoses to all of the referred dyads. Over half of their referred sample met criteria for Axis I disorder. The most prevalent were eating behavior disorders, followed by adjustment disorders, sleep behavior disorders, disorders of attachment, affect, oppositional/aggressive disorder, regulatory disorders, and posttraumatic stress disorder.

Despite the fact that relationship problems accounted for only a small proportion of all reasons for referral (less than 5% of all cases), it was notable that approximately half of the referred sample in the Israeli study met criteria for Axis II (relationship disorder) classification. The majority of those who met criteria for an Axis II disorder were assigned into the "mixed" category, suggesting some limitations to the categorical approach to assessment of problems in this domain. Similarly, very few of the referred participants met criteria for disorder on only one axis, but rather diagnosis on multiple axes was the norm. The most prevalent pattern of multiaxial diagnosis was an Axis I infant diagnosis and an Axis II relationship disorder.

The importance of parents' representations is emphasized in the MFS study, where we found significant associations between parents' reports of infant problems in self-regulation, parental anxiety, and nonbalanced (disengaged or distorted) representations of the infant. Mothers' with nonbalanced representations of their infant were more likely to spontaneously report concerns with infant crying, sleeping, or feeding during the Working Model of the Child Interview (WMCI). These mothers also expressed more feelings of anger, helplessness, depression, or anxiety with respect to parenting their infant, and the problems they experienced were more likely to have begun to affect their acceptance of the infant and other domains of their life (e.g., the marital relationship or work).

Thus it appears that co-occurrence among infant diagnoses with aspects of maternal psychopathology or relationship disturbance is quite common. This "relationship-embedded" feature of infant psychiatric disturbance is not fully reflected in the assignment of single Axis I or II disorder but, rather, in the complex patterning of associations between infant, caregiver, and relationship problems at the behavioral and representational levels.

Illustrating the Diagnostic Challenges: Reported Problems in Infant Sleep or Feeding

Currently available prevalence data highlight several of the key limitations and challenges of our current diagnostic approaches for problems in two of the most commonly referred problems: disturbances in infant sleep and feeding.

Sleep Disorders

The DSM-IV-TR and DC: 0–3 systems provide markedly different diagnostic possibilities for problems in the domain of infant sleep behavior. The DSM-IV-TR provides Axis I sleep disorder diagnoses, but not specifically under the category of disorders usually assigned during infancy, childhood, and adolescence. Distinctions are made between multiple types of sleep disorder, for example, the "dyssomnias" category, which includes insomnia, hypersomnia, and narcolepsy diagnoses, and the "parasomnias" category, which includes sleep terrors and nightmare disorders. The DC: 0–3 system provides a somewhat more limited range of diagnostic options, with only one category of possible sleep disorder— the sleep behavior disorder diagnosis. This broad category has been designed to capture problems in infant sleeping across a range of subdomains.

Estimates of prevalence vary widely (from 15 to 50%), with many studies converging to suggest that approximately one in three infants experience some type of sleep problem, including resisting going to bed and/or settling down to sleep or night waking (Goodlin-Jones, Burnham, & Anders, 2000; Lozoff, Wolf, & Davis, 1985). Concerns regarding sleep are more prevalent in higher-risk populations. For example, two-thirds of the patients of child psychiatrists are described as experiencing problems with sleep (Wolfson, Lacks, & Futterman, 1992). In addition to being fairly common, it appears that problems in this domain are often more than transient perturbations; for example, Zuckerman, Stevenson, and Bailey (1987) observed that approximately 40% of the identified full-term infants with sleep problems had problems that were persistent from infancy into early childhood.

The diagnostic limitations that have been described previously— specifically, the continued need for identification of developmentally appropriate criteria, inclusion of relationship dimensions, and attention to the relationship partners' personal meaning systems—are evident in aspects of both the DSM-IV-TR and the DC: 0–3 systems classification of sleep disorder. There is clearly a need for further refinement of this diagnostic category, as different diagnoses could lead to different interventions.

First, the DSM-IV-TR makes little reference to infant-specific sleep problems; the criteria are almost exclusively phrased in terms of adult manifestation of these disorders. While the DC: 0–3 system aims to address this limitation by providing an infant-relevant diagnosis, unlike the DSM-IV-TR the DC: 0–3 system makes no distinction between types of sleep problems. Furthermore, neither the DSM-IV-TR nor the DC: 0–3 systems provide developmental norms for sleep behavior, despite the accumulation of data describing typical settling and waking patterns across the first 2 years of life (Anders, Goodlin-Jones, & Sadeh, 2000). Anders and colleagues have detailed the limitations of the diagnostic systems for infant sleep disorders and have generated a proposal for a more refined, developmentally appropriate approach to classification of problems in this domain. Their system makes explicit reference to age norms in determining when infant sleep behavior meets criteria for disorder, and they distinguish between several types of infant-relevant sleep problems, including night waking problems, sleep onset problems, parasomnias, and sleep apnea syndromes.

Second, all of the currently available diagnostic systems identify the sleep disorder in the individual infant (i.e., they are Axis I diagnoses), despite accumulating research evidence demonstrating associations between sleep disorders and the caregiving environment (e.g., parenting behavior, parental psychopathology, and attachment insecurity). For example, Paret (1983) found that infants who were night wakers were more likely to have mothers who held and touched them more throughout the day, perhaps indicating less tolerance for independence or autonomy in the infant. Goodlin-Jones et al. (2000) summarize research linking maternal psychopathology, in particular anxiety and depression, with infant sleep problems. For example, mothers who report higher levels of depressive feelings have infants who are less likely to self-soothe during night wakings (Goodlin-Jones, Eiben, & Anders, 1997). Mothers' feelings of depression may be intensified given the loss of sleep, and those feelings of increased depression and exhaustion may further exacerbate interactional difficulties, thus creating a transactional process between caregiver and child that may increase the infant's difficulties with self-regulation (Goodlin-Jones et al., 2000).

Third, the diagnostic systems do not consider representations. Sleep problems have been found to be associated with disturbances in the subjective, or represented, level of the relationship. In our own research on the MFS we have found that mothers' representations of their infant, assessed when infants were 7 months of age via the WMCI, were predictive of subsequent sleep behavior problems, including more night wakings and daytime sleepiness, more than 2 years later when the children were 33 months of age. Similarly, Benoit, Zeanah, Boucher, and Minde (1992) found higher rates of nonbalanced attachment representations, assessed via the Adult Attachment Interview, among the mothers of infants with sleep disorders.

In sum, infant sleep is clearly a dyadically regulated phenomenon with important developmental, behavioral, and representational aspects. Parents often struggle with questions regarding how to manage challenges with infant sleep behavior: Should I go to him when he cries? How often should she wake at night? Problems parents encounter in managing these challenges typically remain in the domain of "relationship perturbations" and resolve over a relatively brief period of time. Yet even in the case of problematic infant sleep that meets diagnostic criteria for disorder, interventions aimed at helping parents manage problems in this domain often focus on supporting parents in the process of helping their child develop more effective regulatory strategies (e.g., Ferber, 1985; McDonough, 2000; Minde et al., 1993). Thus, despite the current diagnostic focus on the individual infant, the caregiving and relational context appears likely to be a central aspect of infant sleep disorder.

Feeding Disorders

The DSM-IV-TR and DC: 0–3 diagnostic systems would also benefit from a more developmental relational approach to the classification of infant feeding disorders. The DSM-IV-TR currently identifies several diagnostic categories for disturbances in eating, including "pica" (i.e., persistent eating of nonnutritive substances), rumination disorder (i.e., repeated regurgitation and rechewing of food), and general feeding disorder (i.e., an unspecified type of feeding disturbance that interferes with growth and weight gain during early childhood). "Failure to thrive" is not described specifically, though would fall under the General Feeding Disorder of Infancy or Early Childhood category. The DC: 0–3 provides one primary infant eating disorder diagnosis: the eating behavior disorder. Failure to thrive is considered under this diagnosis, although the DC: 0–3 system specifies that this category should not be used as a primary diagnosis when a child's eating disturbances are part of a larger symptom picture, associated with other affective or behavioral problems, tactile sensitivity, regulatory disorder, or disturbances in primary relationships.

What do we know about the prevalence of feeding disorders in infancy? Estimates for more extreme disturbances in feeding and nutrition, such as failure to thrive, range from 1 to 5% for infant pediatric hospital admissions and between 4 and 14% of infants in ambulatory care (Lyons-Ruth, Zeanah, & Benoit, 1996). However, much research on feeding problems in infancy has used broader criteria for establishing diagnostic prevalence rates. Lyons-Ruth and colleagues (1996) summarize currently available prevalence data from a variety of studies and determine that feeding disorders affect between 6 and 35% of young children. This is clearly a very broad range of prevalence rates; indeed, feeding and eating disorders were so variably defined across these studies that it is difficult to determine the incidence or prevalence rates of particular types of infant feeding disorders.

Consistent with the need for developmental refinement of the sleep disorder category, it appears that the feeding disorder category may benefit from further refinement of the diagnostic subcategories. Such a system might, for example, distinguish more clearly between specific types of feeding behavior problems that are observed during infancy and toddlerhood (e.g., undernutrition, food refusal, conditioned gagging, conditioned vomiting, or obesity).

Feeding is also a very relationally embedded phenomenon. Infants become increasingly able to self-regulate their feeding efforts, and parents provide the context for these normative transitions to occur (Benoit, 2000; Chatoor, Ganiban, Conner, Plummer, & Harmon, 1998). Yet many of the diagnostic criteria for feeding or eating disorders focus solely on the infant, not the feeding relationship. This failure to incorporate relational phenomenon fails to adequately address an abundance of evidence linking aspects of the caregiving environment with infant feeding and eating disorders. While some controversy exists regarding the causal role of caregiving difficulties, current research has typically revealed a "mixed" etiology for many eating disorders, involving both biological and environmental risk factors (Benoit, 2000; Drotar & Robinson, 2000; Lyons-Ruth et al., 1996). Apparent links between failure to thrive and the caregiving environment, including dramatic weight gain when the infant is removed from a specific relational context, have made this a classic infant mental health condition illustrating the links between infant pathology and problems in the caregiving relationship. Current research has clearly highlighted the need to consider multiple dimensions of causal influences (Benoit, 2000; Crittenden, 1987; Drotar & Robinson, 2000).

Links between feeding problems and problems in caregiving further underscore the need to assess mothers' representations of their relationship with their infants. For example, Coolbear and Benoit (1999) reported that mothers of infants with eating disorders tended to be nonautonomous in their adult attachment relationships and that their representations of their infant tended to be nonbalanced, colored by angry or worried preoccupation or rejection of the infant's needs for autonomy or dependence. Similarly, in our work on the MFS we found that mothers with 7-month-old infants who are described as "difficult to feed" were more likely to have nonbalanced representations of their infant.

The apparent link between problems in the caregiving environment and a variety of eating problems during infancy and toddlerhood suggests that a more appropriate conceptualization for many cases may be a "feeding relationship" versus an "infant eating" disorder.

CASE STUDY: DIAGNOSTIC CHALLENGES
WITH INFANT FEEDING PROBLEMS

A brief case vignette illustrates some of the diagnostic challenges for the assessment of problems with infant feeding. Carol was a 28-year-old European American stay-at-home parent who lived with her husband and their two children, 4-year-old James and 8-month-old Sarah. At the time of referral (into a study focused on infant behavior problems) Sarah was in the low normal range for height and weight, but consistent with her mother's concerns that she was not "taking in" proper nutrition her pediatrician had also noticed that there had been a recent decline in Sarah's rate of growth.

During the initial contact Carol reported no concerns regarding Sarah's sleep or crying, but emphasized that Sarah was difficult to feed and often refused food. This concerned Carol enormously, and it was apparent to the home visitor that she had begun to feel fairly angry and resentful toward Sarah. When asked what about her daughter's behavior concerned her the most, she replied, "Difficult feeding, she's a difficult baby to feed. You have to have a lot of patience, because she'll hold her little mouth shut and you just got to kind of pry it in there. And now I think she thinks that's the way [to eat], because that's what I've been doing. I've just been kind of prying her mouth open, her gums, 'cause she keeps them closed, that or she'll pucker her lips inward. She's just extremely difficult that way."

In response to Carol's reports that feeding was a primary concern, a home visit was timed to include an opportunity for observation of a meal. After a brief "warm-up" period during which the home visitor talked with Carol and observed her and Sarah in free play, Carol indicated that her daughter was ready for lunch. She placed Sarah in an infant seat on the kitchen table. The seat tilted backward, thus preventing Sarah from sitting upright during the feeding. Carol narrated the entire feeding process, describing how the problems typically emerged during a feeding and how Sarah's responses to this observed meal were either similar or different compared to "usual." Between talking with the home visitor and calling out to her son as he ran about the house, Carol only rarely directed her comments toward Sarah.

At the start of feeding Carol indicated to the home visitor that she felt Sarah should already be eating jarred meats, vegetables, and other types of table food, but that she only liked to eat fruit. This greatly concerned her, as she felt Sarah was not getting "proper nutrition." Carol used a spoon to feed Sarah and kept the food coming rapidly, often before Sarah had a chance to swallow completely. Sarah was initially quite compliant, eating at a rapid pace, but after several minutes made efforts to turn away from the spoon for more time to swallow or to avoid the vegetables. In order to get Sarah to eat some of the vegetables, Carol used what she called her strategy of "surprise tactics"—feeding Sarah several spoonfuls of fruit, so that she would open her mouth readily, then filling the next spoonful with vegetables. Whenever this happened, Sarah became distressed, and Carol noted to the home visitor that this was normally the point at which she "tried to make herself gag." Indeed, Sarah did begin to turn her head away and cry, and when Carol persisted in feeding her despite her cries, Sarah gagged on the food placed in her mouth. Carol grew frustrated with Sarah, who was at this point crying, gagging, and attempting to refuse the food her mother continued to try to feed her. This pattern persisted for several minutes before Carol stopped and exasperatedly noted to the home visitor, "You see? She just won't eat. It's done. I don't know how she's going to get the proper nutrition! She won't let me feed her—no matter what I try to do!"

Several days later Carol was seen again at a special developmental playroom. She engaged with her daughter in a series of tasks, including another feeding interaction. The feeding sequence unfolded in much the same fashion, although this time Sarah began to refuse the food much more quickly and Carol again appeared intrusive and frustrated. The interactive tasks were followed by a representational interview focused on Carol's thoughts and feelings about parenting and her relationship with Sarah. During this interview, she revealed that her own mother had been diagnosed with schizophrenia when Carol was young and that she had been in and out of psychiatric hospitals most of Carol's childhood. Carol had often been placed in the role of "caretaker" of both of her younger siblings during her mother's lengthy hospitalizations, as well as of her mother at times when she was at home. She emphasized how much she wanted to be a different type of mother to her daughter, in particular, to be able to provide Sarah the nurturance she herself felt she never had.

Based on these observations, the home visitor provided Sarah's developmental pediatrician with some preliminary feedback, and the pediatrician referred Carol and Sarah for infant mental health services for further assistance with the feeding problems.

Carol and Sarah were seen again approximately 8 months later, when Sarah was almost 1½ years old. At this point Carol reported that Sarah's eating problems had improved significantly; indeed, she was still in the average range for height and weight. However, Carol reported that Sarah was now a very aggressive, "very temperamental" child, and described having problems with disciplining Sarah. As part of the follow-up evaluation, Carol and Sarah participated in a brief separation and reunion task. Following a second brief separation from her mother, Carol returned to reengage with Sarah, who had been quite independent during the separation, exploring the room with apparent glee. When her mother returned Sarah became more reclusive, turning her attention away from her mother and toward a small toy. When her mother tried to interest her in a different toy, Sarah refused to engage. Carol then leaned in towards Sarah's face and asked her daughter to "give her mommy a little kiss," at which point Sarah picked up a block and aggressively swung at her mother's face, loudly asserting, "No! No! No!" Carol retreated from Sarah and watched her play with toys.

Diagnostic Issues

While it should be clear to any practitioner that this is a dyad at risk, it is noteworthy that under stringent application Carol and Sarah would be unlikely to meet the criteria for a specific Axis I disorder using the DSM-IV-TR or the DC: 0–3 systems. The DSM-IV-TR feeding disorder category requires evidence of persistent failure to gain weight or significant weight loss over at least a 1-month period, and the DC: 0–3 eating disorder category rules out problems in feeding that appear to be primarily reflective of disturbances in the relationship.

The DC: 0–3 does, however, provide a reasonable diagnostic alternative for this dyad, specifically, a *relationship disorder* diagnosis on Axis II, most likely an *overinvolved* subtype. Although the disordered behavior appears at the time of referral to be limited to one domain (i.e., feeding), the symptoms appear severe, unlikely to change without intervention, and are clearly beginning to interfere with each partners' developmental and relational tasks, specifically, self-feeding and increased autonomy for Sarah, and feelings of efficacy and opportunities for shared positive affect during feeding for Sarah and Carol. It is thus likely that Carol and Sarah would meet criteria for *disorder* on the PIR-GAS. Although Carol's reports of concern regarding Sarah's eating subsided following treatment and the passing of time, the underlying relationship disturbance remained apparent more than half a year later.

While the DC: 0–3 Axis II relationship disorder seems an appropriate classification, it is important to note that the feeding-specific aspect of their relational disturbance at the initial observation is not captured by this broad category of classification. It is possible that a dimensional approach might have allowed for assessment of both problems in the relationship along the perturbance-to-disorder continuum, as well as assessment of problems in the feeding behavior or aggression/hostility that may not have met criteria for categorical clinical diagnosis.

It is worth noting that while current diagnostic systems may be somewhat limited with respect to diagnoses that fully capture the problems Carol and Sarah experience, current theories of feeding problems in infancy reflect the primacy of the relationship and transactional patterns that unfold over time between individuals. For example, the struggles between Carol and Sarah during feeding interaction closely exemplify a relationship-focused transactional model of feeding disturbance described by Chatoor, Dickson, Schaefer, and Eagan (1985), who have observed that infant feeding disorder is often associated with disturbed relational transactional processes during feeding interactions.

We might wonder about the meaning of these types of interactive sequences in day-to-day life—what consequences will these patterns hold for the infant and caregiver over time? Note that in the case of Sarah and Carol, the developmental pathway of problem behaviors appears to have shifted over the period of observation—from a relationship problem that manifests primarily (or solely) in the feeding domain to aggressive/coercive interactions less than a year later that appeared to be more "fixed" and to cut across a variety of domains. Indeed, when Carol and Sarah were seen for follow-up, Carol's perception of Sarah was no longer simply that she was a "difficult eater" but, rather, that she was now a "difficult child." Sarah's corresponding aggressive and rejecting/avoidant behavior at 1½ may reflect not only problems in the relationship but possible risk factors for later conduct or behavior problems as well. It is possible to imagine, as Stern (1989) has described, the ways in which Carol and Sarah's daily lived interactive moments during feeding routines may have developed over time to create a less than optimal internal representation of the relationship for both partners. What begins as an infant problem, or, perhaps in this case, a maternal "ghost in the nursery," may subsequently truly be a relationship problem in the present that haunts both mother and child (Fraiberg, Adelson, & Shapiro, 1975).

CONCLUSIONS

It is clear that while problems in the individual may be the source of referral, it is often the caregiver–infant relationship that is (or should be) the focus of our assessment and intervention. Our diagnoses, however, often fail to adequately capture the developmental, relational, or representational aspects of problems in infant mental health.

There are high levels of correspondence between infant problems and problems in the caregiving environment. It appears that the most commonly referred problems involve central domains of infant physiological regulation—areas that inherently involve dyadic coregulation between the infant and the caregiver and developmental change over time. These findings underscore the need for diagnostic classification systems that reflect the relational and developmental aspects of disorder. The DC: 0–3 system reflects a clear step in the right direction, incorporating relational components and specifying diagnostic criteria in more age-appropriate terms. However, many of these diagnoses continue to require further refinement, so that they will more adequately reflect the range of infant mental health problems referred and the manifestation of problem behavior during infancy and early childhood.

Furthermore, some of the limitations inherent to categorical diagnostic approaches appear to limit the DC: 0–3 system as well. Dimensional approaches may allow for significant advances in diagnostic conceptualization, permitting the identification of subthreshold risk areas and problems in multiple co-occurring domains. At present, however, the most commonly employed dimensional systems do not directly assess qualities of the caregiver–child relationship. Given the data that so many relationship disorders are classified as the "mixed relationship disorder" type (Emde & Wise, 2003; Keren et al., 2001), it is possible that incorporation of dimensional ratings across all the subpatterns would provide better assessment of the complex patterning of disturbances in parent–child relationships. Finally, relationships often hold powerful subjective meaning for the individuals involved, and assessments of parents' representations of the infant and the relationship with the infant can yield important information regarding the caregiving context and relationship risk. There is a need for more explicit inclusion of subjective, or representational-level, criteria for the diagnosis of parent–infant relationship disorder.

As infant mental health specialists we are often called to intervene not only with infants but also with parent–infant relationships. Subsequent chapters in this volume reflect state-of-the-art relationship-based interventions designed to address problems in a range of infant-relevant domains. It is clearly time for our diagnostic systems to also better address these issues, so that we may continue to refine our assessment, prevention, and intervention services. Only then can we begin to accurately describe the phenomenology of infant mental health disorder, advocate for reimbursement for services provided to relationships at risk, and better tailor our services to the clients we serve.

REFERENCES

Achenbach, T. M. (1985). *Assessment and taxonomy of child and adolescent psychopathology*. Newbury Park, CA: Sage.

Achenbach, T. M. (1994). Child Behavior Checklist and related instruments. In M. E. Marish (Ed.), *The use of psychological testing for treatment planning and outcome assessment* (pp. 517–549). Hillsdale, NJ: Erlbaum.

Achenbach, T. M. (2002a). *Child Behavior Checklist/1½–5 (CBCL 1½ –5)*. Burlington: University of Vermont, Department of Psychiatry.

Achenbach, T. M. (2002b). *Caregiver–Teacher Report Form/1½–5 (C-TRF 1½–5)*. Burlington: University of Vermont, Department of Psychiatry.

American Psychiatric Association. (2000). *Diagnostic and statistical manual of mental disorders* (4th ed., text rev.). Washington, DC: Author.

Anders, T. F. (1989). Clinical syndromes, relationship disturbances, and their assessment. In A. J. Sameroff & R. N. Emde (Eds.), *Relationship disturbances in early childhood: A developmental approach* (pp. 125–144). New York: Basic Books.

Anders, T., Goodlin-Jones, B., & Sadeh, A. (2000). Sleep disorders. In C. H. Zeanah (Ed.), *Handbook of infant mental health* (2nd ed., pp.326–338). New York: Guilford Press.

Angold, A. E., Costello, J., & Erkanli, A. (1999). Comorbidity. *Journal of Child Psychology and Psychiatry and Allied Disciplines, 40,* 57–87.

Bakermans-Kranenburg, M. J., Juffer, F., & van IJzendoorn, M. H. (1998). Interventions with video feedback and attachment discussions: Does type of maternal insecurity make a difference? *Infant Mental Health Journal, 19,* 202–219.

Benoit, D. (2000). Feeding disorders, failure to thrive, and obesity. In C. H. Zeanah (Ed.), *Handbook of infant mental health* (2nd ed., pp. 339–352). New York: Guilford Press.

Benoit, D., Parker, K., & Zeanah, C. H. (1997). Mothers' representations of their infants assessed prenatally: Stability and association with infants' attachment classifications. *Journal of Child Psychology and Psychiatry, and Allied Disciplines, 38,* 307–313.

Benoit, D., Zeanah, C. H., Boucher, C., & Minde, K. K. (1992). Sleep disorders in early childhood: Association with insecure maternal attachment. *Journal of the American Academy of Child and Adolescent Psychiatry, 31,* 86–93.

Briggs-Gowan, M. J., & Carter, A. S. (2001). *Brief Infant–Toddler Social and Emotional Assessment (BITSEA)—Manual Version 1.0*. Unpublished manuscript, Yale University, New Haven, CT.

Briggs-Gowan, M. J., Carter, A. S., Skuban, E. M., & Horwitz, S. M. (2001). Prevalence of social–emotional and behavioral problems in a community sample of 1– and 2–year-olds. *Journal of the American Academy of Child and Adolescent Psychiatry, 40*, 811–819.

Caron, C., & Rutter, M. (1991). Comorbidity in child psychopathology: Concepts, issues and research strategies. *Journal of Child Psychology and Psychiatry and Allied Disciplines, 7*, 1063–1080.

Carter, A. S., & Briggs-Gowan, M. J. (2000). *Infant–Toddler Social and Emotional Assessment (ITSEA)—Manual.* Unpublished manuscript, Yale University, New Haven, CT.

Chatoor, I., Dickson, L., Schaefer, S., & Eagan, J. (1985). A developmental classification of feeding disorders associated with failure to thrive: Diagnosis and treatment. In D. Drotar (Ed.), *New directions in failure to thrive: Implications for research and practice* (pp. 235–258). New York: Plenum Press.

Chatoor, I., Ganiban, J., Conner, V., Plummer, N., & Harmon, R. (1998). Attachment and feeding problems: A reexamination of nonorganic failure to thrive and attachment insecurity. *Journal of the American Academy of Child and Adolescent Psychiatry, 37*, 1217–1224.

Coolbear, J., & Benoit, D. (1999). Failure to thrive: Risk for clinical disturbance of attachment? *Infant Mental Health Journal, 13*, 252–268.

Costello E. J., & Angold, A. (2000). Developmental epidemiology: A framework for developmental psychopathology. In A. Sameroff, M. Lewis, & S. Miller (Eds.), *Handbook of developmental psychopathology* (pp. 57–75). New York: Plenum Press.

Crittenden, P. (1987). Nonorganic failure to thrive: Deprivation or distortion? *Infant Mental Health Journal, 8*, 51–64.

Drotar, D., & Robinson, J. (2000). Developmental psychopathology of failure to thrive. In A. J. Sameroff, M. Lewis, & S. M. Miller (Eds.), *Handbook of developmental psychopathology* (2nd ed., pp. 351–364). New York: Plenum Press.

Emde, R. N., & Wise, B. (2003). The cup is half full: Initial clinical trials of DC: 0–3 and a recommendation for revision. *Infant Mental Health Journal, 24*, 437–446.

Ferber, R. (1985). *Solve your child's sleep problems.* New York: Simon & Schuster.

First, M. B., Bell, C. C., Buthbert, B., Krystal, J. H., Malison, R., Offord, D. R., Reiss, D., Shea, T., Widiger, T., & Wisner, K. L. (2002). Personality disorders and relational disorders: A research agenda for addressing crucial gaps in DSM. In D. J. Kupfer, M. B. First, & D. A. Regier (Eds.), *A research agenda for DSM-V.* Washington, DC: American Psychiatric Association.

Fraiberg, S., Adelson, E., & Shapiro, V. (1975). Ghosts in the nursery: A psychoanalytic approach to the problems of impaired mother–infant relationships. *Journal of the American Academy of Child Psychiatry 14*, 387–421.

George, C., & West, M. (2001). The development and preliminary validation of a new measure of adult attachment: The Adult Attachment Projective. *Attachment and Human Development*, 3, 30–61.

Goodlin-Jones, B. L., Burnham, M. M., & Anders, T. F. (2000). Sleep and sleep disturbances: Regulatory processes in infancy. In A. J. Sameroff, M. Lewis, & S. M. Miller (Eds.), *Handbook of developmental psychopathology* (2nd ed., pp. 309–325). New York: Plenum Press.

Goodlin-Jones, B. L., Eiben, L. A., & Anders, T. F. (1997). Maternal well-being and sleep-wake behaviors in infants: An intervention using maternal odor. *Infant Mental Health Journal*, 18, 378–393.

Keren, M., Feldman, R., & Tyano, S. (2001). Diagnoses and interactive patterns of infants referred to a community-based infant mental health clinic. *Journal of the American Academy of Child and Adolescent Psychiatry*, 40, 27–35.

Lozoff, B., Wolf, A. W., & Davis, N. S. (1985). Sleep problems seen in pediatric practice. *Pediatrics*, 75, 477–483.

Lyons-Ruth, K., Zeanah, C. H., & Benoit, D. (1996). Disorders and risk for disorder during infancy and toddlerhood. In E. J. Mash & R. A. Barkley (Eds.), *Child psychopathology* (pp. 457–491). New York: Guilford Press.

McConaughy, S. H., & Achenbach, T. M. (1994). Comorbidity of empirically based syndromes in matched general population and clinical samples. *Journal of Child Psychology and Psychiatry and Allied Disciplines*, 35, 1141–1157.

McDonough, S. C. (1994). *Preventing mental health problems in multirisk infants*. National Institute of Mental Health RO1 Grant Proposal, University of Michigan, Ann Arbor.

McDonough, S. C. (2000). Interaction guidance: An approach for difficult to engage families. In C. H. Zeanah (Ed.), *Handbook of infant mental health* (2nd ed., pp. 485–493). New York: Guilford Press.

McDonough, S. C., Rosenblum, K., DeVoe, E., Gahagan, S., & Sameroff, A. (1998). *Parent concerns about infant regulatory problems: Excessive crying, sleep problems, and feeding difficulties*. Paper presented at the International Conference on Infant Studies, Atlanta, GA.

Minde, K., Popiel, K., Leos, N., Falkner, S., Parker, K., & Handley-Derry, M. (1993). The evaluation and treatment of sleep disturbances in young children. *Journal of Child Psychology and Psychiatry*, 34, 521–533.

Paret, I. (1983). Night waking and its relation to mother-infant interaction in nine-month-old infants. In J. D. Call & E. Galenson (Eds.), *Frontiers of infant psychiatry* (Vol. 1, pp. 171–177). New York: Basic Books.

Quay, H. C. (1986). Classification. In H. C. Quay & J. S. Werry (Eds.), *Psychopathological disorders of childhood* (pp. 1–34), New York: Wiley.

Rosenblum, K., De Voe, E., McDonough, S. C., Gahagan, S., & Sameroff, A. (1998). *Physiologic regulation problems during infancy*. Paper presented at the International Conference on Infant Studies, Atlanta, GA.

Rosenblum, K. L., Dayton, C., & McDonough, S. C. (in press). Communicating feelings: Links between mothers' representations of their infants and early emotional development. In O. Mayseless (Ed.), *Parenting representations: Theory, research, and clinical implications.* New York: Cambridge University Press.

Sameroff, A. J., & Emde, R. N. (1989). *Relationship disturbances in early childhood: A developmental approach.* New York: Basic Books.

Sameroff, A. J., & Fiese, B. H. (2000). Models of development and developmental risk. In C. H. Zeanah (Ed.), *Handbook of infant mental health* (2nd ed., pp. 3–19). New York: Guilford Press.

Sroufe, L. A. (1989). Relationships, self, and individual adaptation. In A. J. Sameroff & R. N. Emde (Eds.), *Relationship disturbances in early childhood: A developmental approach* (pp. 70–94). New York: Basic Books.

Stern, D. N. (1989). The representation of relational patterns: Developmental considerations. In A. J. Sameroff & R. N. Emde (Eds). *Relationship disturbances in early childhood: A developmental approach* (pp. 52–69). New York: Basic Books.

Wolfson, A., Lacks, P., & Futterman, A. (1992). Effects of parent training on infant sleeping patterns, parents' stress, and perceived parental competence. *Journal of Counseling and Clinical Psychology, 60,* 41–48.

Zeanah, C. H., & Benoit, D. (1995). Clinical applications of a parent perception interview in infant mental health. *Infant Psychiatry. 4,* 539–554.

Zeanah, C. H., Larrieu, J., Heller, S. S., & Valliere, J. (2000). Infant–parent relationship assessment. In C. H. Zeanah (Ed.), *Handbook of infant mental health* (2nd ed., pp. 222–235). New York: Guilford Press.

Zero to Three/National Center for Clinical Infant Programs. (1994). *Diagnostic classification of mental health and developmental disorders of infancy and early childhood.* Arlington, VA: Author.

Zuckerman, B., Stevenson, J., & Bailey, V. (1987). Sleep problems in early childhood: Continuities, predictive factors, and behavioral correlates. *Pediatrics, 80,* 664–671.

PART II

VARIATIONS

CHAPTER 4

INTERACTION GUIDANCE
Promoting and Nurturing the Caregiving Relationship

Susan C. McDonough

The Interaction Guidance (IG) therapeutic treatment model incorporates principles of a family system theory into a multigenerational transactional preventive intervention. The resulting approach focuses therapeutic treatment on the infant–caregiver relationship rather than on either the infant or the caregiver alone apart from the environmental context. *Observable interactions* between the baby and caregiver serves as the early *therapeutic focus* and, as such, serve as the therapeutic port of entry. Caregiver *interactions* with the infant are understood both as *reflection* of family structure and *caregiving nurturance* and as a reflection of the caregiver's and baby's *representational world*.

To faciliate the parents' understanding of growth and development of their child, the caregivers are actively involved in observing both the behaviors of their infant and their own style of interaction and play with their child. The use of videotape in treatment allows for immediate feedback to the parent(s) or family regarding their own behavior and its effect on the infant's behavior. Through viewing samples of parent–child play interaction, family members become more aware of important interactive behaviors that are positive and need to be reinforced, elaborated and extended, and those interactions that were less enjoyable or inappropriate requiring redirection, alteration or elimination. The use of videotape also provides the parents with the opportunity to listen more carefully to what they say to their child and the manner in which they say it.

The IG treatment approach was created specifically to meet the needs of infants and their families who previously were not successfully engaged in mental health treatment or who refused treatment referral. Many of these families could be described as being "overburdened" by poverty, poor education, family mental illness, substance abuse, inadequate housing, large family size, lack of a parenting partner, or inadequate social support. In an effort to reach overburdened families, IG therapists invite each family to take an active role in the creation and evaluation of their family's treatment. The goal was to develop a therapeutic approach that was sensitive to each family's strengths and vulnerabilities.

ELEMENTS OF INTERVENTION PROGRAMS

Successful clinical interventions have both process and structural elements. *Structural elements* are the specific procedures of the intervention. Examples of structural elements of intervention include addressing the unique needs of each family, involving extended family or household members in the treatment plan when appropriate or necessary, offering supplemental assistance when such help is asked or deemed critical to treatment success, providing the option of follow-up services at the conclusion of treatment, and including the family in the evaluation of treatment progress (McDonough, 1995, 2000b). *Process elements* of successful clinical interventions address how the clinician offers the therapeutic assistance, that is, carries out the procedures. These process elements consist of encouraging the family members to define the problem or issue of concern as they see it, emphasizing a family's strengths while recognizing its vulnerabilities and limitations, embracing a nonjudgmental stance in work with families while conveying societal norms for the family's caregiving behavior, using an egalitarian and cooperative approach in the engagement and treatment of families, and offering alternative perspectives to the parents about their child caregiving through individually designed treatment (McDonough, 1995, 2000a).

PROCESSES OF INTERACTION GUIDANCE

IG therapists embrace certain assumptions when working with families. This framework of beliefs is described below as "therapeutic stance." Likewise, there also are specific treatment techniques, or "therapeutic practices," that IG therapists use to facilitate family system change.

Therapeutic Stance

• *Ask, rather than assume, that the family believes that you will be helpful to them.* Simply asking the family the question, "Is there anything you think I can do to be helpful?" can be a powerful message that the ultimate decision to participate in treatment rests with the family. Critical to the success of the helping process are two components: (1) a person offers some assistance or aid, and (2) another person accepts what is offered. Nonacceptance is often conveyed in many indirect ways (e.g., families fail to come to scheduled appointments, no one appears to be at home when the therapist makes a scheduled home visit, or telephone calls go unanswered and outreach efforts are refused). Professionals working with families can increase the likelihood that the offered help will be accepted by encouraging the family members to decide what, if any, assistance they desire or need rather than assuming that a clinician-identified problem is the family's main source of concern. Asking for their opinion also reinforces the role of the parents as decision makers in the family and responsible agents in guaranteeing their child's welfare. Deferring to their expertise as the individuals who know their child "best" affords the parents legitimate power in making or influencing decisions about what's in the best interest for their child. Consider the ramifications of "doing for" a family (including handling the baby) without being asked to do so. Sometimes our "assistance" may be interpreted as the clinician knowing better, taking over, criticizing, or correcting. Therapists offer treatment as a family's opportunity for altering perspectives on the present, understanding the past, and creating possibilities for the future.

• *Embrace a culturally sensitive, nonjudgmental approach in coming to know each family.* Every family has its own unique story to share with people outside the immediate circle of kin. Listening to family stories reveals culturally specific patterns of family interaction and communication that can be acknowledged and sensitively explored. Family stories also convey important information about how the family copes and adapts to typical transitions of family life cycle: marriage, birth, transition to school and work, illness, and death. When the family shares its routines and rituals the therapist is afforded an opportunity to better understand the relevance of certain people, practices, and beliefs in the life of that family. Information gathered through these discussions can provide the therapist with essential knowledge that will guide a therapist's family specific, culturally-sensitive practice.

 • *Take a cooperative, egalitarian stance when identifying problems and generating potential solutions for treatment.* Nearly all parents want to play a meaningful role in their child's life. Often the strategies that overburdened families use do not fulfill this parental desire. Asking the family what they have discovered about what works best and not so well for their own family invites an egalitarian discussion between you and the family. It also offers the possibility for the therapist to share other family's successful efforts to adapt and cope. Using other family's life lessons can be a less threatening way for a family to entertain new ideas or to broaden their perspectives about different ways to think and to behave.

 • *Emphasize family strengths but recognize family vulnerabilities.* The majority of families with whom we work are doing the *best job they know how to do now* in caring for their children and themselves. By emphasizing the phrase "the best they know how to do now," a therapist is able to communicate the belief that parents can acquire new ways of thinking, coping, behaving, and feeling. It also conveys acceptance and respect of where parents are functioning presently without assuming that it is all that they are capable of achieving. No matter how well intentioned, sometimes caregivers' "best job" is not sufficient to guarantee the safety and well-being of their children. In situations where retaining child custody or terminating parental rights are at issue, using existing parental strengths offers the greatest possibility of producing the necessary family change to avoid such extreme family disruption. By acknowledging strengths while recognizing vulnerabilities, therapists provide caregivers with a "reality check" of what changes need to be made. Building on these strengths can instill the confidence and feelings of self-worth to make and maintain the necessary personal and family changes to adequately protect and nurture their young children.

Therapeutic Practice

 • *Work very hard and very quickly to establish a positive working alliance.* When you are working with families who have a history of unproductive contacts with social service professionals, it is useful to acknowledge where the "system" and those working within it have failed them in the past. Clearly many overburdened families have spent years struggling mightily to resolve complex life problems. What needs to be conveyed during an initial family session is that the therapist is asking to join in an alliance with the family members rather than assuming that they will give automatic admission. Because disappointment and failure often characterized past dealing with professionals it seems particularly important to offer concrete assistance that produces some tangible result for the family during your initial family meeting. This may involve arranging a scheduled appointment at the family's convenience rather than during your regular clinical hours. The message to be conveyed is that the therapist intends to work hard toward making this experience a productive one for the family.

• *Address what parents believe to be the problem or issue of concern.* For many professionals working with multiproblem families, it is often frustrating and even heartbreaking to see parents worry excessively about things that they cannot change or fail to take some direct action that could minimize or alleviate some difficulty. Sometimes what appears to be a critical family need is not identified as an area of concern by the family. The family may choose to use its resources differently. Acknowledge and accept the family's negative feelings and attributions about child behavior without feeling as if you need to change them immediately or concur in order to maintain your relationship with the family. Often caregivers are simply seeking to be heard.

• *Make note of parental attitudes and behavior you hope to alter or modify but address only those issues that you believe to be of critical importance.* Often overburdened families come with a plethora of problems and issues of concern. For these families everyday life challenges preoccupy much of their physical and psychic energy. Providing instrumental help, advice, or guidance on how to address a pressing family's concerns may provide some relief, albeit temporary, for the caregivers. Demonstrating a willingness to work with the family members at addressing what they believe to be of critical importance provides concrete evidence of a therapist's commitment to forming an active working alliance. Many worrisome family issues or inadequate problem solving are rooted in longstanding family pathology. Once the therapeutic relationship becomes stronger and the family and therapist experience some satisfaction or success in working together, additional relationship issues can be tackled.

• *Answer questions posed by the family directly; provide informa-*

tion when asked. Many families begin treatment with questions they hope to have answered by the therapist. Occasionally the information requested by the family may be unknown or unanswerable, or the material requested may be too technical to be used by the family. Often families need to have things repeated many times, in many different ways and sometimes by more than one person, before they grasp the meaning of what is being said to them. Even then the family's understanding of the long-term implications of particular circumstances or conditions may change as the family acquires additional information or experiences new insights. Families report that what a professional tells them is not always as important as the manner in which the information is shared. Consequently, minimize your role as the expert with all the answers. Rather, share your expertise in a nonauthoritarian way by providing perspective on caregivers' beliefs and feelings. Several cases are presented below to illustrate these aspects of therapeutic practice.

Case 1: David and His Adolescent Parents

After a second hospitalization for dehydration and failure to thrive during his first 2 months of life, David and his adolescent parents were referred to the hospital's "feeding team." Efforts by the team's nurses and nutritionist to teach the parents what to feed, how to feed, and when to feed their son were judged to be unsuccessful. When the hospital's physicians recommended further nutritional education for the parents, the parents became enraged and refused to cooperate. The physicians felt compelled to report the parents' neglect of their child to the state child protective service agency and sought assistance for the young family from the Interaction Guidance program.

  The IG therapist sought to better comprehend how the parents understood their son's lack of weight gain by asking the parents to describe their son's general daily routine. The therapist inquired about the hours the baby slept and when the baby was awake, and at what times the baby was fed, and which parent generally fed him. The parents replied that their "son was great." He slept throughout the night without waking and rarely fussed or cried during the day. When asked about feeding, the young mother became agitated and asked, "Why don't people believe we feed this kid? He eats whenever we do. You know, like breakfast, lunch, dinner, and sometimes even a bottle before bed." When asked further if the parents ever gave the infant more than three or four 4-ounce bottles a day, both parents looked rather surprised and shook their heads. In answer to the question, "Does the baby ever cry during the night?" the parents reported that whenever they brought David home from the hospital the infant would wake up crying during the night. The parents believed the best way to deal with these awakenings was to ignore them so as not to spoil him, so "David doesn't get used to the idea of getting whatever he wants in the middle of the night."

It seemed clear to the therapist that these parents thought that they were doing the "right" thing for their infant. After all, the parents fed David whenever they were hungry. Both parents believed that David needed to learn the harsh realities of life they had known. That is, a person doesn't always get their needs met, not even if the person is a dependent newborn. Although this style of caregiving seemed the best they knew how to do *now*, it clearly was not enough to sustain their baby.

One of the therapist's immediate tasks was to assist the parents to learn to separate their infant's demands from *their* needs. This can be a challenging issue for mothers and fathers of any age but a particularly difficult task for adolescent parents. The therapist began by recognizing the young couple's dilemma. That is, to follow the doctors' advice, thereby risk "spoiling" their son, or to continue doing what they believed to be the best for their baby and thereby incur the disapproval of the hospital staff. The therapist tried to reframe the issue of "spoiling" for the parents by providing some developmental information about the capacities and abilities of young infants. Night waking at 2 months was explained as their son's way of signaling his parents that he was hungry and needed more nourishment. His signal would need a response from his parents in order for David to learn that his parents were listening and wanted to help him. "Good parents" (what this couple was trying to become) would get up and satisfy his hunger need. Both parents insisted that they wanted to be responsive parents and that they would respond to his cries for food in the future.

TREATMENT PHASES OF INTERACTION GUIDANCE

The treatment phases of IG include engagement visits in the family home or referral source, family video replay treatment sessions, and treatment follow-up and community referral. In each phase of the treatment, the IG therapist embraces the therapeutic stance and uses the therapeutic practices previously mentioned. In this section, the structure and content of each phase are reported more fully.

Assessing the Family Situation and Caregiving Environment

In an effort to understand as vividly as possible the family's experience, the therapeutic process begins with meeting of family household members at the referral source (i.e., at the hospital, human service agency, or in the family home). The child's primary caregiver (often the mother) is asked to invite all family members who assist in the care of the infant to the initial family meeting. The purpose of this household gathering is to gain a clear understanding of how the family members view their situation, to describe the IG program, and to offer the family an opportunity to participate.

Case 2: Melanie and Her Family

Melanie was diagnosed as nonorganic failure to thrive during her second hospitalization in the same month. At 4 months of age, she was the youngest of four children under the age of 3½ born to cognitively limited parents. The therapist met the family members at their home for the first meeting. This family of six shared a noisy, dirty two-bedroom apartment. All four children slept in one cramped room. The kitchen was both the adult conversation area and the children's playroom. As the therapist and parents talked, the children raced around the room, often hitting one another, grabbing toys from each other, and crying when one or the other got hurt. The parents shouted threats at the children but didn't make any attempt to quiet or comfort them or to restructure their play.

It was a full 20 minutes into the visit when the therapist became aware that Melanie neither was present in the room nor did she appear to be sleeping in her bed. When she asked the parents where Melanie was, the parents replied that "Melanie wasn't the *real* problem anyway." The parents identified all the other children as the source of their immediate concern: "They don't mind. They just yell and hit each other. It does no good to try and talk. They just go ahead and do what they want anyway." The therapist expressed acknowledgment of the parents' frustration and concern, then asked again about the whereabouts of Melanie. Mother got up and wheeled a baby carriage from behind the refrigerator. "We just keep her there so she doesn't get hurt by one of these kids." The therapist spoke with the parents on the amount of time it had taken the therapist to recognize the absence of Melanie among all the family activity. The therapist inquired if this ever happened to the parents. The father replied, "She's so good and quiet. Sometimes we even forget she's there!" A formula-crusted bottle from Melanie's earlier morning feeding lay in the carriage as evidence of the parents' "forgetfulness." It appeared that Melanie's struggle to retain the weight she gained while in the hospital was due in part to the parents' inability to find a place for her, both literally and figuratively, in their chaotic lives.

The immediate task for the therapist was to make Melanie more visible within the family while helping the parents address their identified source of concern, the other children's behavior. Once Melanie joined the group, the therapist commented that while she recognized that the parents put Melanie behind the refrigerator to keep her safe, their action resulted in Melanie spending much of her time apart from her family. The therapist asked the parents to think of another place that would keep Melanie safe and visible to the family. After some prompting, the mother suggested putting Melanie's infant seat in the middle of the kitchen table. When Melanie was securely in her seat, she gazed around the kitchen at her parents and siblings. She smiled when her mother spoke to her and kicked her legs when her brother attempted to tickle her feet.

The brother's tickling soon became pulling, then hitting of Melanie. Neither parent attempted to stop the toddler's aggressiveness or to redirect him how to play with his sister. Both parents looked helpless and indicated that this new idea wasn't going to work. With some coaching from the therapist, the father restrained the boy and distracted him from his sister. The therapist then addressed the family's concerns regarding child behavior management. The therapist assisted the family in generating three family rules that could be followed by the children and enforced by the parents: no hitting, no biting, and no throwing toys. With prompting from the therapist, the parents made plans for what to do if a family rule was broken. The visit concluded with the parents expressing a willingness to keep Melanie in a safe and visible place, to follow the child management plan, and to evaluate its effectiveness during the next week.

Who Comes to Treatment?

A common aspect among many relationship-based treatments is the focus on working with at least two family generations (Sameroff & Emde, 1989; Stern, 1996). In IG treatment, the infant's caregiver is encouraged to invite a parenting copartner into the treatment sessions. Treatment "families" can be the child's biological parents and siblings, a single parent and friend, or an adolescent mother and her own mother. The treatment session always includes at least two family generations: caregiver and child. Although families often bring siblings to the sessions, there are some cases where it is advisable to work initially with the caregiver(s) and a single child. For example, in the case of a fragile infant who easily becomes overstimulated, it may be more advantageous to work with the parent and child alone until the caregiver is confident of being able to soothe and calm the infant. Gradually other family members can join the treatment session.

Interaction Guidance Family Treatment Sessions

Families generally are seen weekly for hourly treatment sessions. The treatment sessions usually are held in a specially designed playroom equipped with developmentally appropriate toys, a play mat, comfortable chairs or a sofa, and a diapering area. A video camera is available to record the play session for viewing by the family and therapist. The room is arranged to comfortably meet the needs of both adults and very young children.

The sequence of activities during each family session remains fairly consistent throughout treatment. Families whose own lives are disorganized and chaotic seem to find this predictable routine comforting. Once the family is welcomed into the playroom, the therapist inquires about what has occurred in the family's life since the last visit. This is an opportunity to learn about the issues and topics with which the family members have dealt and how comfortable they are with what has transpired. This is also a time of information solicitation and exchange early in the treatment process. The family shares information from the time of the last contact, offers opinions, and asks questions of the therapist. As the family members display more trust in the therapeutic relationship, they spontaneously share a wider range of affects with the therapist. Family members speak of the frustration and disappointment they encounter in their efforts to make changes in their lives or, conversely, express the increased enjoyment and satisfaction they receive from their interactions with one another. Consequently as treatment evolves, the therapist spends more time initially listening to and speaking with the family.

In each session, once the therapist judges that the family members appear satisfied that their concerns were heard or addressed, the therapist invites them to play with the infant the way they would if they were home. While the family interacts, the therapist videotapes a short period of the play sequence, approximately 5 minutes. Following family–infant play, the family and therapist will view this "movie." The therapist remains in the treatment room but sits apart from the family and tries not to interact with family members. Whether videotaping or observing the family in the treatment room, the therapist makes particular note of existing positive caregiving behavior and examples of parental sensitivity that will become the basis for elaborating and extending nurturing caregiving behavior during the video replay period. The therapist also makes note of behaviors that need to be modified or altered because of their critical importance (e.g., caregivers failing to adequately provide for infant's safety).

Reviewing the Videotape

After the taping of the play interaction session, the videotape is viewed by the family and the therapist. The therapist stays in a position to simultaneously watch the family view the "movie" and see the video herself. Initially, the therapist listens for spontaneous comments or reflections from the family. Then the therapist gently solicits comments from the parent(s) concerning their perception of the session and their thoughts and feelings regarding their infant and their role as parents. A series of systematic probes are posed to the family to facilitate the conversation, such as "Was this play session typical of what happens at home?" or "Were you surprised by anything that happened during the session?" These questions often stimulate discussion among the caregivers and the therapist about what the family members saw on the screen, what it meant to them, how they felt about what they saw, how they thought their children felt, and how they felt about themselves as parents. Although the initial focus of the therapy is on the present, caregivers' reflections of their own past parenting experience often invite a discussion of how the past can influence the present.

Following the caregivers' comments, the therapist highlights specific examples of positive parenting behavior and parental sensitivity in reading and interpreting their infant's behavior. Focusing on what family and therapist agree is mutually satisfying and enjoyable to all interactive partners seems to convey a sincere sense of caring and concern on the part of the therapist. During these repeated occasions, most families begin to realize that the focus of treatment is positive in nature and that the therapist will address family-identified problems through the use of family competence and strength.

The videotape viewing and feedback aspect of the sessions can be especially meaningful to the family at the beginning of treatment. As families become more comfortable in spontaneously verbalizing their thoughts and concerns with the therapist, they seem to view the video-tape feedback as an opportunity to reflect on what the taped event represents to them in a broader context. For example, some families will use the videotape viewing as a stimulus to discuss events of the past week whereas others will reflect on experiences from years past and the feelings that accompany these memories. Another advantage of videotaping is the opportunity it affords both the family and therapist to review the changes that occur across sessions. In situations where change is subtle and progress is slow, a retrospective viewing of previous tapes can emphasize progress over time and can often encourage a family's effort at continuing treatment.

Case 3: Samuel and His Young Mother

The case of 4-month-old Samuel and his young mother, Lisa, may illustrate how a well-intentioned but insensitive caregiver can be "coached" to engage in more contingently responsive and sensitive communicative play. Both Samuel and his mother presented as depressed and irritable when they were seen in the playroom. Samuel had been diagnosed as nonorganic failure to thrive after a second hospitalization for weight loss during the first 4 months of his life. His mother reported that he continued to vomit almost everything that she fed him despite her attempts to explicitly follow the hospital staff's recommendations. Lisa expressed feelings of failure as a parent and of resentment toward Samuel for causing her all these problems.

During the initial play period, Lisa sat behind her son and presented Samuel with one toy after another. Samuel fussed and whimpered throughout the time and only showed momentary regard to any of the objects placed before him. Lisa appeared oblivious to his apparent lack of interest and continued to mechanically present each toy. During the video viewing and feedback session, Lisa said that they didn't have many toys at home and Samuel preferred playing games such as peek-a-boo and tickling. Lisa volunteered to show the therapist their family games. During the peek-a-boo game, Lisa, with her hands covering her face, lunged at Samuel as he lay on his back. She repeatedly exclaimed, "Peek-a-boo! Peek-a-boo! Peek-a-boo!" without pause to note his reaction. Samuel lay staring wide eyed and looking somewhat frightened. Lisa looked up at the therapist and said disappointedly, "I guess he's not going to do it for me today."

The therapist observed that although Samuel appeared to be watching his mother's efforts, he almost seemed too startled to react. The therapist invited the mother to play the game once again but this time to pause when she said "Peek-a-boo" and look at Samuel's face before continuing the game. Lisa tried again, waiting for her son's response before continuing. Samuel cooperated by kicking his legs vigorously. The therapist said to Lisa, "Well, it seems as if he's very happy to play this time." Lisa nodded and tried the game again. This time Samuel's response included waving his arms and kicking his legs. Lisa smiled broadly and repeated the game several more times. As Samuel's interest waned, Lisa again became more intrusive. The therapist suggested that Samuel's lack of response might be his way of telling his mother that he wished to play something else. As Lisa sat back, Samuel's body relaxed and he made eye contact with his mother and smiled.

Concluding the Play Session

After the videotape is reviewed and discussed, the therapist continues talking with the family members while they play with the infant. Sometimes issues raised by the family during the video replay are discussed for the remainder of the session. Other times the conversation expands into other aspects of family life beyond the caregiver's parenting role. The therapist attempts to follow the client's lead in exploring areas of concern and conflict but also raises issues the therapist believes are interfering with the growth and development of family members, particularly the infant.

The session concludes with a therapist-led discussion regarding treatment progress or lack of progress. The family is encouraged to comment candidly on the treatment process. The parents are then asked if they would like to schedule a visit for the coming week. The purpose of offering another appointment to family members rather than assuming a standing meeting is to convey the importance of their active decision making concerning their treatment participation and progress.

Therapeutic Considerations for Video Use

At the end of treatment, the clinician prepares an edited copy of the videotape that documents the changes that occur in parent–infant interactions and family transactions over the course of the treatment. This "family movie" is given to the parents as a record of their evolving patterns of sensitivity, responsiveness, and nurturance toward the infant and to one another. The edited video provides a visual narrative of the family's story that can be viewed and shared with others. There are several situations where offering a copy of the videotape to the family before the completion of treatment may assist in treatment progress. Sometimes a spouse or coparent (friend, relative, household member) is unable or refuses to participate in the treatment sessions. Sharing a movie of what happens during a play session often alleviates unspoken concerns or fears by the resistant party about what actually occurs during the treatment hour. Also, having other household members view and hear what is done and said by the therapist often provides a source of validation for the client in their attempt to restructure or to change previous ways of thinking or behaving. Finally, viewing the videotape is a very concrete way for the family to share the experience with other persons interested and concerned about the infant's well-being and happiness.

INTERACTION GUIDANCE INTERVENTION TECHNIQUES

In each of the cases described earlier, the IG therapist sought to provide perspective to the family's beliefs and feelings. The therapist also explored and clarified distortions in the caregivers' attributions of their infant's behavior and intent. When asked, the therapist provided instrumental help to the family. In Case 1, the therapist shared information on infant behavior and development; in Case 2, the therapist assisted the parents in developing a plan to manage their children's behavior.

The therapist tried to highlight what the families were doing well before attempting to address problem areas. In each case, the therapist provided guidance but did not undermine the parents' role as primary caregivers by acting as an authority figure. Rather, an effort was made to convey the therapist's expertise in a nonjudgmental way.

In all cases the therapist tried to elaborate and extend positive family interactions and help the parents more accurately interpret their infants' cues and signals. In Case 3, the therapist altered the parent's interactions with her son through the use of video replay and by helping the caregiver reframe her attributions of Samuel's behavior and intent.

In each case, the therapist modeled a supportive, nurturing, and caring interactive style with the infant and family. The therapist conveyed that the family's negative feelings, thoughts, and comments would be heard fully and nonjudgmentally. With the therapist's support the family could explore these emotions and ideas in the context of the therapeutic play session. The therapist's approach to the family remained positive regardless of the nature of the family's problems.

TREATMENT EFFICACY

The evaluation of individual family treatment and overall program progress can be assessed in several ways depending on the circumstances of
preventive intervention treatment. Because each treatment session is
videotaped, measures can be employed to examine treatment efficacy by
impartial evaluators. The IG approach has proven to be a promising
treatment for parent–infant relationship disturbances (Cramer et al.,
1990; McDonough, 1993, 1995; Robert-Tissot et al., 1996; Stern, 1995).
Treatment efficacy studies currently are continuing in the United States
and Switzerland.

The most objective source of information regarding the treatment
progress is the videotapes. However, the most clinically meaningful
source of information concerning treatment efficacy may be the family
exit interviews completed at the conclusion of the follow-up home visits.
In these the families have the opportunity to reflect on the elements of
the treatment that had the most positive impact and what they saw as
turning points in their understanding or behavior.

When the IG therapist is discussing treatment efficacy with multiproblem, multirisk families, it seems important to clearly define what is
meant by treatment success. Unfortunately, the vast majority of these
families will never be free from the problems caused by poverty, lack of
education, family mental illness, substance abuse, large family size, or
lack of adequate social support or an interested coparent. However,
many of these families have used their relationship with the IG therapist
to help make meaningful changes in their lives (McDonough, 1992,
2000a). In many cases, the families were able to reallocate their limited
resources more effectively to meet their infant's needs. Sometimes this
involved helping the caregivers restructure their family so that one person was free to adequately nurture and care for the infant (McDonough,
1993, 1995). Other instances called for the therapist to help a caregiver
redefine his or her own mental health issues in a way that permitted the
infant to grow and develop along a more appropriate developmental
course (Cramer et al., 1990, Stern, 1995).

INTERACTION GUIDANCE
THERAPIST TRAINING PROGRAM

Training for individuals wishing to implement the IG approach has been
conducted during intensive 2-month sessions and short-term, intensive

follow-up workshops. Many cohorts of IG therapists have been trained to administer the treatment in a variety of sites in the United States and abroad. The training consists of didactic teaching, group discussions, video case presentations, self-study materials, observations of ongoing clinical treatment cases, and supervised practice of the IG with families.

Emphasis is placed on both the theory and the practice of IG techniques. Each trainee accompanies an experienced IG therapist on a home visit to observe an initial intake and family assessment. During the final portion of training every participant conducts IG play sessions with a nonclinical volunteer family. Every case is observed by the IG supervisor and discussed with fellow trainees. During the treatment supervision that follows a family's playroom visit, the supervisor focuses on positive aspects of the trainee's efforts to arrange the playroom, engage the family in the play session, videotape the caregiver–infant play interactions, provide feedback and commentary to the family, and comfortably conclude the family play session.

In addition to the *Interaction Guidance Treatment Manual*, each participant in the training program receives a collection of background readings that covers each phase of the treatment process: assessment of the infant, family, home environment, and cultural context; family engagement process, treatment implementation, and monitoring treatment progress; and evaluation of treatment efficacy. A videotape library of select treatment cases is available for the trainees' viewing throughout the session. To illustrate special characteristics of the IG approach, the supervisor presents videotaped examples from clinical treatment cases for group discussion. Trainees also are encouraged to bring videotapes of their work with families at their employment site and to videotape themselves working with one volunteer family at the training site. By watching and listening to the videotapes, the trainees gain a better understanding of what they say and the manner in which they say it. Just as the IG treatment is positive in its approach and nurturing of individual development, so too is the training of IG therapists.

MONITORING FIDELITY
OF INTERACTION GUIDANCE TREATMENT

Criteria have been developed to "certify" the therapists in the implementation of the IG preventive intervention. We have found it useful to use the Interaction Guidance Treatment Adherence Scale as an ongoing part of training. Early in the training experience, trainees rate experienced clinicians as they work with treatment families. Later the trainees self-administer the scale as they watch themselves on tape interacting with volunteer families. In the final weeks, supervisors rate the trainees and use this information in individual trainee clinical supervision.

A specific Interaction Guidance Treatment Adherence Scale uses 18 subscales in five categories to rate interventionists' use of therapeutic principles and techniques (see Table 4.1).

SUMMARY

Parents and infants experience relationship problems that seriously compromise the growth and development of the baby and minimize parental feelings of pride, self-confidence, and enjoyment in their parenting. The IG treatment approach addresses family relationship problems by observing ongoing parent–infant interactive behavior and by providing guidance to the caregivers in their effort to gain a more complete understanding of their infant's and their own feelings, thoughts, and actions. In doing so, the IG therapist improves the parent–infant relationship, which in turn reduces the infant's symptoms and increases the mutual satisfaction both caregiver and child obtain from one another. By emphasizing family strengths and empowerment as overarching constructs and employing videotape feedback to facilitate development-promoting relationships, IG has proven to be a valuable adjunct to the treatment of early relationship problems.

TABLE 4.1. Interaction Guidance Treatment Adherence Scale

I. Defining treatment
  1. Family defines problem
  2. Family defines intervention success

II. Interventionist's role
  3. Offers assistance
  4. Monitors treatment progress
  5. Enhances parent–infant interaction

III. Acknowledging parents
  6. Emphasizes instances of positive parenting
  7. Accepts negative family feelings
  8. Uses therapeutic approach
  9. Provides new perspectives

IV. Using videotape feedback
  10. Uses videotape
  11. Provides salient feedback
  12. Increase awareness of family interactions

V. Therapist problems
  13. Sets own agenda
  14. Uses critical comments
  15. Overreliance on modeling behavior
  16. Excessive focus on child
  17. Excessive focus on caregiver
  18. Disparagement of treatment model

REFERENCES

Cramer, B., Robert-Tissot, C., Stern, D. N., Serpa-Rusconi, S., DeMuralt, M., Besson, G., Palacio-Espasa, F., Bachmann, J., Knauer, D., Berney, C., & D'Arcis, U. (1990). Outcome evaluation in brief mother-infant psychotherapy: A preliminary report. *Infant Mental Health Journal, 11,* 278–300.

McDonough, S. C. (1992). Treating early relationship disturbances with Interaction Guidance. In G. Fava-Vizziello & D. N. Stern (Eds.), *Models and techniques of psychotherapeutic intervention in the first years of life* (pp. 221–233). Milan: Raffaello Cortina Editore.

McDonough, S. C. (1993). Interaction Guidance: Understanding and treating early relationship disturbances. In C. H. Zeanah (Ed.), *Handbook of infant mental health.* New York: Guilford Press.

McDonough, S. C. (1995). Promoting positive early parent–infant relationships through interaction guidance. *Child and Adolescent Psychiatric Clinics of North America, 4,* 661–672.

McDonough, S. C. (1996). Models of interaction for parents and children. In J. Gomes-Pedro & M. Folque Patríco (Eds.), *Bebě XXI: Infants and families in the next century* (pp. 227–239). Lisbon: Fundacao Calouste Gulbenkian.

McDonough, S. C. (2000a). Interaction guidance: An approach for difficult to engage families. In C. H. Zeanah (Ed.), *Handbook of infant mental health* (2nd ed., pp. 485–493). New York: Guilford Press.

McDonough, S. C. (2000b). Preparing infant mental health personnel for 21st century practice. In J. D. Osofsky & H. E. Fitzgerald (Eds.), *WAIMH handbook of infant mental health* (pp. 538–548). New York: Wiley.

Robert-Tissot, C., Cramer, B., Stern, D. N., Serpa, S., Bachmann, J., Besson, G., Palacio-Espasa, F., Knauer, D., DeMuralt, M., Berney, C., & Mendiguren, G. (1996). Outcome evaluation in brief mother–infant psychotherapies: Report on 75 cases. *Infant Mental Health Journal, 17,* 97–114.

Sameroff, A. J., & Emde, R. (1989). *Relationship disturbances in early childhood: A developmental approach.* New York: Basic Books.

Stern, D. N. (1996). *The motherhood constellation: A unified approach to mother–infant psychotherapy.* New York: Basic Books.

CHAPTER 5

CHILD–PARENT PSYCHOTHERAPY

A Relationship-Based Approach to the Treatment
of Mental Health Disorders in Infancy
and Early Childhood

Alicia F. Lieberman

The treatment of mental health disorders in the first years of life has focused primarily on enhancing the quality of the emotional relationship between the young child and the parents. Approaches to treatment give primacy to a variety of factors that contribute to the child's clinical condition. These include the parent's unresolved psychological conflicts as these are reenacted in the relationship with the child (Fraiberg, Adelson, & Shapiro, 1975; Fraiberg, 1980; Lebovici, 1988; Cramer & Palacio-Espasa, 1993), the mutually reinforcing impact of reality-based stresses and psychological conflicts as obstacles to effective parenting (Fraiberg, 1980; Lieberman & Pawl, 1993), the transactional nature of the parent–child contributions to the child's mental health problems (Lieberman, 1991, 1998; Lieberman, Silverman, & Pawl, 2000), and parental strengths as a scaffold for building new parental competencies and alleviating maladaptive parenting practices (McDonough, 2000).

The present chapter describes child–parent psychotherapy as a relationship-based treatment approach for infants, toddlers, and preschoolers who are experiencing mental health problems or whose relationship with the parent is negatively affected as a result of parental factors such as mental illness, child constitutional characteristics that interfere with the formation of a secure attachment, and/or discordant temperamental styles between the parent and child.

Child–parent psychotherapy emphasizes the child's centrality as an active partner in the treatment by focusing on the child's emotional experience and embedding this experience in the child–parent relationship. The goal is to promote a psychological partnership where the child's modulation and integration of affect and accurate reality testing are supported by the parent's increasing ability to provide concrete protection and developmentally appropriate responses. Using the format of joint child–parent sessions, the therapist relies on play, behavioral interventions, and verbal interpretation to translate the emotional experience of the child to the parent and to explain the parent's behavior to the child in order to promote empathic understanding and encourage emotional reciprocity. The approach supports and reinforces child and parent perceptions and behaviors that convey mutuality of positive affect, age-appropriate self-assertion, and constructive conflict resolution. It targets for change dysregulated child and parent behaviors, including externalizing problems such as excessive control, punitiveness, aggression, defiance, and recklessness, and internalizing problems such as somatization, emotional withdrawal, and fear. Individual sessions with the parent and/ or the child may be added when clinically indicated as an adjunct to the joint child–parent sessions.

CONCEPTUAL ORIGINS
AND DEVELOPMENTAL CONSIDERATIONS

Child–parent psychotherapy is an extension to the first 6 years of life of infant–parent psychotherapy (Fraiberg, 1980; Lieberman & Pawl, 1993; Lieberman et al., 2000), a form of intervention developed by Selma Fraiberg to address mental health problems in infants from birth to the age of 3 years. The theoretical target (Stern, 1985) of infant–parent psychotherapy is the web of mutually constructed meanings in the infant–parent relationships (Pawl & St. John, 1998; Lieberman et al., 2000). While the infant's mental health is the ultimate goal, the primary therapeutic focus of infant–parent psychotherapy involves the uncovering of unconscious links between the parent's psychological conflicts and parenting practices that are gravely misattuned to the baby's needs and derail the infant's normative development. In this approach, the parent's enduring conflicts have the role of "ghosts in the nursery" that must be exorcised in order to free the baby from their malignant influence (Fraiberg et al., 1975; Fraiberg, 1980).

Infant–parent psychotherapy is based on the premise that, because behavioral patterns are not internalized as part of the personality structure before the age of 3 years, infants and toddlers can regain their momentum toward normal development when they are no longer the recipients of maladaptive parenting practices (Fraiberg, 1980). However, intimate relationships influence mental health well beyond infancy. Profound personality changes can occur across the lifespan through the vehicle of a deep and transformative relationship with another person. This perspective forms the basis for relational approaches to psychotherapy with children and with adults (Bowlby, 1988; Emde & Robinson, 2000; Holmes, 2001; Kohut, 1971).

As Fraiberg commented on numerous occasions, a sustained therapeutic focus on the links between the parent's unresolved, often childhood-based psychological conflicts and current feelings toward the child is most feasible in the first 12 months of the child's life, when parents are relatively free to use the session for their own needs in the presence of a baby who is neither mobile nor verbal. While each baby's unique individuality is an integral element of infant–parent psychotherapy, the child's claim for separate attention becomes increasingly more insistent during the active and demanding toddler and preschool years, necessitating important modifications in the conceptualization and implementation of therapeutic modalities (Lieberman, 1991). These modifications, in turn, open up the use of a relationship-based therapeutic approach to the treatment of toddlers, preschoolers, and older children by incorporating therapeutic techniques that are developmentally appropriate for these older ages.

Toddlers and preschoolers are not infants. Their increasing capacity to move autonomously and to say what is in their minds profoundly transforms their sense of self, emphasizing their autonomous agency in their transactions with the world. At the same time, as during infancy, they continue to be profoundly influenced by the responses they evoke from others, and most particularly by the emotional quality of their attachments. These characteristics must inform the approach to treatment. Like infant–parent psychotherapy, child–parent psychotherapy targets the web of mutually constructed meanings between the child and the parent, but it differs from infant–parent psychotherapy in emphasizing the growing child's autonomous agency during the treatment, with a concomitantly lesser emphasis on uncovering the parents' childhood conflicts or helping them reflect on their individual experience. In child–parent psychotherapy, the therapeutic focus is placed on the child's subjective experience of the self through the lens of the child–parent relationship, with the goal of enhancing the child's mental health by promoting reliance on the parents as sources of protection and safety, more accurate reality testing, and modulation and integration of positive and negative affect.

The relationship between infant–parent psychotherapy and child–parent psychotherapy is best understood in terms of the developmental continuum determined by the child's stage-appropriate capacities. Both treatments target the system of meanings constructed by the parent and the child to understand themselves and each other, with different emphases on either the parent's or the child's contributions. As a rule, infant–parent psychotherapy targets for change the parent's maladaptive parenting practices by focusing on the parent's behaviors and mental representations of the self and the baby (Lieberman et al., 2000). Child–parent psychotherapy targets for change the child's maladaptive behaviors and perceptions of the self and others, engaging the parent as an indispensable partner in this therapeutic endeavor. Within each approach, the degree of relative emphasis on parental or child contributions may vary with the individual clinical situation and is guided by the salience of the parenting problems, the child's symptoms, and the child's role as an agent in the parent–child constellation. Individual sessions with the parent or the child may be used as adjuncts or even substitutes for joint child–parent sessions for weeks or months at a time when the parent is so self-absorbed, destructive, or antagonistic toward the child that progress toward building a parent–child partnership calls for a preparatory period of individual attention to one or both parties involved.

WHY A THEORETICAL TARGET ON INTERPERSONAL MEANINGS BEYOND INFANCY?

Given very young children's capacity to benefit from individual psychotherapy, it is reasonable to ask why a therapist may choose a joint parent–child format as the vehicle for therapeutic intervention when a toddler or preschooler is showing mental health problems. It may be argued, for example, that child–parent psychotherapy is "neither fish nor fowl" because the clinician works with split attention between the parent and the child. As a result, this approach does not encourage uninterrupted exploration of the child's subjective experience, because the parent's presence and subjective experience need to be recognized and addressed during the session. Neither does it offer the parent an unencumbered opportunity to express and explore the range of feelings evoked by the child, because the child's presence and subjective experience need to be likewise acknowledged and addressed. Rather than being free to be fully available to either partner, the child–parent psychotherapist is constantly searching for the most parsimonious "port of entry" (Stern, 1985) into the constellation of feelings, attributions, and behaviors that constitute the web of meanings between the parent and the child. This includes always being attentive to the impact on one partner of the therapist's attention to the other. As a result, the child–parent therapist may often feel that no single theme is pursued fully enough or deeply enough with either therapeutic partner because the needs and wishes of the other partner routinely assert themselves into the process. In this sense, the quandaries presented by child–parent psychotherapy recall those faced by practitioners of couple therapy and family therapy.

Why, then, adopt a relationship-based approach to the mental health problems of young children who are no longer infants? The most concise answer can be phrased as follows: "We take this approach because young children learn about subjective meaning from how their intimate relationships feel to them." In other words, relationships, both in the form of concrete real-life interactions and in the form of abstract mental representations, are the bedrock for the experience of self in young children, and deriving self-affirming meanings from these relationships is the most expeditious route to the formation and consolidation of a solid and integrated sense of self. In the first years of a child's life, parents and primary caregivers are the most pervasive influences in this process. A therapist may have a transformational impact on a young child's sense of self through individual psychotherapy, but when the therapy comes to an end the child will no longer have a steady partner helping to negotiate the emotional upheavals of family relationships. The child will then need to rely on the "shadow of the object" (Bollas, 1987) cast by the departed therapist, but this shadow may not be long enough to counterbalance the continuing impact of maladaptive parenting. Of course, collateral meetings with the parents can help to modify pathogenic parenting practices, but the scope of collateral sessions is curtailed by the individual therapist's commitment to confidentiality regarding the child's clinical material. Therapists working individually with a very young child may also develop a protective identification with the child's portrayal during the sessions of the parents' behavior and may find it difficult to be equally accepting of the parents' point of view simply due to the lack of opportunity to understand them at similar depth. These constraints are not present in child–parent psychotherapy, because its aim is to transform the child–parent relationship by promoting reciprocal perceptions and interactions that support and expand each partner's sense of self-worth in relation to the other, so that these new meanings remain mutually reinforcing after the therapy has ended.

BASIC PREMISES FOR THE CREATION OF A TREATMENT PLAN

Child–parent psychotherapy is guided by three basic premises, which are described below.

1. Mental health problems in infancy and early childhood, regardless of their etiology, need to be addressed in the context of the child's primary relationships, because the child's sense of self unfolds and is sustained by those relationships (Fraiberg, 1980; Lieberman et al., 2000; Lieberman & Zeanah, 1995; Sameroff & Emde, 1989). Even when the child's mental health problems are the sequelae of constitutionally based factors, the quality of the child's closest interpersonal relationships plays an important role in exacerbating or alleviating the child's difficulties (Greenspan & Wieder, 1998; Sameroff & Emde, 1989).

2. Mental health risk factors in the first 5 years of life operate in the context of transactions between the child and his or her social environment, including the family, neighborhood, community, and larger society (Cicchetti & Lynch, 1993). The child's parents may live in circumstances that tax their resources and may be beyond their control, such as poverty, discrimination, low education, unemployment, violent neighborhoods, inadequate housing, transportation and health services, substance abuse, and/or mental health problems. Such circumstances affect the child's development both directly, through the negative conditions they create, and indirectly, by impairing the parents' capacity to provide adequate care. These negative circumstances have a cumulative effect on the child's development (Sameroff, 1993; Sameroff & Fiese, 2000). Faced with such stressors, parents are often unable to support their children's development unless the intervention includes a concerted effort to help them improve their own circumstances and well-being (Henggeler, Schoenwald, Borduin, Rowland, & Cunningham, 1998).

3. Childrearing mores and parenting practices are imbued by deeply held and often unconscious cultural values about who is a worthy human being and which characteristics should be encouraged or discouraged in raising a child. In countries characterized by a preponder-

ance of ethnic and cultural diversity as well as high rates of immigration such as the United States, mental health intervenors must be particularly cognizant of the importance of learning about and incorporating culturally appropriate therapeutic practices in their work. This includes the therapist's interest in learning about the cultural outlook and traditions of the specific family being treated, and how these are expressed in childrearing values and practices.

The three premises described above provide the foundation for child–parent psychotherapy and guide the clinical application of knowledge in several domains. These include developmental processes in infancy and early childhood, the contribution of different etiological factors in the child and the parent, the intergenerational mechanisms of transmission of psychopathology, and the range of therapeutic interventions that ameliorate different pathogenic factors and maladaptive conditions.

DEVELOPMENTAL PROCESSES IN INFANCY AND EARLY CHILDHOOD

As development unfolds beyond the first year of life, the child's primary relationships become increasingly complex because parents must not only maximize the chances for the child's survival and healthy development but must also socialize the child into cultural, community, and family values regarding what is expected, permitted, and forbidden in the child's behavior. This protracted and often emotionally trying process calls into play the entire repertoire of behavior-changing mechanisms available to humans, including education, negotiation, persuasion, compromise, and assertion versus abrogation of power in various combinations of tactfulness, authoritativeness, and—as all parents know—occasional authoritarianism when all else fails in enforcing strongly held family values and expectations.

Children and parents have complementary but different developmental agendas in the socialization process. The growing child strives to explore, learn, and individuate; the parent endeavors to protect and socialize. These agendas complement each other when children are motivated to please and to emulate adult standards, and when adults are motivated to help children learn and derive satisfaction from the child's achievements.

Developmentally expectable parent–child conflicts emerge from differing values regarding what is desirable, both in a particular situation and in the long run. Young children want things in the moment. They lack the future orientation and understanding of causality needed to delay gratification and foresee the possible consequences of their actions. The power of young children's convictions and their zeal in pursuing their goals often surpass their parents' energy level and emotional investment in the outcome of an exchange, with the result that parents may give up on a demand or may become inconsistent in their enforcement of rules in the face of the child's determined refusal to comply. Alternatively, parents may become harshly punitive in pursuing their goals and children may become provocatively defiant in response (Lieberman, 1991, 1993). The quick acquisition and differentiation of emotions in the second and third years of life adds to the intensity of these parent–child exchanges around appropriate and inappropriate behavior (Mahler, Pine, & Bergman, 1975; Sroufe, 1979).

The etiological picture of mental health disorders of toddlerhood and early childhood often involves the failure of the parent and child to establish a partnership that enables them to find acceptable solutions to the routine conflicts posed by incompatible agendas (Bowlby, 1973). When this happens, the inevitable and routinely surmountable conflicts of everyday life become hardened into rigidly entrenched patterns of maladaptive interactions, where neither partner understands or responds contingently to the communications of the other (Sameroff & Emde, 1989; Zero to Three/National Center for Clinical Infant Programs, 1994). Regardless of their etiology (whether in the parent's distorted perceptions of the child, the child's challenging constitutional characteristics, or the interplay between both sets of factors), these maladaptive interactions can become pathogenic in their own right, setting up negative mutual perceptions and self-fulfilling expectations of a negative outcome when the parent and child face any one of the myriad challenges of everyday life. Child–parent psychotherapy involves a search for the recurrent parameters of these maladaptive interactions, including the environmental circumstances that trigger them and the mechanisms that perpetuate them, for the purpose of providing alternative pathways for conflict resolution.

THE CHILD'S CONTRIBUTION

As infants grow into toddlers and preschoolers, improving parental attitudes and parenting practices may no longer suffice to create or restore the child's developmental momentum toward health. Focused efforts to change the child's behavior and internal representations are often needed as well.

The emerging knowledge that children can suffer from mental health disorders even in the absence of significant environmental stressors or parenting problems adds to the importance of a sustained focus on the child's individual contribution to interactional difficulties with the parents (Zero to Three/National Center for Clinical Infant Programs, 1994). Likewise, an understanding of how disordered attachments affect the child's functioning in domains outside of the parent–child relationship provides important guidelines for conceptualizing the treatment approach.

Current knowledge about the classification of mental health disorders in the early years has been organized in DC: 0–3, *Diagnostic Classification of Mental Health and Developmental Disorders of Infancy and Early Childhood* (Zero to Three/National Center for Clinical Infant Programs, 1994). This instrument provides a multiaxial framework to assess the individual child in the context of his or her primary relationships, environmental circumstances, and developmental functioning (see Rosenblum, Chapter 3, this volume). A survey of clinical cases reported by infant mental health clinicians showed that many children showed symptoms of mental health disorders in the absence of clinically significant relationship problems (Lieberman, Barnard, & Wieder, in press). In other words, maladaptive parenting practices and attachment disorders were not necessarily the primary factor in the etiology and evolution of mental health disorders in the young children surveyed. This evidence suggests that the child's symptomatology, whatever its origins, needs to be addressed directly in order to alleviate the child's individual suffering as well as to contain its contribution to the self-perpetuation of maladaptive parent–child interactions.

THE PARENTS' CONTRIBUTION

A review of the extensive empirical and clinical literature documenting the contribution of parents to the child's developmental course is beyond the scope of this chapter, but comprehensive recent reviews and theoretical formulations can be found in Bradley (2000), Cassidy and Shaver (1999), Cichetti and Cohen (1995), Fonagy (2001), Osofsky and Fitzgerald (2000), Shonkoff and Phillips (2000), Stern (1985), and Zeanah (2000). The bulk of the literature focuses on the mother's role, although there is increasing recognition of the importance of the father as a primary contributor to the formation of the child's personality (Fonagy & Target, 1995; Lamb, 1999; Thompson, 1999). The available literature examines the centrality of the parents' input in the infant's and young child's regulation of bodily rhythms (e.g., eating, sleeping, or elimination), expression and modulation of affect, formation and socialization of interpersonal relationships (including the internalization of cultural values about appropriate and inappropriate social behavior), and learning about age-appropriate and culturally appropriate patterns for exploration of the environment.

The parent's individual functioning is a key factor in how the child copes with and resolves the specific challenges posed by these separate but converging developmental tasks. For example, there is extensive empirical and clinical evidence that mothers who are depressed have children who manifest less self-control, more aggression, poorer peer relationships, more difficulties in school, and greater risk for psychopathology than matched controls raised by nondepressed mothers (Campbell, Cohn, & Meyers, 1995; Cummings & Davies, 1994; Dawson & Ashman, 2000; Downey & Coyne, 1990). The pathways linking maternal depression with child outcome involve the interaction between mother and child, with depressed mothers showing greater incidence of the polar states of withdrawal/lethargy and intrusiveness/hostility than do nondepressed mothers (Frankel & Harmon, 1996; Tronick & Weinberg, 1997; Zeanah, Boris, & Larrieu, 1997). Infants of depressed mothers, in turn, have higher rates of anxious attachment, lower activity level, and greater negative affect than do babies of nondepressed mothers (Cummings & Davies, 1994; Frankel & Harmon, 1996; Seifer & Dickstein, 2000).

Taken as a whole, this body of research illustrates how one specific environmental condition, in this case maternal depression, is linked to interactive patterns that in turn affect the infant's immediate functioning as well as later developmental outcomes. At the same time, mothers (even depressed ones) do not exist in a vacuum. Perhaps it is time to paraphrase Winnicott's (1965) much quoted dictum that "there is no such thing as a baby" and point out with equal forcefulness that there is no such thing as a mother: there is only a mother operating in a particular interpersonal, social, economic, and cultural context where different elements may converge to provide support for her mothering or may conspire to make her feel alone, incompetent, and overwhelmed. The same thing may be said, of course, for fathers. The impact on the child of even well-established single risk factors such as a maternal depression can be significantly modified by the presence or absence of other risk or protective factors (Sameroff, 1993, 1995; Cicchetti & Lynch, 1993). For example, a depressed mother who has the internal and external re-sources to seek treatment for her depression may be more emotionally available to her baby than an equally depressed mother who has no hope for improvement because she cannot access appropriate treatment. As-sessing the parent's strengths as well as the stresses and vulnerabilities that constrict or distort the parent's ability to parent must be an essential component of developing a treatment plan.

THE INTERGENERATIONAL TRANSMISSION OF PSYCHOPATHOLOGY

Child–parent psychotherapy is based on the premise that patterns of mental health and mental disturbance are transmitted from generation to generation, a topic that has generated considerable clinical and re-search interest in recent years (e.g., Fonagy, Steele, & Steele, 1992; Ly-ons-Ruth, Bronfman, & Atwood, 1999; Main & Hesse, 1990; Silverman & Lieberman, 1999; Slade, 1999; Stern, 1985). This is an area where the contributions of different theoretical orientations converge to help eluci-date the transmission mechanisms, including the growing rapproche-ment between attachment theory and psychoanalysis (Fonagy, 2001; Lieberman, 2000; Slade & Aber, 1992).

From the perspective of attachment theory, a young child who is treated by the parent in a harsh, unpredictable, or arbitrary manner can-not form or sustain an internal representation of that parent as a secure base. On the contrary, it is the parents themselves who may engender fear, while simultaneously eliciting a strong wish for their protection (Main & Hesse, 1990). When these patterns are unrelieved by sustained enough experiences of nurturing, the child develops "a model of himself as unloveable and unwanted, and a model of attachment figures as likely to be unavailable, or rejecting, or punitive" (Bowlby, 1980, p. 247).

A converging explanation for the mechanisms of transmission of re-lationship patterns involves an integration of the cognitive concept of pa-rental attributions (Dix & Grusec, 1985) and the psychoanalytic concept of projective identification, particularly as used by Ogden (1982). Par-ents routinely make attributions to their children, and these attributions are essential for the child's healthy development when they are flexible and predominantly positive ("he's so cute"; "she's so smart"). On the other hand, when parental attributions become rigid, disconnected from the child's developmental stage, and negative in their emotional tone, they can ensnare the child's evolving sense of self and of intimate rela-tionships into what Fraiberg (1980) called "engulfment in the parental conflicts." In the early years of life, negative parental attributions constrict the child's range of emotions and coerce compliance with these attributions because of the young child's developmentally appropriate need to please the parent in order to preserve the parent's love. Ogden's (1982) three-phase description of the process of projective identification applies to this phenomenon. In this description, projective identification involves, in the first phase, the projection of an unwanted part of the self on to another person. In the second phase, there is pressure on the recipient of the projection to behave in ways consistent with the projection. Finally, in the third phase, the recipient yields to the pressure and behaves in ways that are consistent with the projection. The example that follows illustrates how this mechanism is thought to operate.

A 3-year-old boy was referred for treatment because his mother reported that the child was excessively aggressive with her. When mother and child arrived for the first assessment session, the boy was dressed in a black leather jacket with a skulls-and-bones insignia on the back and his hair was cut in a "punk" style. He looked like a diminutive gang member, although his demeanor was shy and withdrawn. Throughout the session, the mother described him as being out of control, mean, and dangerous. He looked at her forlornly while she spoke. When she left to go to the bathroom, he cried and tried to follow her, but she rebuffed him harshly. He was still crying when she came back, and she made fun of him by saying that he was putting up a big show for the therapist's benefit. When he tried to climb on her lap, she pushed him back. He then hit her while continuing to cry. The mother turned to the therapist and said, as if finally proven right, "See? What did I tell you? He just pretends to need me, but he is really mean."

This example illustrates the mother's attribution to her child of aggressive traits that she denied in herself. She had a history of relationships with violent men, and her son had been conceived when she was raped at gunpoint by her boyfriend, who subsequently left her. This mother saw herself as the helpless victim of dangerous men but was unable to recognize her own anger in her behavior toward her child. Instead, she pressured him to become a bully by dressing him up as a gang member, treating him in ways that would trigger his anger, and dismissing his signals of anxiety as an effort to manipulate her. When the child complied to this pressure to be aggressive by hitting her when she rejected his approach, the mother interpreted his behavior as a confirmation that her perceptions of him as intrinsically aggressive were accurate.

We can find here a bridge where attachment theory and psychoanalysis meet through the interface between internal working models and projective identification. Rigid parental attributions and the behaviors expressing those attributions describe the cognitive, affective, and behavioral manifestations of working models of attachment and of the self in relation to attachment. The term "projective identification" (Klein, 1946/1975) describes the preverbal, inchoate psychic experiences attendant to the coercive or misattuned exchanges between the parent and the child and existing in the levels of somatic experience and unconscious fantasy. Parental attributions and their unconscious substrate, projective identifications, are facets of the parent's working model of the self and of attachment relationship that are transmitted to and internalized by the child in the course of day-to-day interactions (Lieberman, 1997, 2000; Silverman & Lieberman, 1999). By their very nature, negative parental attributions detract from the parent's empathic understanding of the child's motives and behavior, a parental frame of mind with empirically demonstrated links to the child's quality of attachment (Oppenheim, Koren-Karie, & Sagi, 2001).

Other theoretical perspectives on mechanisms of transmission are essential as well. For example, social learning theory provides a persuasive rationale for the link between coercive parenting practices and aggressive behavior in children (Patterson, 1982). Imitation and the wish to emulate important and admired others are basic learning mechanisms throughout the lifespan but particularly in infancy and early childhood, because during the early years children have not yet acquired reliable internal constructs that guide their perception of what is happening, the meaning they attribute to it, and their inferences about how the event relates to their own behavior. For example, a child who regularly watches his father yelling at and hitting his mother is likely to imitate this behavior when he wants something from his mother, and such imitation may well be the first building block on which more complex mechanisms of transmission (such as projective identification, cognitive attributions, and internal working models of the self and other) are built. In the process of treatment, the different mechanisms for the transmission of maladaptive relationship patterns need to be addressed as clinically indicated.

TREATMENT PARAMETERS IN CHILD–PARENT PSYCHOTHERAPY

Child–parent psychotherapy usually takes place during weekly sessions lasting between 60 and 90 minutes. The main participants are the child and at least one parent, although other family members may be present as well depending on clinical considerations and practical need. For example, both parents may participate when clinically indicated, such as when both parents are experiencing difficulties in their relationship with the child. Siblings may also be involved when sibling rivalry is a central issue. The child–parent psychotherapist may have a Master's degree or more advanced degree in a variety of disciplines, including psychology, social work, psychiatry, occupational therapy, or nursing. The duration of treatment is geared to clinical considerations and may range from a few months to 1 or 2 years. The sessions may take place in the home, a clinic-based playroom, or a community agency such as a childcare center, a family resource center, or a battered women's shelter. When the session occurs outside of the clinic playroom, the therapist brings to the session a bag of toys that are selected according to the child's developmental stage and psychological needs. The basic toy selection includes a family of dolls belonging to the same ethnicity as that of the family members, wild and domestic miniature animals, a medical kit, kitchen utensils, miniature cars and trucks, and drawing implements. If the child has been exposed to a traumatic situation, evocative toys such as a police car, police dolls, and an ambulance are often included.

A treatment manual is available that provides guidelines for child–parent psychotherapy with young children traumatized by witnessing domestic violence (Lieberman & Van Horn, 2001). Preliminary research findings indicate that 68 preschoolers referred for treatment because they witnessed severe domestic violence showed significant decreases in externalizing and internalizing problems and significant increases in cognitive performance when compared to baseline scores after 1 year of weekly child–parent psychotherapy. Their mothers showed significant decreases in symptoms of posttraumatic stress, depression, and anxiety. A randomized clinical trial is in process, comparing child–parent psychotherapy with a comparison group receiving case management and referral to community-based therapeutic intervention in a setting selected by the mother.

PORTS OF ENTRY IN CHILD–PARENT PSYCHOTHERAPY

"Port of entry" (Stern, 1985) refers to the basic element of the parent–child system that is the immediate object of clinical attention—the road that leads to the theoretical target of the intervention. Given that in child–parent psychotherapy the target of the treatment is the web of meanings mutually constructed by the child and the parent, the ports of entry need to be versatile in response to the many pathways that humans use to construct, express, and decode meaning. The choice of a port of entry is guided by the therapist's clinical judgment of what needs attention in the moment, either because it is charged with emotional meaning or because it has implications for the emotional health of the child.

Play as a Context for Choosing Ports of Entry

Child–parent psychotherapy encourages the spontaneous unfolding of play because children use play to enact their innermost experiences (Erikson, 1950; Slade & Wolf, 1995). Through play, children can set up models of reality and then experiment with them at will, suspending the rules and constraints of physical and social reality, operating within a safe space where unspeakable fears and wishes can be expressed, and trying out different avenues for the management of anxiety.

Child–parent psychotherapy builds upon these functions of play by encouraging play between the child and the parent. When the sessions take place in the clinical playroom, toys are carefully selected to be developmentally appropriate and to evoke emotionally central themes, including daily caregiving, aggression, danger, and protection. When the sessions take place in the home, the therapist takes a bag of toys selected with the same principles in mind.

The child–parent therapist's role is to help the child and the parent create joint meaning by playing together. When timely, the therapist may step out of the play and reflect on it. This process often involves helping the parent understand and tolerate the painful experiences that the child conveys through play. The therapist serves as the mediator between the child's play and the parent's understanding of it, providing a steady presence that speaks for the legitimacy of the child's play as it moves through the inevitable periods of chaos, unclarity, rigidity, or disorganization that characterize the therapeutic process. The parent's quality of participation in the child's play provides a useful barometer for therapeutic progress because it reflects the parent's degree of empathic attunement with the child's subjective experience and readiness to meet the child's developmental needs.

Action and Language as a Context for Choosing Ports of Entry

Life intrudes into the therapeutic sessions, and this is as it should be. A parent may speak about tensions at work, describe a disagreeable encounter at day care involving the child's behavior, or yell at the child for engaging in a forbidden behavior. The child may hit the parent or hide under a chair while telling the therapist about an upsetting experience. All these events constitute potential ports of entry for child–parent psychotherapy because they provide windows into how the parent and the child perceive themselves, each other, and their individual and joint place in the world. By responding flexibly to the child's and the parent's behavior and narrative, the child–parent psychotherapist conveys the message that everything has meaning and everything the parent and child say and do is deserving of careful attention. Behavior can be the shortest avenue to understand mental representations, and mental representations are routinely accessed through behavior. Reality and the perception of reality are equally genuine fodder for therapeutic intervention. The richness of child–parent psychotherapy resides in the fact that nothing is excluded on principle from the realm of therapeutic attention.

Commonly Used Ports of Entry

The range of potential ports of entry is quite large. A list of commonly used ports of entry and examples is provided in Table 5.1. This list is by no means exhaustive. Relationships affect relationships, and this influence is manifested through behavior and through mental representations, opening up many possibilities for intervention. The specific port of entry is less important for the treatment outcome than the match between the therapist's chosen port of entry and the child's or parent's receptiveness to the intervention (Lieberman et al., 2000; Lieberman, Van Horn, & Ozer, 2001). For this reason, the timing of the intervention needs to be carefully calibrated to the feeling tone of the working relationship between the therapist and the child and parent, both as individuals and as a dyad.

MUTATIVE FACTORS: THE THERAPEUTIC RELATIONSHIP AS THE MATRIX FOR TREATMENT

Much attention has been devoted to the question of what constitutes the mutative factors in dyadic parent–child interventions (Stern, 1985). In infant–parent psychotherapy and child–parent psychotherapy, salience is given to three major factors: parental insight into how intrapsychic conflicts are expressed in ambivalence toward the child, that is, the par-

TABLE 5.1. Commonly Used Ports of Entry

Commonly used ports of entry	Examples
1. The child's behavior, including the child's play	A toddler has a tantrum.
	A preschooler at play makes a dinosaur angrily eat the baby zebra while the mother zebra looks helplessly on.
2. The parent's behavior	A mother complains of fatigue about having to keep track of her toddler's whereabouts.
3. The parent–child interaction	A parent is unresponsive to a toddler's destructive behavior.
4. The child's self-representation	A preschooler says, "Nobody likes me."
5. The child's representation of the parent	A preschooler says to the parent, "You are crazy."
6. The parent's representation of the self	A parent says, "I hurt my children by not leaving their father earlier."
7. The parent's representation of or attribution to the child	A parent says of her toddler, "She is too sexy."
8. The child–mother–father interaction	A preschooler says to his mother, "My dad says you are bad."
9. The parent–therapist relationship	A parent tells the therapist, "I dreamed that you came to live with us."
10. The child–therapist relationship	A toddler clings to the therapist at the end of the session and cries, "No bye-bye."
11. The child–parent–therapist relationship	A preschooler says to the parent about the therapist, "I want to stay with her."
12. The parent–child–therapist relationship	A parent says to the therapist, "My child prefers to be with you rather than with me."

ent's understanding of the child's role as a negative transference object (Fraiberg, 1980); the corrective attachment experiences provided to the child and to the parent by the therapeutic relationship (Lieberman, 1991); and the power of learning and practicing mutually satisfying forms of interaction both between the parent and the therapist and between the parent and the child (Pawl & St. John, 1998). These mechanisms of change do not necessarily operate through verbal interpretation or explicit forms of knowing; the "something more" than interpretation has a powerful mutative role in psychotherapy with young children and their parents, just as it does in individual psychotherapy with adults (Stern et al., 1998).

The relative weight of different mutative factors may differ from case to case depending on the psychological characteristics and sociological circumstances of the parent and the child. Another factor is the length of treatment, which may or may not allow the deepening of certain forms of intrapsychic and interpersonal ways of knowing. It is certain, however, that the quality of the therapeutic relationship is a necessary condition for a successful outcome, although it may not be a sufficient one. A treatment outcome study of infant–parent psychotherapy with toddlers found, for example, that the mother's relationship to the therapist was related to some measures of improvement in both maternal and child behavior, but that maternal psychological mindedness during the therapeutic process was associated more strongly with improvement in both mother and child (Lieberman, Weston, & Pawl, 1991).

Parental readiness to engage in a therapeutic relationship on behalf of the child varies widely and is strongly influenced by the circumstances of the referral, particularly whether the parent perceives the referral as judgmental and coercive or as well-meaning and benign (Lieberman & Pawl, 1993). Depending on the parent's motivation, the treatment may begin with a sense of mutual engagement or it may need a prolonged preparatory period where the therapist cultivates the parent's trust in the therapist's motives and in the goals of the therapeutic process.

Young children in need, on the other hand, seem to be almost invariably eager for treatment. A recurrent finding in child–parent psychotherapy with toddlers and preschoolers is the child's capacity to bring the parent into the treatment through his or her clear enthusiasm for the process. A 4-year-old said it well when she greeted her therapist with an ebullient "I love coming here!" Her mother added, "She keeps asking me how long until it is Tuesday; she keeps waiting to come here the whole week." The child's investment in the work of getting better is often an irresistible inducement for the parent to join in the therapeutic enterprise. Although some parents may become jealous of the child's emotional investment in the therapist, this is a treatable situation provided the therapist remembers that the focus of the work is on the child–parent relationship and not, as is the case in individual psychotherapy with children, on the child–therapist relationship.

CLINICAL EXAMPLES

Two clinical vignettes are now presented to illustrate the versatility of points of entry in child–parent psychotherapy.

Vignette I

This session involves Khalil, age 3, whose mother sought treatment for him because he is very aggressive in childcare and has many fears at home. In this session, Khalil says that he is scared of monsters and adds, "The tiger and the monster will come and eat me." The mother says to the therapist, "I keep telling him that monsters don't exist, but he is still scared of them. He doesn't believe me." The intervenor answers, "I think Khalil wants to believe you, but his fear is so strong that he can't. Most children at this age believe in monsters. He wants you to believe that his monsters are real because he really believes in them." The mother says, "But they are not real." The intervenor replies, "You know how some things can be real for us but not for other people? That is how it is with children. They really believe in monsters and see them in their imagination. How about if you tell him that you will make sure the monsters won't come close to him because you will scare them away?"

Amused and seeing a way out of the impasse with Khalil, the mother says, "I can do that." The intervenor encourages her to tell this to Khalil. The mother says to Khalil, "I will kick the tiger and the monster out so they can't eat you." Khalil asks, very seriously, "How?" Hesitating, the mother says, "I will lock the door." Khalil asks again, "And what more?" The mother answers, "I will lock the windows." Khalil says, "Will you say, 'Go away, monster, don't bother my little boy'?" The mother promises she will do that. Increasingly enjoying the exchange, Khalil and his mother continue in this way for a while until Khalil changes the topic, clearly satisfied that his mother will take effective action to protect him.

In this episode, the therapist made use of two ports of entry: Khalil's mental representation of himself as endangered and the mother's mental representation of Khalil as misguided in feeling himself endangered. By building a bridge between the two incompatible mental representations held by the mother and the child, the therapist encouraged a sense of partnership between them in the goal of finding common ground on how to handle Khalil's fear. The mother expanded her understanding of young children's magical worldview and engaged in behavior that led to a satisfying exchange between herself and her child. Khalil found himself protected and expanded his mental representation of his mother as receptive to his needs and effective in providing protection.

Note that the therapist addressed the mental representations through behavior. She stayed at the concrete level of monsters that needed to be kept at bay, without addressing the possible symbolic meaning of the images or the psychodynamic meaning of the mother's initial refusal to take Khalil's fear seriously and promise protection. Instead, she made use of straightforward developmental guidance to let the mother know about the prevalence of the fear of monsters among preschoolers and the importance of providing concrete reassurance rather than debating the merits of the child's fear. This approach was the simplest possible intervention, and its success made clear that it was sufficient, at least for the time being. Both the child's and the mother's initial responses are common enough that it was worthwhile exploring whether a developmentally informed intervention would suffice. The therapist would have moved on to a more specific exploration of the roots of the impasse if the mother had refused to go along with the therapist's suggestion or if Khalil had refused to believe the mother's assurance that she would protect him.

Vignette 2

This session involves a 3-year-old child, Jamala, who witnessed her father being taken to jail by the police after an episode of violence with her mother. In this session, Jamala ties the therapist's wrists with ropes and says, "You are going to jail! You are bad!" The therapist responds by saying that she is scared, that she is not so bad, asking for forgiveness and in other ways expressing fear, sorrow, and remorse. Jamala is unmoved and escalates the punishment, although never doing anything that can actually hurt the therapist or herself. Jamala's mother watches uncomfortably at first but becomes increasingly fascinated by her child's accurate portrayal of the scenes Jamala witnessed during episodes of domestic violence. The mother's efforts to participate are met by the child's refusal to let her play: "You stay out, Mommy. You are ugly." The therapist says to Jamala, "I think you are angry at your mommy because your daddy went away." Jamala asks the therapist to tie her wrists and send her to jail. The therapist says, "I don't want to do that. It's OK to be angry at your mom. I will be too sad if you go away." Jamala screams: "Do it!" The therapist ties up Jamala's wrists hesitantly, checking with Jamala in a stage whisper to see if she still wants this to happen at each stage of the play.

When Jamala "goes to jail," the therapist and the mother loudly call out for her, telling each other how much they miss her. Jamala reenters, smiling, and is greeted with great joy by the mother and the therapist. Similar play takes place for many weeks. In another session, 3 months later, Jamala says to the therapist, "Even when I am angry with you, I love you," and sighs as if realizing something very important.

In this intervention, the therapist goes along with Jamala as the child enacts in play the victim and the victimizer roles of the drama she had witnessed routinely between her mother and her father. Jamala could not tolerate bringing her mother into the play because, if she did, the play would come much too close to the terrifying reality she had witnessed. The therapist provided a safe alternative that allowed the mother to watch and gain progressively deeper understanding of what her daughter had gone through. The repeated symbolic enactment of the violence, and the therapist's and mother's capacity to tolerate the range of feelings expressed by the child, enabled Jamala to reach a beginning integration of love and hate, anger and vulnerability, first with the therapist and later, very progressively, with her mother.

Importantly, the mother was gradually able to move from the harsh suppression of Jamala's aggression that characterized her relationship with the child at the beginning of treatment to a verbal acknowledgment of Jamala's legitimate reasons for being angry. Jamala and her mother began to speak with each other about "being angry" as a state of mind that could be addressed instead of succumbing to violent action as a way of giving expression to it. The child's intense separation anxiety declined significantly as her ability to modulate aggression improved, suggesting that the separation anxiety was a response not only to the loss of her father but also a reflection of Jamala's fear that her anger would be punished by the loss of her mother, just as her father's anger had been.

CONCLUSION

Child–parent psychotherapy is a relationship-based form of intervention for toddlers and preschoolers that emphasizes the growing child's centrality as an active partner in the intervention by making play and the child's behavior the foci of the sessions. It is intended for situations where the child is experiencing mental health problems or where the relationship between the young child and the parent is negatively affected by the family's difficult circumstances, including parental depression or other mental illness, bereavement, or chronic stress; child constitutional or developmental characteristics that interfere with the formation of a secure attachment; and discrepancies in temperamental style between the child and the parent. Child–parent psychotherapy uses behavior-based strategies, play, and verbal interpretation as agents of therapeutic change. The approach supports and reinforces child and parent perceptions, attitudes, and behaviors that convey positive affect, age-appropriate assertion or discipline, reciprocal play, joint exploration of the world, and constructive conflict resolution. Using a variety of ports of entry that move flexibly between behaviors and mental representations, it targets for change dysregulated child and parental behaviors, including externalizing problems such as excessive punitiveness, aggression, defiance, noncompliance, and recklessness, and internalizing problems such as somatization, social and emotional withdrawal, and multiple fears. A manualized set of guidelines is available, and preliminary research findings show significant improvements in child clinical symptoms and cognitive functioning, maternal psychological functioning, and quality of the mother–child relationship.

REFERENCES

Bollas, C. (1987). *The shadow of the object*. New York: Columbia University Press.

Bowlby, J. (1973). *Attachment and loss: Vol, 2. Separation*. New York: Basic Books.

Bowlby, J. (1980). *Attachment and loss: Vol. 3. Loss, sadness and depression*. New York: Basic Books.

Bowlby, J. (1988). *A secure base: Parent–child attachment and healthy human development*. New York: Basic Books.

Bradley, S. J. (2000). *Affect regulation and the development of psychopathology*. New York: Guilford Press.

Campbell, S. B., Cohn, J. F., & & Meyers, T. (1995). Depression in first-time mothers: Mother–infant interaction and depression chronicity. *Developmental Psychology, 31*, 349–357.

Cassidy, J., & Shaver, P. R. (Eds.). (1999). *Handbook of attachment: Theory, research, and clinical applications*. New York: Guilford Press.

Cicchetti, D., & Cohen, D. J. (1995). Perspectives on developmental psychopathology. In D. Cicchetti & D. J. Cohen (Eds.), *Developmental psychopathology: Vol. 1. Theory and methods* (pp. 3–20). New York: Wiley.

Cicchetti, D., & Lynch, M. (1993). Toward an ecological/transactional model of community violence and child maltreatment: Consequences for children's development. *Psychiatry, 56*, 96–118.

Cramer, B., & Palacio-Espasa, F. (1993). *La pratique des psychothérapies mères–bébés: Études cliniques et technique*. Paris: Presses Universitaires de France.

Cummings, M., & Davies, P. T. (1994). Maternal depression and child development. *Journal of Child Psychology and Psychiatry, 35*, 73–112.

Dawson, G., & Ashman, S. (2000). On the origins of vulnerability to depression: The influence of the early social environment on the development of psycho-biological systems related to risk for affective disorder. In C. A. Nelson (Ed.), The effects of adversity on neurobehavioral development. *Minnesota Symposium on Child Psychology* (Vol. 31). Hillsdale, NJ: Erlbaum.

Dix, T. H., & Grusec, J. E. (1985). Parent attribution in the socialization of children. In I. E. Sigel (Ed.), *Parental belief systems: Psychological consequences for children* (pp. 231–237). Hillsdale, NJ: Erlbaum.

Downey, G., & Coyne, J. C. (1990). Children of depressed parents. *Psychological Bulletin, 108,* 50–76.

Emde, R., & Robinson, J. (2000). Guiding principles for a theory of early intervention: A developmental–psychoanalytic perspective. In J. P. Shonkoff & S. J. Meisels (Eds.), *Handbook of early childhood intervention* (pp. 160–178). Cambridge, UK: Cambridge University Press.

Erikson, E. H. (1950). *Childhood and society.* New York: Norton.

Fraiberg, S. (1980). *Clinical studies in infant mental health.* New York: Basic Books.

Fraiberg, S., Adelson, E., &. Shapiro, V. (1975). Ghosts in the nursery: A psychoanalytic approach to the problems of impaired infant–mother relationships. *Journal of the American Journal of Child Psychiatry, 14,* 387–422.

Frankel, K. A., & Harmon, R. J. (1996). Depressed mothers: They don't always look as they feel. *Journal of the American Academy of Child and Adolescent Psychiatry, 35,* 289–298.

Fonagy, P. (2001). *Attachment theory and psychoanalysis.* New York: Other Press.

Fonagy, P., Steele, M., & Steele, H. (1991). Maternal representations of attachment during pregnancy predict the organization of infant–mother attachment at one year. *Child Development, 62,* 880–893.

Fonagy, P., & Target, M. (1995). Understanding the violent patient: The use of the body and the role of the father. *International Journal of Psycho-Analysis, 76,* 487–502.

Greenspan, S., & Wieder, S. (1998). *The child with special needs.* Reading, MA: Addison-Wesley.

Henggeler, S. W., Schoenwald, S. K., Borduin, C. M., Rowland, M. D., & Cunningham, P. B. (1998). *Multisystemic treatment of antisocial behavior in children and adolescents.* New York: Guilford Press.

Holmes, J. (2001). *The search for the secure base: Attachment theory and psychotherapy.* London: Brunner Routledge.

Klein, M. (1975). Notes on some schizoid mechanisms. In *Envy and gratitude and other works, 1946–1963* (pp. 1–24). New York: Basic Books. (Original work published 1946)

Kohut, H. (1971). *The analysis of the self.* New York: International Universities Press.

Lamb, M. E. (1999). *Parenting and child development in nontraditional families.* Mahwah, NJ: Erlbaum.

Lebovici, S. (1988). Fantasmatic interactions and intergenerational transmission. *Infant Mental Health Journal, 9,* 10–19.

Lieberman, A. F. (1991). Attachment theory and infant–parent psychotherapy: Some conceptual, clinical and research considerations. In D. Cicchetti & S. Toth (Eds.), *Models and integrations. Rochester Symposium on Developmental Psychopathology* (Vol. 3, pp. 261–287). Hillsdale, NJ: Erlbaum.

Lieberman, A. F. (1993). *The emotional life of the toddler.* New York. Free Press.

Lieberman, A. F. (1997). Toddlers' internalization of maternal attributions as a factor in quality of attachment. In L. Atkinson & K. J. Zucker (Eds.), *Attachment and psychopathology* (pp. 277–291). New York: Guilford Press.

Lieberman, A. F. (1998). The satisfactions and tribulations of clinical consultation to child protective services. *Zero to Three: Bulletin of the National Center for Infants, Toddlers and Families,*

Lieberman, A. F. (2000). Negative maternal attributions: Effects on toddlers' sense of self. *Psychoanalytic Inquiry, 19*(5), 737–757.

Lieberman, A. F., Barnard, K. E., & Wieder, S. (in press). In A. Carter & R. Del Carmen–Wiggins (Eds.), *Handbook of infant and toddler mental health assessment.* New York: Oxford University Press.

Lieberman, A. F., & Pawl, J. H. (1993). Infant–parent psychotherapy. In C. H. Zeanah (Ed.), *Handbook of infant mental health* (pp. 427–442). New York: Guilford Press.

Lieberman, A. F., Silverman, R., & Pawl, J. H. (2000). Infant–parent psychotherapy: Core concepts and current approaches. In C. H. Zeanah (Ed.), *Handbook of infant mental health* (2nd ed., pp. 472–484). New York: Guilford Press.

Lieberman, A. F., & Van Horn, P. J. (2001). *Guide to child–parent psychotherapy.* Unpublished manuscript.

Lieberman, A. F., Van Horn, P., & Ozer, E. (2001). *The impact of domestic violence on preschoolers: Predictive and mediating factors.* Unpublished manuscript.

Lieberman, A. F., Weston, D., & Pawl, J. H. (1991). Preventive intervention and outcome with anxiously attached dyads. *Child Development, 62,* 199–209.

Lieberman, A. F., & Zeanah, C. H. (1995). Disorders of attachment in infancy. In K. Minde (Ed.), Infant psychiatry. *Child and Adolescent Psychiatric Clinics of America, 4,* 579–588.

Lyons-Ruth, K., Bronfman, E., & Atwood, G. (1999). A relational diathesis model of hostile–helpless states of mind: Expressions in mother–infant interaction. In J. Solomon & C. George (Eds.), *Attachment disorganization* (pp. 33–70). New York: Guilford Press.

Mahler, M. S., Pine, F., & Bergman, A. (1975). *The psychological birth of the human infant: Symbiosis and individuation.* New York: Basic Books.

Main, M., & Hesse, E. (1990). Parents' unresolved traumatic experiences are related to infant disorganized attachment status: Is frightened and/or frightening parental behavior the linking mechanism? In M. Greenberg, D.

Cicchetti, & M. Cummings (Eds.), *Attachment in the preschool years: Theory, research and intervention* (pp. 161–182). Chicago: University of Chicago Press.

McDonough, S. C. (2000). Interaction guidance: An approach for difficult-to-engage families. In C. H. Zeanah (Ed.), *Handbook of infant mental health* (2nd ed., pp. 485–493). New York: Guilford Press.

Ogden, T. H. (1982). *Projective identification and psychotherapeutic technique.* New York: Academic Press.

Oppenheim, D., Koren-Karie, N., & Sagi, A. (2001). Mother's insightfulness of their preschoolers' internal experience: Relations with early attachment. *International Journal of Behavioral Development, 25,* 16–26.

Osofsky, J., & Fitzgerald, H. (Eds.). (2000). *WAIMH handbook of infant mental health: Vol. III. Parenting and childcare.* New York: Wiley.

Patterson, G. R. (1982). *Coercive family process.* Eugene, OR: Castalia.

Pawl, J. H., & St. John, M. (1998). *How you are is as important as what you do.* Washington, DC: Zero-to-Three/National Center for Clinical Infant Programs.

Sameroff, A. J. (1993). Models of development and developmental risk. In C. H. Zeanah (Ed.), *Handbook of infant mental health* (pp. 3–13). New York: Guilford Press.

Sameroff, A. J. (1995). General systems theories and developmental psychopathology. In D. Cicchetti & D. J. Cohen (Eds.), *Manual of developmental psychopathology: Vol. 1. Theory and methods* (pp. 659–695). New York: Wiley.

Sameroff, A. J., & Emde, R. N. (1989). *Relationship disturbances in early childhood: A developmental approach.* New York: Basic Books.

Sameroff, A. J., & Fiese, B. H. (2000). Transactional regulation: The developmental ecology of early intervention. In J. P. Shonkoff & S. J. Meisels (Eds.), *Handbook of early childhood intervention* (pp. 135–159). Cambridge, UK: Cambridge University Press.

Seifer, R., & Dickstein, S. (2000). Parental mental illness and infant development. In C. H. Zeanah (Ed.), *Handbook of infant mental health* (2nd ed., pp. 145–160). New York: Guilford Press.

Shonkoff, J. P., & Phillips, D. (2000). *From neurons to neighborhoods: The science of early childhood development.* Washington, DC: National Academy Press.

Silverman, R., & Lieberman, A. F. (1999). Negative maternal attributions, projective identifications, and the intergenerational transmission of violent relational patterns. *Psychoanalytic Dialogues, 9*(2), 161–186.

Slade, A. (1999). Attachment theory and research: Implications for the theory and practice of individual psychotherapy with adults. In J. Cassidy & P. R. Shaver (Eds.), *Handbook of attachment: Theory, research and clinical applications* (pp. 575–594). New York: Guilford Press.

Slade, A., & Aber, J. L. (1992). Attachments, drives, and development: conflicts and convergences in theory. In M. Barron, D. Eagle, & D. Wolitzky (Eds.),

Interface of psychoanalysis and psychology. Washington, DC: APA Publications.

Slade, A., & Wolf, D. P. (Eds.). (1995). *Children at play: Clinical and developmental approaches to meaning and representation*. New York: Oxford University Press.

Sroufe, L. A. (1979). The coherence of individual development: Early care attachment, and subsequent developmental issues. *American Psychologist, 34*, 834–841.

Stern, D. N. (1985). *The motherhood constellation: A unified view of parent–infant psychotherapy*. New York: Basic Books.

Stern, D. N., Sander, L. W., Nahum, J. P., Harrison, A. M., Lyons-Ruth, K., Morgan, C., Bruschweiler-Stern, N., & Tronick, E. Z. (1998). Non-interpretive mechanisms in psychoanalytic therapy: The "something more" than interpretation. *International Journal of Psycho-Analysis, 79*, 903–921.

Thompson, R. A. (1999). Early attachment and later development. In J. Cassidy & P. R. Shaver (Eds.), *Handbook of attachment* (pp. 265–286). New York: Guilford Press.

Tronick, E. Z., & Weinberg, M. K. (1997). Depressed mothers and infants: Failure to form dyadic states of consciousness. In L. Murray & P. J. Cooper (Eds.), *Postpartum depression and child development* (pp. 54–81). New York: Guilford Press.

Winnicott, D. W. (1965). The theory of the parent–infant relationship. In D. W. Winnicott (Ed.), *The maturational processes and the facilitating environment* (pp. 37–55). New York: International Universities Press.

Zeanah, C. H. (Ed.). (2000). *Handbook of infant mental health* (2nd ed.). New York: Guilford Press.

Zeanah, C. H., Boris, N. W., & Larrieu, J. A. (1997). Infant development and developmental risk: A review of the past 10 years. *Journal of the American Academy of Child and Adolescent Psychiatry, 36*, 165–178.

Zero to Three/National Center for Clinical Infant Programs. (1994). *Diagnostic classification of mental health and developmental disorders of infancy and early childhood*. Arlington, VA: Author.

CHAPTER 6

THE PRIMARY TRIANGLE

Treating Infants in Their Families

Elisabeth Fivaz-Depeursinge
Antoinette Corboz-Warnery
Miri Keren

In this chapter, we present a new method of structured therapeutic assessment of family relationships based on a developmental systems approach. It evolved from a program of research of the Lausanne University Centre for Family Studies on the development of "triangular"—namely, three-person—relationships between new parents and their first child (Fivaz-Depeursinge & Corboz-Warnery, 1999). The project aimed in particular at designing a method of therapeutic assessment for families with parental psychopathology around birth and through early childhood. It was extended to systems consultations for therapists and other professionals working with infants suffering functional problems and their parents. Lately, the model was used in training professionals in a nationwide early childhood psychiatry program in Israel (Keren, Fivaz-Depeursinge, & Tyano, 2001).

Before we state and illustrate the basic tenets of the method, it is necessary to describe the Lausanne trilogue play (LTP) paradigm because it constitutes the cornerstone of the family assessment. The LTP situation allows the systematic observation of family interactions in a three-way relationship between the father, the mother, and the infant. Trilogue play is the analogue of dialogue play, but between three persons instead of two. As with dialogue play, the goal of trilogue play is to enable three-person families to share moments of pleasure and reach moments of intersubjective communion. The LTP scenario is divided into four parts:

1. One parent plays with the infant, while the other parent is the third party (2+1).
2. The parents reverse roles (2+1).
3. The three partners play together (3-together).
4. The parents interact with each other, and the infant is the third party (2+1).

The three different 2+1's and the single 3-together are what it takes to systematically observe the face-to-face interactions in a three-person family. A videotape is made of the procedure to be used later by the therapist.

The three family members sit in a triangular formation. The infant is in a special seat adjustable for size and inclination. The seat can be turned so the infant faces either parent or can be oriented in between them in such a way that the baby faces both parents and all three can play together. Note that the four-part paradigm can be adapted to later age levels. The toddler is seated in a high chair at a table and is provided with toys appropriate for symbolic play. The young child sits in a regular chair with a set of play dolls, and the parents are instructed to help the child tell a story around a significant theme, for example, a story in which the parents leave for the weekend and the child remains at home with other caretakers. A prenatal version allows one to assess the coparenting alliance in formation, with the parents enacting their first meeting with their infant (represented by a doll) right after birth.

It is important to remember that trilogue play, like dialogue play, specifically targets affect regulation and sharing and empathic responsiveness as they relate to the motivations of warmth, affection (MacDonald, 1992), or intersubjectivity. It does not assess other domains of functioning, such as security of attachment, with its specific target of fear and exploration, or learning and teaching or control and discipline with their specific goals (for details see Emde, 1989; Hirschberg, 1993). However, it is possible to apply the LTP paradigm to assess these other domains by asking the parents to engage in the different configurations of 2+1 and 3-together as they teach the child or set limits, for instance.

BASIC TENETS OF THE METHOD

There are a number of basic tenets underlying the therapeutic assessment of family interactions. These emphasize the family as a unit and the relationships between its members.

Family Practices Are the Port of Entry

In working with an infant in his or her family, the port of entry can only be through the interaction and, what's more, bodily communication between the infant and the parents. First, the mere presence of a baby in the session inevitably calls attention to such interactions. Secondly, as clinicians in the domain of infancy well know, a few minutes of feeding, diapering, play, and separation–reunion provide more information than might be inferred from long conversations. It follows that having a family enact interactions rather than just talk about them is only logical. These principles are in line with the perspective of the practicing family as defined by Reiss (1989).

Observation and Assessment Cannot Be Dissociated from Intervention

Indeed, a family enacting trilogue play or any other clinically meaningful situation is transforming itself—for better or for worse (Sameroff & Emde, 1989). Chances are for the better when the situation is carefully formatted and integrated in a clinical context so designed as to facilitate growth and change. Then it can strengthen the family members' implicit relational knowledge of their three-way relationship (Lyons-Ruth et al., 1998).

A well-known way of enhancing this type of experience is by means of video feedback to support awareness of positive and negative interactive patterns (Bakermans-Kranenburg, Juffe, & van IJzendoorn, 1998; Downing & Ziegenhain, 2001; McDonough, 1993, and Chapter 4, this volume). Direct intervention on interactions is another way to make the experience a growth-enhancing one. It consists of triggering changes in the problematic patterns of interaction, and it may be conducted immediately within the interactive setting and/or by means of prescriptions or rituals to be carried out at home in between sessions (Imber-Black & Roberts, 1992). It is particularly indicated when parents are not prone to reflection or when enacting the procedure has not been sufficiently positive for them. Then intervention itself takes an interactive form be-

tween the consultant and the family and is based on the observable behaviors, not necessarily on the verbalized representations that underlie
them.

We should stress, however, that in addressing the behavior of the
practicing three-person family we also touch on their triangular intersubjective experience, whether implicitly or explicitly.

Relationships Are Wholes

Members of a three-person family establish "threesome" relationships,
distinct from "twosome" ones. As Sroufe has argued, the systems perspective on relationships is that "relationships are wholes . . . with
unique properties not reducible to characteristics of individuals" (1989,
p. 102). We further argue that individuals in families not only establish twosome relationships but also threesome relationships. Moreover,
threesome relationships are distinct from twosome ones. In systems
terms, threesome relationships cannot be reduced to the sum of their
constituent twosome parts. In other words, it is not possible to extrapo-
late from threesome relationships to twosome ones, and reciprocally
"each level of social complexity has properties not relevant to that below" (Hinde & Stevenson-Hinde, 1988, p. 366).

Relationships Have Two Sides, the Interactive
and the Intersubjective

The interactive is the behavioral–observable side, and it is made up of
patterns of actions and signals between the partners. The intersubjective
is the intimate psychic side, and it is made up of the intentions, feelings,
and meanings shared between the family members. The two sides are
indissociable. When the interactive coordination of actions and signals
and the corresponding intersubjective communion are insufficient, negative affective patterns and experience dominate, engendering pain and
misery in family members.

Families Constitute Alliances

Relationships at the level of the family as a unit may be characterized in
terms of alliance, that is, the degree of coordination that the family members attain in working jointly toward realizing a task. In the case of
trilogue play, the goal is to reach moments of playful affective communion. It is the extent to which the partners coordinate their actions and

their signals and in parallel align their subjective experiences to reach that goal which defines their type of family alliance, from most coordinated to least coordinated.

Therapeutic Relationships Affect Family Relationships

It is widely believed that it is through the relationship with the therapist that the relationships within the family are likely to change. We see this process as creating a "good enough holding environment" for the family (see Stern, 1985; also Chapter 2, this volume), as Winnicott (1965) would put it metaphorically, analogous to the "good enough holding" of the parent in relation to the infant. It is also close to the Vygotskian concept of how parents facilitate their child's development as they work in the proximal zone of development (Vygotsky, 1979), Bruner's concept of "scaffolding" (1985), or Fogel's concept of "framing" (1977). Yet these concepts lack the formalization of the influence of children on their parents. The systems model we describe here defines both influences. In addition, it draws a parallel between the mutual influences parents and child exert on each other to promote developmental change and the influences therapists and families exert on each other to facilitate such change (Fivaz, Fivaz, & Kaufmann, 1982).

Let us take an example from normal development. In early gaze interaction during dialogue or feeding, the mother provides a spatio-temporal frame for the infant by looking for long episodes at him or her (Fogel, 1977). Within this frame, the infant will freely alternate between engaging and pausing but will almost invariably meet the mother's gaze when looking at her. Gaze contact will in turn sustain the motivation of the baby for social engagement and promote its differentiation (framing influence), a development that in turn will further sustain the mother's framing. The infant's behavior that maintains the mother's framing involvement has been called an "implicative influence" (Cronen, Kenneth, & Lannamann, 1982) .

In a problematic situation, say, of an infant having sleeping difficulties, at the level of the family the infant's implicative influence is exerted through the intense driving force of the symptom, in spite of its paradoxical nature. This indicates the possibility of a problematic framing by the parents because this framing is maladjusted and/or insufficiently predictable. At the level of the therapeutic group, the family members' influence is exerted by their engagement in therapeutic work. The therapist's framing influence vis-à-vis the family will have to integrate all the family elements to help reestablish a normal developmental course (see

Fivaz, Fivaz, & Kaufmann, 1981, for a detailed description). Figure 6.1 is an illustration of the model.

In sum, in "framing-implicative" interactions, the "framing" party (parents or therapists) creates a context that is adjusted to the direction of change in which the child is moving or the family is straining; this context is sustained as long as necessary. Thus, adjustment and predictability are the two conditions for a productive framing influence. In return, the implicative party (child or family) indicates in which direction development or change is aiming and works toward it. Thus engagement in the relationship and motivation for development and change are the two conditions for a productive implicative influence.

The parallel between parents and therapists may go further in interventions with families of infants. It is known that parents activate intuitive parenting behaviors that are specifically adjusted to their child's level of development (Papousek & Papousek, 1987). With parents unable to activate these parenting behaviors in interacting with their infants, therapists may find themselves activating their own intuitive parenting

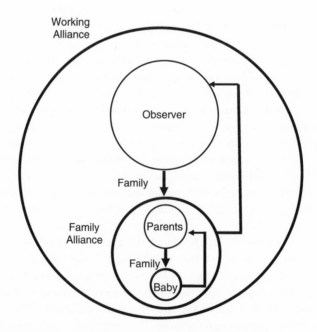

FIGURE 6.1. Framing–developing interactions in the clinical system (working alliance) and in the family system (family alliance). Large arrows depict framing influences, and small arrows depict implicative influences.

behaviors in relation to these parents by constructing a vocal envelope to appease anxious parents faced with a nervous baby, sometimes actually holding a mother whose holding of her infant is maladjusted, or sitting on the floor with a father who fails to join his child at his level. In other words, this method actually draws on the therapist's own intuitive parenting inheritance and implicit relational knowledge (Lyons-Ruth et al., 1998); it also helps elucidate how modeling might work.

An example of a systems consultation will best illustrate the above basic tenets. The concept of systems consultation was put forward by Wynne, McDaniel, & Weber (1986) to refer to a special assessment session, possibly repeatable, in which a therapist asks a consultant for assistance in order to identify or clarify a situation and consider different options for intervention.

USING THE LTP PARADIGM IN A SYSTEMS CONSULTATION

Suzan, a 9-month-old with a sleeping problem, and her parents were brought to our family center by a family therapist after two sessions (for a more extensive description, see Fivaz-Depeursinge & Corboz-Warnery, 1999). The therapist asked for a consultation with an infant specialist about the socioaffective development of the child and her communication with her parents. The parents had agreed to be videotaped playing with their baby and knew that they would receive feedback during video replay in the presence of the therapist. They also knew that the consultant preferred not to hear about the motive for the consultation nor to learn about the clinical data until she had made her observations in order to prevent any bias on her part. The therapist and the family came at the time of the infant's feeding. This rather informal time allowed them to get acquainted with the consultant and provided information about the way the parents cared for their daughter. It was visible from the outset that they were extremely invested in parenting. However, the coparenting cooperation was suffering from competition between the father and mother in the face of a very demanding child. Having changed Suzan's diapers, the parents declared themselves ready to play. They were introduced to the LTP procedure described above. They were to play as a family, in four parts: (1) one of them would begin playing with Suzan, while the other one would be simply present; (2) they would change roles; (3) they would play together with Suzan; and (4) it would be Suzan's turn to be simply present, and they would talk together.

Then, the consultant joined the family in the LTP setting. She was prepared to do a direct intervention. On the one hand, she had noted the parents' high level of motivation in parenting; but, on the other hand, she had noted problematic patterns in their interactions and wanted to test their flexibility to change.

These problematic patterns were hyperregulation of the infant's affects, competition between the parents for the child's attention, and displacement of their tension onto the outside as well as onto the child (S. Minuchin, 1974). For instance, the mother kept presenting the girl with a lighted cigarette lighter; she showed Suzan how the flame hurt the mother's hand—but with much misleading enthusiasm. The father kept trying to calm things down, but he did it in a self-defeating way by abruptly presenting other toys to Suzan, interfering in the mother's play. He was promptly dismissed by both of them. He then withdrew and turned to the observing team's window with a look of complicity in a demonstration of his disagreement with the mother. Thus Suzan kept getting contradictory signals from her parents, in the context of boundary distortions between the family's generations (Sroufe, 1989).

The consultant wondered above all else how the parents felt about the "playing with fire" game and was ready to work on this theme. But when she returned to the playroom and asked the parents how they felt about the play, they answered that it had been all right and quite representative of home play, but they felt bad about the fourth part, when they were supposed to talk together and leave the child on her own. They felt they were unable to do it, assuming that Suzan would not allow them to be on their own.

Indeed, the consultant had observed that during this last part the parents did not turn to each other to engage in a dialogue. They simply sat back and looked at their child, who obviously did not understand what was happening, began fussing, and was given a bottle. She calmed down, but they still did not engage with each other.

To go along with the parents' feelings and wishes, the consultant decided to focus her trial intervention on the last part of the LTP by trying to draw a boundary between the couple and their daughter. She asked them whether they wanted to try the last part again. They said no, it was useless; it was like that at home too—Suzan did not want to be left alone. The consultant accepted their refusal and asked them to describe how they would have done it if Suzan had allowed them to do so.

Eventually the parents sat facing each other, talking about their troubles with Suzan, while the consultant listened with empathy. At some point, the father exclaimed, "But this is what is happening now!"

and the three of them laughed together. And the parents agreed to try a dialogue. However, they sustained eye contact for only a few seconds and kept averting their eyes from each other and turning toward the child. Suzan had kept quiet throughout, apparently happy to get a rest.

The consultant thanked them for having worked so hard with her and asked the therapist to return and formulate her request. She learned that the parents sought help because Suzan cried every hour at night. How could the therapist get the parents to believe in their own competence so that they would finally give themselves the right to make mistakes? Her request also implicitly indicated her concern for the pattern of overstimulation of the child and the tension displaced onto her. Note the parallel process between the parents asking for help from a therapist and the therapist asking for help from a consultant.

They watched the videotape of the session together. The consultant emphasized at length the competence and the strength of the child as well as the parents' resourcefulness and their working so hard in order to be good parents. Then she stated emphatically that she was concerned for them—she felt they were exhausted. She thought they could afford to give themselves a break and why not their baby, too. She wondered how come they had learned to work themselves so hard, asking if perhaps they had to care a lot for their own parents.

Referring to the basic tenets of the method described above, the assessment had revealed that in Suzan's family the partners had an intense threesome relationship, but it was marked with negative interactive patterns. Presumably, it was a frustrating subjective experience for everyone involved; the sharing of intentions, feelings, and meanings that makes up intersubjective communion was failing. This failure was related to a lack of coordination between the parents in relation to their child. Their interactions were typical of "collusive alliances."

In terms of intervention, great care had been taken throughout the session to establish a positive relationship with the parents and the child. Carrying out the trilogue play procedure allowed the parents to precisely experience and indicate the change they were straining for together (their implicative influence). The consultant's direct intervention was adjusted to this goal and was sustained until it was reached. Her framing influence consisted in drawing the necessary boundary between the parents and the baby. Moreover, it led to the father's insight about the change they were achieving unaware ("But this is what is happening now!"), giving the parents hope concerning their ability to change and motivation to continue treatment.

Video feedback was used to strengthen the positive experience and indicate how the change could translate in the context of the larger family, and was continued in the therapy. Interestingly, the technique of intervention was deceptively simple. Sitting with the family in the LTP setting, listening empathetically, and establishing a vocal envelope were the ingredients of the framing. As the parents and the baby actively collaborated, they progressively relaxed and came to realize their goal.

A systems consultation is thus but a piece of a wider therapeutic program. Therapists find it useful as an anchor for their work with difficult family interactions. They may sometimes repeat it to check on the progress of the therapy.

The therapist reported later that the sleeping problems had receded. She had been using the above observations to work with the parents on the boundary distortions between themselves and the baby as well as between themselves and their families of origin. In particular, they had worked on the father's increased support of the mother in respect to his own mother, who was living in the same house. She reported that as this work progressed the pattern of overstimulation of the child weakened, so that "playing with fire" was of no more concern.

ASSESSING AND INTERVENING
WITH THE FAMILY ALLIANCE

The analysis of the task of trilogue play has revealed that there are four necessary and embedded conditions that must be met in order to reach the goal of trilogue play—defining different types of family alliance. Each type has specific strong and weak points that indicate the exact target of intervention. They are represented in Figure 6.2.

Participation

First, is everyone included? If any of the three partners is excluded, there is no possibility of attaining the goal of trilogue play. An example of exclusion of the infant by the parents is setting up the baby with insufficient support in her seat, for instance, by setting the seat too straight, an equivalent of inappropriate holding, so that the infant is made unable to interact. It frequently occurs in a context of covert divergence between the parents. It leads them to overlook the discomfort of the child, interpreting it as resulting from mishandling by the other parent or as rejection on the part of the infant. Exclusion of an adult may result when a third-party parent stonewalls (Gottman, 1994). In such situations, a

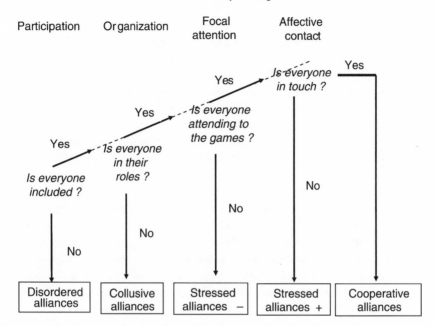

FIGURE 6.2. Assessing family alliances.

young infant may get a glazed look or systematically avert his or her gaze, thus reinforcing the negative subjective experience of the parents.

When there is a family pattern of exclusion, the alliance is categorized as "disordered." This is often observed in families with serious parental psychopathology, whether it is diagnosed or not, with the child being caught in a role reversal, a "parentified" position. For instance, an 18-month-old toddler was continuously confronted with contradictory attitudes of his parents. During the 2+1 with his mother, she forbade him to throw down objects while his father kept picking them up. During his 2+1 with his son, the father was lenient and the mother silently blaming, stonewalling. As time came for playing the 3-together, the boy took it upon himself to release the tension between his parents. He took charge by putting on a show, leading them in applauding together, saving them from having to actively coordinate games together.

A pattern of exclusion calls for a specific intervention directed at the exclusion. Suppose it is the baby who is excluded by being seated in an inappropriate position for engaging with the parents. A direct trial intervention might consist of creating an empathic, reassuring vocal envelope in which the parents are quietly led to perceive and change the position of the baby. This would in all probability result in the infant's engagement in the interaction and in turn trigger positive feedback on the part of the parents, helping to build trust in the possibility of change. Or, when an infant's glazed look or head aversion occurs in the context of parental intrusiveness, the direct intervention might consist of triggering change by having the parents follow the infant's initiatives rather than lead them (Malphurs et al., 1996).

When parents exclude themselves, for instance, by means of stonewalling, it is obviously more difficult to trigger change. Here, the techniques elaborated by family therapists to deal with family and coparenting conflict are essential tools. For instance, during video feedback, the therapist might reframe the parents' self-exclusion and their ensuing disengagement from the child as being the result of their "invisible loyalty" to their families of origin (Boszormenyi-Nagy & Sparks, 1973). In brief, such patterns of exclusion often indicate the necessity of long-term treatment that may require home visits and intensive work on the network by all the professionals involved (Grasset, Fivaz-Depeursinge, & Rougemont, 1989).

In contrast, when everyone is included in trilogue play, this constitutes an essential resource of the family's interactions. It is thus part of the intervention to emphasize this, as was the case in Suzan's family.

Then the second condition should be examined.

Organization

Is everyone keeping to their roles, or is someone interfering or abstaining ? Again, if not, then the possibility of attaining the goal of trilogue play is prevented. Examples are (1) the parent in the third-party role interferes by moving forward and addressing the infant instead of keeping back, (2) the parent in the active position abstains from engagement, or (3) the parents fail to coordinate in the 3-together. In these situations, the infant's attention may be "monoparental"; that is, he or she engages with one parent only. When there is a pattern of failing to keep to assigned roles, the alliance is categorized as "collusive." Such a pattern is observed in families with nonnegotiable conflict between the parents, with the child being imprisoned in a scapegoat or go-between position (McHale & Fivaz-Depeursinge, 1999; Vogel & Bell, 1960).

Direct intervention in these situations may be productive, again in a context of the holding of the family, namely, remaining close to the parents as they engage in a game with their baby, thus putting pressure on them to stay in their roles, or by helping them in the last 2+1 configuration to establish a boundary with respect to the baby, such as occurred in Suzan's family. When the patterns of interference are not too severe, video feedback may allow the parents to perceive their negative implications, voice their subjective experience, and find ways to change.

When the second condition is met, roles are sufficiently respected. Then the third condition should be examined.

Focalization

Do the partners share the same focus, or is someone attending elsewhere? Here we examine whether the partners co-construct a joint focus of attention (the games in trilogue play) and sustain it. Suppose the active parent fragments the games she is proposing to the baby, or the parents during their own discussion in the fourth part keep interrupting their dialogue to interact with the baby, and perhaps in addition the baby has difficulty in focusing his or her attention, then again the goal is not fully attainable. When the focus is not sufficiently shared and sustained, the alliance is categorized as "stressed plus (+)." Our observations of nonclinical families lead us to consider this as part of the normative range.

When everyone is included and keeps to his or her roles, work on negative patterns of joint attention is comparatively easy, provided that the therapeutic alliance is positive enough. Encouragement of the parents to persist in a game, to follow more closely the lead of the child, and to let themselves be more animated and playful may be achieved by the therapist's direct intervention or during video feedback.

When a joint focus is co-constructed and sustained, an additional resource of importance is to be emphasized. Then the fourth condition should be examined.

Affective Contact

Are the three partners emotionally in touch, or are they out of tune with each other? Here we examine whether warmth and empathic understanding are dominating or whether the affective climate is too negative. Suppose the parents fail to sufficiently help the baby to regulate his or her affects by hyperstimulating or hypostimulating him or her; then it is not possible to reach moments of shared pleasure on a regular basis, or the parents' affects tend to vary according to the infant's affects. In this case the alliance is categorized as "stressed minus (–)."

It is at this level that one enters most naturally the intersubjective side of the relationship. This may be achieved during video replay of brief microsequences, where processes of coordination, miscoordination, and repair (Tronick & Cohn, 1989) are made visible through slow motion. For instance, a mother in the third-party position failed to validate her infant daughter's bid for sharing a moment of pleasure she was experiencing in playing with father. After three unsuccessful attempts, the baby became distressed and avoided making other bids.

When the partners are in tune, they share moments of affective communion as a threesome, mostly pleasurable, and in each of the configurations. Then the alliance is categorized as "cooperative"; cooperative alliances are observed at the upper end of the normative range.

Enacting the LTP procedure may be of great benefit to families with cooperative alliances. Some of them are able to benefit by themselves through the enactment of the LTP. For instance, during the fourth part of the LTP parents may discuss whether they actually play as a threesome at home and reflect on why they do not do it more. In our experience, the more coordinated the family, the more it is able to learn and to change.

TRIANGULAR MICROPROCESSES

Triangular microprocesses may appear in infants as early as 3 months of age, if not earlier—albeit in less differentiated, more context-bound forms than at age 9 months (Fivaz-Depeursinge & Frascarolo, 1999). We consider them as part of primary intersubjectivity (Stern, 2000). It is extremely interesting to follow microprocesses as they differentiate past secondary intersubjectivity up to the domain of moral emotions and then of narratives in Stern's scheme.

Triangular microprocesses are also very revealing in families with problematic interaction patterns but are much more difficult to work with, because the parents may not be ready to open up to experiencing them. Basically, they are more often negative and tend to function to regulate the parents' relationship rather than to primarily establish intersubjective communion in the threesome.

For instance, in a family with high competition between the parents, one may observe a pattern of "chase and dodge" (Beebe & Stern, 1977). In an interaction between a father and his 3-month-old son, the baby briefly orients to his father, who immediately looms over him. The baby averts his gaze and orients to his mother, looking at her and protesting. This is where the mother takes advantage of the situation to show that she is the better parent and thus interferes with the father by trying to rescue the baby. Chances are that her turn will come to be interfered with too. The baby will be caught in a negative triangular pattern—or, as often referred to in the family clinical domain, in a scapegoat position.

In Suzan's family, there was one dramatic instance of this infant's social referencing with her parents that illustrates the difficulty in this type of family interaction in sharing meanings as a threesome. At the height of the "playing with fire" sequence, the mother recruited the father to burn his finger too. He voiced his refusal but then did it anyway. The mother exclaimed, "Ouch, that hurts!"—but with a broad smile. Suzan looked at her father with a mixed expression of perplexity and excitation; he validated her feeling by making a grimace of pain and then smiling at her in a reassuring way. Then Suzan turned to her mother who was taking her turn at putting her finger in the flame, again with the same enthusiasm. The mother exclaimed, "Ouch!"but once more she smiled engagingly. The combined effect of the parents' contradictory signals and ways of validating Suzan's feelings could not be anything but confusing.

We have observed other families' problematic interactions where the infant hardly made triangular bids. The infant seemed to learn to avoid the triangle, systematically averting attention from the parents or interacting with one parent only or taking refuge in objects. In such a case a few triadic person–person–object interactions, more cognitively oriented but almost devoid of affect, might have been observable. Thus the parents were spared being faced with the triangular process.

USING THE LTP PARADIGM
IN AN EXTENSIVE THERAPEUTIC ASSESSMENT

In the following example, we show how the LTP paradigm may be used to inform a longer-lasting therapeutic assessment. It also illustrates how the method is applied in early childhood. It consists in the therapeutic assessment of the family triad and of the three dyads separately. We conduct this type of assessment whenever it is indicated and when it is possible to work for a longer term with a family—in particular, when parental psychopathology is associated with rigid family coalitions that put the child right in the troubled middle.

Andrew's family sought help because the 3-year-old boy was "excluding his mother." After two sessions with the couple, the therapists offered an extensive therapeutic assessment.

First Session: Narrative LTP

The parents were invited to help Andrew tell and enact a story with play dolls on the following theme: Mom and Dad are leaving for the weekend, and the child is cared for by other adults. The narrative is divided into four parts: (1) one of the parents begins the story with Andrew while the other parent is simply present; (2) the other parent continues the story while the first parent takes the third-party role; (3) the three of them terminate the story; and (4) the parents talk together about the enactment and the child is in the third-party position, drawing or playing by himself.

Mother–Andrew, with Father as the Third Party

The mother started, helping Andrew to select the characters and enact the first part of the story, namely, in which Mom and Dad are leaving. Of note was that during Andrew's story the child insisted that Mom and Dad simply say good-bye and leave, while his mother insisted that Andrew provide for the child numerous explanations about leaving ("What would you like Mom and Dad to say before leaving?"). In the meantime, the father kept distant, immobile, visibly restraining himself in order not to interfere. Thus, the exclusion pattern was manifested by the father (self-exclusion), but not by Andrew in relation to the mother.

Father–Andrew, with Mother as the Third Party

The father's attitude in the first part contrasted with his very close interactive style as he took over the role of active parent and enacted Mom and Dad's departure. He was soon taking over complete control of the narration, developing wilder and wilder fantasies about the child's activities over the weekend that had only a loose connection with the main theme. Andrew followed with pleasure but refused to take any initiative. The mother oscillated between sitting back and reengaging and interfering, but neither the father nor the child seemed to take notice of any of her moves. The pattern of exclusion was jointly manifested by the father and Andrew with respect to the mother. The latter's oscillations between withdrawal and engagement only reinforced her being excluded.

Father–Mother–Andrew

Eventually the father signaled the mother to reengage for the 3-together part and to enact Mom and Dad's return. The father briefly closed Mom and Dad's weekend story by stating that they had done what they had to do. He continued to assume complete control of the narrative, with the mother following with good grace. However, as the doll family reunited, she insisted on having the child doll kiss Mom. Her initiative was ignored by the father as well as by Andrew. Overall, Andrew did not interact directly with his mother. Thus the pattern of the mother's exclusion by the father and son was continued.

Father–Mother, with Andrew as the Third Party

The fourth part with the dialogue between the parents was almost skipped. The parents decided they had done enough in the previous parts and quickly put a stop to the play session.

In conclusion, the LTP revealed a disordered alliance during this session. Andrew indeed excluded his mother, but the pattern was a family one, led by the father with respect to the mother. The mother colluded with her own exclusion by alternating between interfering and withdrawing. Andrew colluded in excluding his mother when his father was active but not when interacting in the 2+1 with her. Finally, the parents' skipping the last part confirmed their avoidance of facing their coparenting conflict.

Furthermore, exclusion prevented the partners from keeping to their roles and sharing a joint focus as a threesome. There was not a single moment of triangular sharing of affects, so that intersubjective communion as a threesome was utterly failing. This 3-year-old child's lack of initiative and submission to his father were alarming. They contrasted sharply with his advanced speech development. The other side of this disorder was manifested during the video replay. Indeed, the replay was made almost impossible due to Andrew's extreme opposition. He began yelling and running around as soon as the therapists addressed the parents. Several direct trial interventions failed to reestablish order.

In brief, on the one hand, the therapists were impressed by the parents' motivation to work on the problem of Andrew excluding his mother; on the other hand, they were concerned by Andrew's relational disorders, as well as by the father's extremely seductive/intrusive style and the mother's distant style with Andrew. They felt it was necessary to assess the dyadic interactions separately, in spite of the parental dyad's avoidant stance toward conflict, in order to measure the extent of the problematic interactions.

Second Session: Therapeutic Assessment of Parent–Child Dyads

Mother–Andrew

The therapists started to work with the mother and child, while the father filled out questionnaires in a separate room. Upon observing the mother's distant, cold attitude during free play, the female therapist came in and asked her to take her son on her lap. The mother did so skillfully. She also complied skillfully when asked to sing with him. These positive results led the therapist to emphasize her maternal competence and affection, which she had in some ways kept hidden. She was asked to continue the process at home without telling her husband about it.

Father–Andrew

Work with the father revealed difficulties in spite of his good will. On observing the very same extremely intrusive style, the male therapist asked him to try following the child's initiatives rather than leading, staying with him in the room. There followed a "silence," with the child manifesting few initiatives. Soon the father was leading again, even though he wondered aloud how come he hyperstimulated his child so much. The therapist felt utterly powerless in helping father, as if faced with an impenetrable bubble. Congratulated for trying in spite of the difficulty, the father was told to continue the process at home without telling his wife.

Thus, the dyadic interaction between the mother and the child was better coordinated and became less distant and warmer when assessed and worked with separately than in the context of the family triad. In contrast, the dyadic interaction between the father and the child was similar in both contexts and revealed resistance to change even under direct intervention.

Third Session: Therapeutic Assessment of the Parental Couple

The parents came to the third session alone. They reported that life at home with Andrew was even more difficult. He had become physically aggressive with his mother and also with his maternal grandmother who lived in the same house. He refused to separate from his father and dictated every move in the home. The therapists empathized with the parents but urged them to hold on, arguing that Andrew was undergoing a painful process of loss in relation to his father. But his socioaffective development was at stake, especially regarding triangular and group relationships.

The couple was asked to enact a conflict discussion about a disagreement concerning their child. They were first at a loss, reacting as if conflict was a dirty word. Exclusion was the child's problem, not the couple's. Eventually, they found a superficial divergence and gracefully went along with the instructions of working toward a resolution. They settled it in a few minutes, insisting that they never had such a disagreement or needed to be in conflict.

The therapists decided to break what they felt was pseudomutuality (Wynne, Ryckoff, Day, & Hirsch, 1958) and to intervene. Standing by each spouse, they announced they would role-play the feelings they figured they themselves would experience in this situation, that is, the wife feeling excluded by the husband and the husband feeling that his wife did not understand the depth of his relationship with his son. Moved, the mother confirmed the therapist's perception, but the father looked utterly perplexed. They left with the task of demonstrating to their boy that they formed a couple—by sticking together, putting him to bed together—in as many ways as possible. In addition, the father was to prevent the boy from hitting his mother and the mother was to help the father in following the boy's initiatives rather than leading.

Fourth Session: Elaboration

The parents came alone for further reviewing of the work at home and during the sessions. They reported an alleviation of Andrew's conduct and of his sleeping problems. The therapists stressed again that the problem was serious but that the parents were to be congratulated for having come early and for working with such devotion. Different options for further treatment were suggested—couple therapy, working with their families of origin, and individual therapy for the father—but to no avail. The couple felt no need to work on their relationship. The mother vetoed working with the families of origin. She said that they were able to handle on their own the admittedly difficult relation between her own mother, living in the same house, and her husband. Further instructions were elaborated with the parents about how to work with their child at home.

Fifth Session: Therapeutic Assessment in Free Family Interaction

The parents came with Andrew. The situation had improved. The therapists started the session by addressing the boy, thanking him for bringing the family to the center and telling him they knew how hard he was working, too. Andrew was visibly impressed. Direct interventions were aimed, on the one hand, at furthering solidarity and cooperation between the parents with respect to Andrew and, on the other hand, at providing Andrew with a positive experience of being in the third-party position as well as of threesomeness. The parents sang together to their child and Andrew agreed to listen to them with the help of the therapists, then joined them. He oscillated between letting the adults address each other and yelling, between cooperating with his mother and excluding her by clinging to his father. The therapists commented on Andrew being in transition and on the necessity for the parents to continue their work with him. The parents insisted on continuing to try working by themselves. The date for the video reviewing of that session was set for 2 months later.

Sixth Session: Video Feedback

The parents reported ups and downs in Andrew's evolution. Work with the couple was focused on supporting family threesomeness. The microepisodes of triangular affect sharing observed during free family play were reviewed, and the context of inclusion in which they occurred was contrasted with the context of exclusion in the first LTP in which no threesome affect sharing had been observed. The next session was planned as a follow-up a few months later, when Andrew would turn 4 years old.

Follow-Up: Narrative Trilogue Play

The theme of the narrative to be enacted was negotiated with the parents. The topic was a disagreement that had occurred between the parents the day before. The Mom and Dad dolls were to ask the child doll to go play in his room while they were trying to resolve their disagreement.

The similarities and differences in the family interactive patterns were to provide a measure of the progress and difficulties experienced by the three members in establishing a more favorable family alliance.

The pattern of exclusion had markedly decreased. Andrew no longer excluded his mother, nor did the mother collude with being excluded by interfering or abstaining to engage. However, the father still had to exclude himself during the 2+1 between the mother and Andrew in order not to interfere. Of note was the change in the 3-together, where the father and mother were acting in a more coordinated way.

Another important change was that Andrew actively cooperated and took initiatives. He stated at the outset that he had carefully listened to the instructions and insisted throughout on sticking to them. For instance, he repeatedly stated that the boy was to go to his room and play by himself while the parents discussed things. Likewise, he was the one who initiated the transitions between the parts. As the mother insisted that he enact a parent role, Andrew stated, "We said each one in his turn. . . . Now Dad . . .," " thus escaping that role by initiating the transition to the second part. Likewise, it was he who introduced his mother in the 3-together, by inviting her, "Mom, come too!," when Dad called for the child to return to eat dessert.

However, the parents were not ready to validate Andrew's new attitudes. During their dialogue in the last part, they stated that he had not been true to himself. Normally, at home, he would have refused to play by himself, whereas in the enactment the boy did so without a problem. The father went on to state that he did not feel in the action himself, that actually he did not feel well that day. Andrew immediately declared that the drawing he was making was for his father. A few seconds later, his mother, short of ideas for conversation with the father, leaned toward Andrew and asked, "What are you doing?" He replied sharply that this was for Dad. At this, his mother declared, "Need we say more?"—and the father signaled the end of the play session.

The last part had not lasted longer than during the first LTP. It showed that Andrew was not yet free enough of having to regulate his parents' relationship and to repair his father's vulnerability and assume a role reversal position with respect to him. However, he was on his way, as shown by his enthusiastic cooperation with the therapists during the following intervention.

One of the therapists came in and asked the parents to enact with the dolls the discussion about the parents' disagreement. Andrew immediately announced that he could play by himself. As always, the parents went along with good grace. Andrew monitored them with extreme attention as they tried to enact a conflict. As his name was mentioned, he exclaimed with surprise and pleasure, "You have named the child after me?"

Eighth Session: Video Feedback

Video feedback was focused on showing the parents that Andrew's behaviors in the LTP were progressive, even if not yet representative of his
usual behavior at home. The therapists stressed again that the child was
in transition and that it was important to validate his moves toward
drawing a boundary between himself and his parents. They also showed
in detail a microsequence of repair after an exclusion move in order to
reinforce the parents' own sense of making progress. This sequence occurred after Andrew had invited his mother to begin the 3-together. He
had played out that Mom had invented a new recipe for chocolate cream
and his mother and Andrew had shared a moment of pleasure, but his father had broken in with "But the child does not like chocolate!" The
mother and Andrew had looked at him with a dismayed expression. A
minute later, father had repaired this by proposing to close the game by
their eating chocolate together and the threesome had shared a moment
of pleasure.

In summary, in this session the pattern of exclusion was much less
pronounced, with the mother assuming a more engaged stance, the father working hard, if not very effectively, toward a less intrusive interactive style, yet allowing the child to slowly evolve out of the tension-
displacing coalition of the parents. Andrew himself was a key driving
force in "bringing the parents along" in letting him grow out of it
(Brazelton, Koslowski, & Main, 1974). In the light of the significant but
partial changes the family made, it was expected that other phases would
take place at key developmental stages of the child.

DISCUSSION AND CONCLUSION

This example illustrates in a detailed way the basic tenets of family relationship therapeutic assessment. Whether at the triadic or dyadic level
of the family, it invariably focuses on relationships as wholes, with their
two sides, the interactive and the intersubjective. The importance of taking into account the family unit, the "realistic context" in which infants
grow, is widely acknowledged (P. Minuchin, 1988; see also Crockenberg,
Lyons-Ruth, & Dickstein, 1993; Parke, 1988). Yet, the LTP paradigm is
the first systematic, detailed procedure for assessing threesome interactions available for clinicians as well as reserachers. It is part of a new
trend in research focusing on family-level variables in infancy, which
emphasizes in particular the coparenting alliance as distinct from the

marital alliance (Belsky, Rovine, & Fish, 1989; McHale & Rasmussen, 1998). Of note is that family-level variables, especially warmth and cooperation, account for child development outcomes distinct from those predicted by attachment variables. Not surprisingly, they concern in particular child sociability with peers. These results confirm the systems concept of dyadic and triadic levels making distinct contributions to family functioning (for reviews, see McHale & Cowan, 1997; McHale & Fivaz-Depeursinge, 1999).

As already emphasized, specifically targeting on interaction as a port of entry cannot but make sense when therapists are working with infants and young children in their families. Infants communicate via interaction and their parents respond in kind, even if they do also speak to each other in parallel. Likewise, young children enact as much as they speak. Thus having a family enact a task rather than only talk about it is plain common sense, making interaction the port of entry of choice when working with infants and older children in their families. But this by no means excludes taking into account the indissociable intersubjective side of the relationship, from the outset of infancy on.

The use of relatively standardized research procedures such as the LTP for assessing the interaction has several advantages, provided that they are sufficiently like real life (Crosswell & Fleischmann, 1993). They allow for systematic, detailed assessments. They may be repeated in later sessions, thus providing precise measures of change. However, the standardization of the task is less a concern than that the task be pertinent to the domain to be assessed. In our clinical experience, some young parents who have still unresolved issues around their own parents' authority perceive the LTP as an imposed procedure and resist it in more or less explicit ways. In these cases, it is often helpful to start with an unstructured session, and after the parents feel they have some control, to have them do the LTP.

Videotaping, as long as it is used for the clients' benefit too, is also essential. Video feedback provides the subjects with a double perspective on their functioning (Bateson, 1979): interaction as experienced in real time and later reexperienced from a distance. It is the same for the therapist: interaction as observed in real time and interaction as reviewed, often in slow motion so as to sharpen the observation. And last but not least, videotaping lends itself to research purposes. Thus it has become an integral part of many intervention methods (see McDonough, 1993, and Chapter 4, this volume; Hedenbro, 1997).

The ideal setting for this type of treatment is the typical family clinic laboratory with videotaping facilities and a one-way mirror. However, it is possible and sometimes desirable to video record interactions at home (Hedenbro, 1997) or even have the families video record themselves (Downing & Ziegenhain, 2001). With thorough knowledge of the observation situations, the experienced developmental systems therapist may work in real time. Yet, it is always more productive to take time between sessions to study the interactions and select pertinent sequences for video feedback.

The importance of detecting and working with strengths has been stressed by many authors (for a review, see Stern, 1995). Thanks to its hierarchical nature, the model of alliances as exemplified by the LTP provides a step-by-step procedure by which therapists can face the complexity of threesome relationships and precisely detect where there are resources and difficulties.

Yet, we should note that the alliance is a high-level construct; in particular, it does not differentiate between over- and underregulation (Anders, 1989) or between different styles of coparenting, such as symmetry versus complementarity. For instance, along a coordination axis from low to high coordination, one may obtain overregulation as a style at the upper end or as a problematic process at the lower end. Or, in collusive alliances, one may have two parents competing actively or competing covertly, or overengagement of one parent and underengagement of the other (see McHale & Fivaz-Depeursinge, 1999). These and other dimensions give key information for clinical purposes and thus must be added to the assessment of the family alliance.

We have operationalized for research and clinical purposes the model of alliances for trilogue play. But it applies as well to dyadic play interactions (Fivaz-Depeursinge, 1987). We are presently on the way to extending it to tetradic play in order to assess four-member family interactions—a realistic family context as soon as a second child is born, with the relationship between siblings coming to the fore (Dunn, 1983). There is again a step function between the triadic and the tetradic family interactions, engendering a new systemic level with distinct properties. In our experience, the model is readily applicable to free-play interactions, although with less precision. It awaits operationalization for other tasks. Finally, it is also possible to use it to assess children in other family constellations where caretaker roles are taken on by grandparents or other persons.

Likewise, the model has been applied to the working alliance between the consultant-therapist and the family, as well as to the working alliance within the team of professionals. In each of these groups, a preliminary but key issue is to determine whether each partner is included, keeps to his or her roles, focuses on the same goal, and stays in tune with the others (see Fivaz-Depeursinge & Corboz-Warnery, 1999; Keren et al., 2001).

We have stressed the therapeutic benefits that can take place within an assessment procedure, provided that care is taken to create a good enough "holding environment" (Winnicott, 1965) or "clinical relational matrix" (Hirschberg, 1993; see also Clark, Paulsen, & Conlin, 1993; Parker & Zuckerman, 1990). The systems model we have advanced has the advantage of formalizing the "effect of relationships on relationships" (Emde, 1988) in this particular domain. As mentioned above, the model explicitly defines the implicative influence of the developing party (the family) in relation to the contextual influence of the framing party (the therapist) within the working alliance. Thus, the direction of influences between them is defined as both hierarchical and circular in conformity with the principles of systems theory (see Fivaz-Depeursinge, 1991). Moreover, it enlightens the analogy between the framing–developing interactions in therapy and in family development. Finally, like other systems models, it is a metamodel and thus applies equally to the different methods of therapeutic interventions.

To return to the clinical domain, it is of note that the implicative influence of the child in respect to his or her parents is particularly strong in infancy. As stated by Hirschberg, "very little evokes as much intense emotion in most people as troubles with a baby" (1993, p. 176). This is similar to the implicative influence of the family with respect to the therapist: "Most parents want desperately to do well by their babies" (Selma Fraiberg, cited by Hirschberg, 1993, p. 177). This may be one of the grounds for the rapidity of therapeutic work in infancy and early childhood and thus legitimate the brevity of therapeutic assessment methods.

The LTP method was originally designed to deal with parental psychopathology. The primary aim was to free the baby from the effects of parental conflict (Lieberman & Pawl, 1993). It was extended to families with infants suffering functional problems, such as feeding, sleeping, and separation difficulties. As yet, it has not been extended to infants suffering psychopathology. Indeed, in our research up to this point, we have studied only firstborn, medically intact children. The systematic study of families with infants with difficult temperaments, special sensitivities, or more severe disabilities would greatly help to further highlight the implicative influence of the child on the family alliance. We assume that the LTP method would then readily apply to many different populations.

REFERENCES

Anders, T. (1989). Clinical syndromes, relationship disturbances and their assessment. In A. J. Sameroff & R. N. Emde (Eds.), *Relationship disturbances in early childhood* (pp. 125–144). New York: Basic Books.

Bakermans-Kranenburg, M., Juffer, F., & van IJzendoorn, M. (1998). Intervention with video feedback and attachment discussions: does type of maternal insecurity make a difference? *Infant Mental Health Journal, 19,* 202–219.

Bateson, G. (1979). *Mind and nature.* Toronto: Bantam Books.

Beebe, B., & Stern, D. N. (1977). Engagement–disengagement and early object experiences. In N. Freedman & S. Grand (Eds.), *Communicative structures and psychic structures: A psychoanalytic interpretation of communication.* New York: Plenum Press.

Belsky, J., Rovine, M., & Fish, M. (1989). The developing family system. In M. R. Gunnar & E. Thelen (Eds.), *Systems and development* (Vol. 22, pp. 110–165). Hillsdale, NJ: Erlbaum.

Boszormenyi-Nagy, I., & Sparks, G. (1973). *Invisible loyalties.* New York: Harper & Row.

Brazelton, T. B., Koslowsky, B., & Main, M. (1974). The origins of reciprocity: The early mother–infant interaction. In M. Lewis & L. Rosenblum (Eds.), *The origins of behavior: The effect of the infant on its caregiver* (Vol. 1, pp. 49–76). New York: Wiley.

Bruner, J. (1985). Vygotsky: A historical and conceptual perspective. In J. V. Wertsch (Ed.), *Culture, communication and cognition: Vygotskian perspectives* (pp. 21–34). New York: Cambridge University Press.

Clark, R., Paulsen, A., & Conlin, S. (1993). Assessment of developmental status and parent-infant relationships: The therapeutic process of evaluation. In C. H. Zeanah (Ed.), *Handbook of infant mental health* (pp. 191–209). New York: Guilford Press.

Crockenberg, S., Lyons-Ruth, K., & Dickstein, S. (1993). The family context of infant mental health: II. Infant development in multiple family relationships. In C. H. Zeanah (Ed.), *Handbook of infant mental health* (pp. 38–55). New York: Guilford Press.

Cronen, V. E., Kenneth, M. J., & Lannamann, J. W. (1982). Paradoxes, double binds, and reflexive loops: An alternative theoretical perspective. *Family Process, 21,* 91–112.

Crosswell, J., & Fleischmann, M. (1993). Use of structured research procedures in clinical assessments of infants. In C. H. Zeanah (Ed.), *Handbook of infant mental health* (pp. 210–221). New York: Guilford Press.

Downing, G., & Ziegenhain, U. (2001). Besonderheiten der Beratung und Therapie bei jugendlichen Müttern und ihren Säuglingen: Die Bedeutung von Bindungstheorie und videogestüztern Interventionen. In G. J. Suess, H. Scheuerer, & W.-K. P. Pfeifer (Eds.), *Bindungstheorie und*

Familiendynamik: Anwendung der Bindungstheorie in Beratung und Therapie (pp. 271–295). Giessen: Psychosozial.

Dunn, J. (1983). Sibling relationships in early childhood. *Child Development, 54,* 787–811.

Emde, R. N. (1988). The effects of relationships on relationships: A developmental approach to clinical intervention. In R. A. Hinde & J. Stevenson-Hinde (Eds.), *Relationships within families* (pp. 354–364). Oxford, UK: Clarendon Press.

Emde, R. N. (1989). The infant's relationship experience: developmental and affective aspects. In A. J. Sameroff & R. N. Emde (Eds.), *Clinical syndromes, relationship disturbances and their assessment* (pp. 33–51). New York: Basic Books.

Fivaz, E., Fivaz, R., & Kaufmann, L. (1981). Dysfunctional transactions and therapeutic functions: An evolutive model. *Journal of Marital and Family Therapy, 7,* 309–320.

Fivaz, E., Fivaz, R., & Kaufmann, L. (1982). Encadrement du développement, le point de vue systémique: Fonctions pédagogique, parentale, thérapeutique. *Cahiers Critiques de Thérapie Familiale et de Pratiques de Réseaux, 4–5,* 63–74.

Fivaz-Depeursinge, E. (1987). *Alliances et mésalliances dans le dialogue entre adulte et bébé: La communication précoce dans la famille.* Neuchâtel and Paris: Delachaux & Nestlé.

Fivaz-Depeursinge, E. (1991). Documenting a time-bound, circular view of hierarchies: A microanalysis of parent–infant dyadic interaction. *Family Process, 30*(1), 101–120.

Fivaz-Depeursinge, E., & Corboz-Warnery, A. (1999). *The primary triangle: A developmental systems view of fathers, mothers and infants.* New York: Basic Books.

Fivaz-Depeursinge, E., & Frascarolo, F. (1999). *Three-month-old infants share their attention and affects with both parents during triadic play.* Paper presented at the annual meeting of Society for Research in Child Development, Albuquerque, NM.

Fogel, A. (1977). Temporal organization in mother–infant face-to-face interaction. In H. R. Schaffer (Ed.), *Studies in mother–infant interactions* (pp. 119–152). London: Academic Press.

Gottman, J. (1994). *What predicts divorce?: The relationship between marital process and marital outcomes.* Hillsdale, NJ: Erlbaum.

Grasset, F., Fivaz-Depeursinge, E., & Rougemont, T. (1989). Thérapie familiale de longue durée et processus de développement. *Thérapie Familiale, 10,* 147–162.

Hedenbro, M. (1997). Interaction, the key to life: Seeing possibilities of children through videopictures. *Signal, 4*(2), 9–15.

Hinde, R. A., & Stevenson-Hinde, J. (Eds.). (1988). *Relationships within families.* Oxford, UK: Oxford Science.

Hirschberg, L. (1993). Clinical interviews with infants and their families. In C. H. Zeanah (Ed.), *Handbook of infant mental health* (pp. 173–190). New York: Guilford Press.

Imber-Black, E., & Roberts, J. (1992). *Rituals for our times.* Northvale, NJ: Aronson.

Keren, M., Fivaz-Depeursinge, E., & Tyano, S. (2001). Using the Lausanne family model in training: An Israeli experience. *Signal, 9*(3), 5–10.

Lieberman, A., & Pawl, J. (1993). Infant–parent psychotherapy In C. H. Zeanah (Ed.), *Handbook of infant mental health* (pp. 427–442) . New York: Guilford Press.

Lyons-Ruth, K., Bruschweiler-Stern, N., Harrison, A. M., Morgan, A. C., Nahum, J. P., Sander, L., et al. (1998). Implicit relational knowing: Its role in development and psychoanalytic treatment. *Infant Mental Health Journal, 19*(3), 282–289.

Malphurs, J., Field, T., Larraine, C., Pickens, J., Pelaez-Nogueras, M., Yando, R., & Bendell, D. (1996). Altering withdrawn and intrusive interaction behaviors of depressed mothers. *Infant Mental Health Journal, 17*(2), 152–160.

McDonald, K. (1992). Warmth as a developmental construct: An evolutionary analysis. *Child Development, 63,* 753–773.

McDonough, S. C. (1993). Interaction guidance: Understanding and treating early infant-caregiver relationship disorders. In C. H. Zeanah (Ed.), *Handbook of infant mental health* (pp. 414–426). New York: Guilford Press.

McHale, J., & Fivaz-Depeursinge, E. (1999). Understanding triadic and family group interactions during infancy and toddlerhood. *Clinical Child and Family Psychology Review, 2,* 107–127.

McHale, J., & Rasmussen, J. (1998). Co-parental and family group-level dynamics during infancy: Early family predictors of child and family functioning during preschool. *Development and Psychopathology, 10,* 39–58.

McHale, J. P., & Cowan, P. A. (Eds.). (1996). *Understanding how family-level dynamics affect children's development: Studies of two-parent families* (New Directions for Child and Adolescent Development, No. Vol. 74). San Francisco: Jossey–Bass.

Minuchin, P. (1988). Relationships within the family: A systems perspective on development. In R. A. Hinde & J. Stevenson-Hinde (Eds.), *Relationships within families: Mutual influences* (pp. 7–26). Oxford, UK: Clarendon Press.

Minuchin, S. (1974). *Families and family therapy.* Cambridge, MA: Harvard University Press.

Papousek, H., & Papousek, M. (1987). Intuitive parenting: A dialectic counterpart to the infant's integrative competence. In J. D. Osofsky (Ed.), *Handbook of infant development* (2nd ed., pp. 669–720). New York: Wiley.

Parke, R. D. (1988). Families in life-span perspective: A multilevel developmental approach. In E. M. Hetherington, R. M. Lerner, & M. Perlmutter

(Eds.), *Child development in life-span perspective* (pp. 159–190). Hillsdale, NJ: Erlbaum.

Parker, S., & Zuckerman, B. (1990). Therapeutic aspect of the assessment process. In S. J. Meisels & J. P. Shonkoff (Eds.), *Handbook of early child intervention* (pp. 350–369). New York: Cambridge University Press.

Reiss, D. (1989). The represented and practicing family: Contrasting visions of family continuity. In A. J. Sameroff & R. N. Emde (Eds.), *Relationship disturbances in early childhood* (pp. 191–220). New York: Basic Books.

Sameroff, A. J., & Emde, R. N. (Eds.). (1989). *Relationship disturbances in early childhood*. New York: Basic Books.

Sroufe, L. A. (1989). Relationships and relationship disturbances. In A. J. Sameroff & R. N. Emde (Eds.), *Relationship disturbances in early childhood* (pp. 97–124). New York: Basic Books.

Stern, D. N. (1985). *The interpersonal world of the infant*. New York: Basic Books.

Stern, D. N. (1995). *The motherhood constellation: A unified view of parent–infant psychotherapy*. New York: Basic Books.

Stern, D. N. (2000). Introduction to the paperback edition. *The interpersonal world of the infant* (pp. xi–xxxix). New York: Basic Books.

Tronick, E. Z., & Cohn, J. F. (1989). Infant–mother face-to-face interaction: Age and gender differences in coordination and the occurrence of miscoordination. *Child Development, 60,* 85–92.

Vogel, E. F., & Bell, N. W. (1960). The emotionally disturbed child as the family scapegoat. In N. W. Bell & E. F. Vogel (Eds.), *A modern introduction to the family* (pp. 382–397). New York: Free Press.

Vygotsky, L. (1979). *Mind in society: The development of higher psychological process*. Cambridge, MA: Harvard University Press.

Winnicott, D. W. (1965). The theory of the parent–infant relationship. In D. W. Winnicott (Ed.), *The maturational processes and the facilitating environment* (pp. 37–55). New York: International Universities Press.

Wynne, L. C., McDaniel, S. H., & Weber, T. T. (Eds.). (1986). *Systems consultation: A new perspective for family therapy*. New York: Guilford Press.

Wynne, L. S., Ryckoff, I. M., Day, J., & Hirsch, S. I. (1958). Pseudo-mutuality in the family relationships of schizophrenics. *Psychiatry, 21*(2), 205–220.

CHAPTER 7

A SENSORY PROCESSING APPROACH TO SUPPORTING INFANT–CAREGIVER RELATIONSHIPS

Winnie Dunn

There are many factors that we must consider when examining the characteristics of and influences on the infant–caregiver relationship. An emerging perspective involves examining the ways that the infants and caregivers respond to sensory experiences in their everyday lives—a sensory processing perspective. We receive information through our senses, and the nervous system interprets this input so we can respond. As the infant and caregiver begin to interact, the infant's responses to sensory experiences begin to affect the emotional reactions of the caregiver. Some mothers report on the sensations their unborn babies generate for them from the womb, for example, "I feel the baby pressing against my diaphragm," or "The baby seems to move when I lay down." These very early experiences provide the mother with information about the baby's responsiveness and can begin to generate early interpretations about how the baby will be after birth. Then, when the baby is born, the baby and caregivers accumulate additional information about each other, including how each responds to touch, sounds and light in the environment.

Sensory processing refers to the way that the nervous system receives, interprets and responds to sensory input. The way a person responds to sensory input is very personal, and develops based on both genetic and environmental variables. Both infants and parents in the same family have individualized responses to the same sensory events. For example, some family members may not notice noise in the background, whereas other family members become distracted or irritable by it, for example, music, TV, or others talking.

It is helpful to understand the infant and caregiver's sensory processing patterns as a means for interpreting both positive and challenging interactions. There is also some preliminary evidence linking a young child's patterns of sensory processing with specific temperament characteristics (Daniels & Dunn, 2003), suggesting that these early interactions are also informing the caregiver about the infant's emerging personality.

When caregivers understand both the meaning of the infant's behaviors and their own responses to the sensory aspects of everyday life, they can anticipate how to construct activities to make interactions and performance successful. As caregivers anticipate their own and their infant's sensory processing needs and limits, they experience success at constructing daily living rituals and begin to feel more competent, which generates more interest in interacting. Simultaneously, as infants experience just the right amounts of sensory input during activities, they can participate and interact more positively—they are not overwhelmed with too much stimulation nor lethargic from too little input. The relationship becomes generative because both partners are able to focus on the interaction and the activity, rather than on protection (from too much sensory input) or arousal (when too little sensory stimulation is available). By understanding the possible patterns of sensory processing, including what triggers particular responses, caregivers can increase their feelings of competence and satisfaction and infants can get their basic needs met. Therefore, knowledge about sensory processing increases insights that can enhance the infant–caregiver relationship.

If an infant is very sensitive to sounds, movement, and touch experiences, for example, the infant is likely to become fussy during a family gathering with lots of talking and passing the baby around to take turns holding her. In this situation, Mom might have difficulty calming the baby. Although the baby's irritability is due to being overwhelmed from all the sounds and touch experiences, Mom might interpret the baby's responses as rejecting her attempts to calm the infant. This feeling of being rejected can contribute to a sense of incompetence and interfere with the Mom and baby's bonding. On the other hand, if mom understood the baby's sensory sensitivity to touch and sounds, she could begin to anticipate her baby's needs. For the family gathering, the mother might be sure to gravitate toward a quieter part of the house and limit the number of people holding the baby, preferring to hold the baby herself in a way that others could see. They could then interact with the baby without all the jostling that goes with passing a baby around. Sensory processing knowledge can be a powerful tool in supporting strong infant–caregiver relationships.

A MODEL FOR A SENSORY PROCESSING APPROACH

Dunn (1997) introduced a model for sensory processing that can be used to inform caregivers about their infants' sensory processing patterns and can also assist the caregivers in understanding their own sensory processing needs. Using this model, we can begin to interpret behaviors and make adjustments that are supportive of the infant's and caregiver's needs in their emerging relationship. We have studied sensory processing patterns across the lifespan and these same patterns occur in infants and adults. Therefore, as we discuss the impact of this model on the infant–caregiver relationship, it is important to consider both the infant's and the caregiver's patterns of sensory processing. Both partners in this relationship must get their sensory processing needs met for a successful outcome. Figure 7.1 summarizes this model using two dimensions.

The vertical continuum on the model represents the *neurological threshold*. Within the nervous system, there is a balance between excitation and inhibition; these inputs combine to determine whether there is

	SELF-REGULATION STRATEGY CONTINUUM	
NEUROLOGICAL THRESHOLD CONTINUUM	PASSIVE Act in accordance with thresholds	ACTIVE Act to counteract thresholds
High neurological thresholds (habituation)	LOW REGISTRATION	SENSATION SEEKING
Low neurological thresholds (sensitization)	SENSORY SENSITIVITY	SENSATION AVOIDING

FIGURE 7.1. Dunn's conceptual model of sensory processing. From Dunn (1997). Copyright 1997 by Lippincott Williams & Wilkins. Reprinted by permission.

enough excitation to fire the neurons, sending a message to the brain. There is a continuum of responding, with "sensitization" at one end of the continuum representing low threshold activation, or responding more often to stimuli. At the other end of the continuum is "habituation," representing high thresholds or less responding to stimuli. At both extremes, thresholds can interfere with daily life. With too much sensitization the person might be overly distracted by stimuli, whereas with too much habituation the person might not notice important stimuli.

The horizontal continuum on the model represents the person's responding, or *self-regulation strategies*. At one end of this continuum persons have a more "passive" responding strategy. This means that the person allows sensory events of daily life to occur without interference. At the other end of this continuum is an "active" responding strategy. This means that the person engages in particular behaviors to manage or regulate the input. As with the neurological threshold continuum, extremes of the response continuum can also interfere with daily life. When a person is too passive, stimuli can be overwhelming, and when a person is too active, the approach or avoidance behaviors can become the focus rather than the developing relationship.

When these two continua intersect,four quadrants emerge to reflect the possible combinations of thresholds and self-regulation strategies: *Low registration* reflects high neurological thresholds and a passive self-regulation strategy. (2) *Sensation seeking* reflects a high neurological threshold with an active self-regulation strategy. (3) *Sensory sensitivity* reflects a low neurological threshold with a passive self-regulation strategy. (4) *Sensation avoiding* reflects a low neurological threshold with an active self-regulation strategy.

Impact of Infant Patterns of Sensory Processing on the Relationship: The Quadrant Model

Low Registration

When persons have low registration, they miss a lot of stimuli that others notice readily. Typical sensory events may not be strong enough for these persons to notice what is going on. They may appear oblivious, dull, have a flat affect, or may seem self-absorbed. Because people with low registration tend not to notice stimuli, they have a high capacity for sticking with a task in a busy environment because they are not as easily distracted as others might be. Table 7.1 contains examples of common observations that can indicate challenges with sensory registration.

TABLE 7.1. Common Observations of Infants and Toddlers That Suggest Challenges with Each Pattern of Sensory Processing from Dunn's Model

Low Registration

- Takes a long time to focus on your face.
- Needs more support for sitting than others.
- Seems oblivious to activity in groups such as family gatherings or trips in the community.
- Doesn't notice when touched on arm or back.
- Doesn't notice clothing twisted on body.
- Doesn't react to drool or food on face.
- Doesn't notice people coming in the room.

Sensation Seeking

- Mouths objects more than other children.
- Chews on nonfood objects.
- Craves movement and roughhousing.
- Frequently asks you to look at things noticed in environment.
- Plays well even with lots of background noise.
- Bangs toys more than other children do.
- Makes noise for its own sake.
- Rocks when sitting.

Sensory Sensitivity

- Fusses during hair washing.
- Easily distracted from activities.
- Notices toilet flushing down the hall.
- Pulls at clothing throughout the day.
- Stops eating when someone moves or talks.
- Cries when hands get messy.
- Gets agitated with vacuum cleaner noise.
- Is a picky eater.
- Easily gets cranky with the caregiver when running errands.
- Struggles to settle down for rest.
- Indicates strong preferences for being held a certain way.

Sensation Avoiding

- Only tolerates a narrow range of clothing choices.
- Will only eat a few foods prepared in a specific way (e.g., a certain temperature).
- Pushes washcloth away during bath time.
- Pulls hats off and becomes angry when the caregiver is putting them on.
- Gags easily.
- Refuses messy activities.
- Hates roughhousing.
- Holds body in stiff positions.
- Covers eyes/ears in busy environments.

Note. Copyright by Winnie Dunn. Reprinted by permission.

As with all the patterns of sensory processing, there are helpful and challenging influences on the infant–caregiver relationship. When infants have low registration, they seem very calm and you might observe that they are passive. They may not respond to voices or movement as quickly as other babies and therefore might be harder to arouse after sleep. Because babies with low registration notice less, they are also easygoing and therefore are easier to include in busy family and community environments. This baby is easy to have around; indeed, he or she is so inactive that busy caregivers might well interpret this baby's behaviors as adaptive and calm. On the other hand, this baby is likely to respond slowly to interaction attempts and therefore may not provide the caregiver with enough feedback to encourage the parent to continue the interactions. In this case, caregivers might think the baby doesn't like them and bonding might be difficult. This can then lead to a feeling of incompetence in caregiving, which can erode the relationship.

Sensation Seeking

Persons who are sensory seekers enjoy sensory stimuli. Even though they have high thresholds like persons with low registration these persons want to have sensory experiences, and so find ways to get extra sensory stimuli throughout the day. Babies might babble, wiggle around, rub on clothing or blankets, and respond enthusiastically to roughhousing. A key feature is their pleasure with sensation, so they are likely to demonstrate creativity in generating ideas about alternative methods for engaging with the environment. Table 7.1 contains examples of common observations that can indicate challenges with sensation seeking.

When babies are sensation seekers, they are likely to be very active and engaging both by themselves and with their caregivers. These babies will entertain themselves, for example, by playing in their cribs and finding alternative things to do with their toys and their food. As they become more mobile, these babies will get interested in things both in and out of reach, and they may even get into danger by focusing on the interesting new object rather than on a safe path to get to the object.

So again there are both helpful and challenging aspects of the caregiving relationship when babies are sensation seekers. Because these babies are so active, caregivers might interpret all this seeking behavior as a sign of creativity and intelligence. Caregivers who are also sensation seekers will likely delight in having a sensation-seeking partner to experience the world with. However, sensation-seeking babies also need more supervision, since they are interested in many things. This may be frustrating for caregivers and may be interpreted as deliberate attempts to be defiant or difficult. When caregivers themselves are more sensitive to stimuli (see below), babies with sensation-seeking tendencies might be more challenging and overwhelming, causing the caregiver to withdraw or feel resentful about all the time and attention required to meet the baby's needs.

Sensory Sensitivity

When persons have sensory sensitivity, they have low neurological thresholds and a passive self regulation strategy. People with such sensitivity notice many more stimuli than do others. They hear faint sounds in another room, notice when someone is rustling papers, get distracted by cluttered spaces, or get fussy about the texture of clothing. Because they are so vigilant, persons with sensory sensitivity are typically very good at keeping track of details and notice smaller changes in people and the environment.

Babies who have sensory sensitivity will react to many things in everyday life. They will be light sleepers, will turn to look at sounds and movements around them, may only settle into one or two outfits, and are likely to make a rough transition to eating pureed and solid foods. Table 7.1 contains examples of common observations that can indicate challenges with sensory sensitivity. Babies with such sensitivity are also likely to notice very small mood changes in caregivers, probably because the caregivers handle and interact with the baby a little bit differently when they are in different moods. Caregivers will quickly begin to catalog their baby's likes and dislikes, which is easy to do, since these babies will react to even small differences. For some caregivers, beginning to know the baby's tolerances and intolerances will make them feel competent to meet the baby's needs. For other caregivers, the baby's high rate of noticing even small changes will seem overwhelming and lead to a sense of hopelessness to meet the baby's needs.

Sensation Avoiding

When persons are sensation avoiders, they have low neurological thresholds and an active self-regulation strategy. They notice stimuli similarly to persons who have sensory sensitivity, that is, low thresholds for noticing, but the stimuli are so uncomfortable for persons who are sensation avoiders that they construct strategies to keep from encountering new, unfamiliar stimuli. Therefore, rituals are quite important for sensation avoiders, most likely because rituals create recognizable patterns of sensory input that reduce the possibility of encountering other stimuli that are less familiar. It is important to recognize that this rigidity in following rituals and patterns is an adaptive strategy for regulating sensation avoiders' own input. Figure 7.1 contains examples of common observations that can indicate challenges with sensation avoiding.

Babies who have sensation-avoiding patterns will also notice a lot of things about their clothing, food, and environment, just like babies with sensory sensitivity. These babies, however, are more likely to withdraw from activities to cope with the overwhelmed feeling that all the sensory input generates. So this baby might be more quiet, but it will be from withdrawing from sensations, rather than from lack of noticing sensory stimuli as with babies who have low registration. Sensory-avoiding babies will be more tense and rigid even in their quietness, suggesting some anxiety about activities and surroundings. These babies will respond more positively to strict routines, and so caregivers are more likely to fall into exacting schedules and patterns to try to keep the baby content. As with babies who have sensory sensitivity, some caregivers will feel competent and successful at meeting this exacting schedule whereas other will feel overwhelmed at trying to meet the baby's needs.

The Impact of Caregiver Patterns of Sensory Processing on the Relationship

Low Registration

When a caregiver has low registration, the caregiver may not notice cues from the baby as quickly as do others. Small cues, like a little fussiness, may occur without this caregiver's awareness. Being slower to notice and respond can be helpful in the sense that it may encourage the baby to develop adaptive strategies, but it can also increase the baby's distress signals to get the caregiver's attention. Caregivers with a low registration pattern of sensory processing can set up reminders for themselves, like an alarm watch to provide cues to interact with the baby periodically as a strategy for checking on the baby's status on a regular basis.

Sensation Seeking

When a caregiver has a sensation-seeking pattern of sensory processing, the caregiver will be interested in interacting a lot with the baby. This caregiver will talk with the baby, offer toys, sing, carry the baby, and will want to engage with the baby throughout the day. For babies with low registration and sensation seeking, these repeated interactions will provide the high level of sensory input the baby needs to remain engaged in the relationship. The active engagement of a sensation-seeking caregiver may be overwhelming for babies that have sensory sensitivity and sensation-avoiding patterns because these babies can reach their limit of sensory input very quickly. In these cases, it is important for the caregiver to recognize that fussiness (sensitivity) or withdrawal (avoiding) are not indications of disliking the caregiver, but rather are behaviors that indicate the baby has had enough for that moment in time. The active self-regulation strategy of sensation seeking will enable this caregiver to notice the baby's responses and adjust interaction strategies to meet the baby's needs without providing too much input.

Sensory Sensitivity

When caregivers have sensory sensitivity, they will be very vigilant about noticing the baby's condition at all times. These caregivers will be attentive to even small changes in the baby's status and may appear overly concerned from other people's point of view. This heightened attentiveness provides a protection for the baby in the sense that potential difficulties will be noticed very quickly, for example, a few bumps developing into a rash, or small body temperature changes, and then can be acted upon. These caregivers give their babies lots of attention, but it can take the form of anxiety and concern, which can interfere with the developing relationship between the caregiver and the baby. The caregiver with sensory sensitivity may need to check with others to gauge the level of action that needs to be taken when noticing small changes to guard against overreacting.

Sensation Avoiding

With a sensation avoiding pattern of sensory processing, caregivers may be more cautious about interacting with their babies. These caregivers are likely to prefer following routines for caregiving, using these rituals as a structure for interacting with the baby because the baby's responses may be more predictable and therefore manageable within the rituals. Babies with sensitivity and avoiding patterns will respond positively to such routines because the predictable patterns lessen the baby's need to confront new and unfamiliar sensory stimuli. Babies who have sensation-seeking patterns may be more challenging to the relationship because the caregiver may feel overwhelmed more easily and the baby won't get input needs met. The caregiver can participate in the routines of care, while including other care providers in less structured interaction time to meet the baby's needs and keep the caregiver from feeling overwhelmed. This caregiver will be able to establish pleasant routines with babies who have low registration, since these babies are more easygoing. It is important to remember that babies with low registration will need additional sensory input, so including other care providers or creating other situations may be helpful, for example, mother's day out.

EVIDENCE REGARDING
THE SENSORY PROCESSING MODEL

Dunn and colleagues (Brown, Cromwell, Filion, Dunn, & Tollefson, 2002; Brown, Tollefson, Dunn, Cromwell, & Filion, 2001; Daniels & Dunn, 2002; Dunn, 1997, 1999; Dunn & Brown, 1997; Dunn & Daniels, 2002; Dunn & Westman, 1997; Ermer & Dunn, 1998; Kientz & Dunn, 1997) have studied infants, toddlers, children, adolescents, and adults with and without disabilities. Factor analytic studies have provided evidence that the quadrants in this model are reflected in the factor structures in each age group. Comparison studies also indicate that persons with various disabilities, including autism, attention-deficit/hyperactivity disorder (ADHD), schizophrenia, and Asperger syndrome have distinctly different patterns of sensory processing when compared to their peers. The details of the studies are reported elsewhere. Below we review overall findings from the infant and toddler data.

Overall Developmental Features of Sensory Processing in Infants and Toddlers

For the low threshold quadrants described above (sensation avoiding and sensory sensitivity), the average performance remains at the same level across the 7- to 36-month age range. Dunn (2002) hypothesizes that the constancy of these scores reflects the nervous system's vigilance for keeping track of what is going on around the infant or toddler.

In regard to sensation seeking, younger infants notice more stimuli than do older infants and toddlers. There is a steady change across the birth to 36-month period, with responses being more frequent when the babies are younger and becoming less frequent as the babies get older. Dunn (2002) hypothesizes that the myriad of stimuli available outside the womb engenders high attention at first and then the baby begins to habituate to certain stimuli as he or she becomes more familiar with the patterns of sensory events in everyday life. Dunn also hypothesizes that the continuous shift in the sensation-seeking pattern reflects the baby's way of gathering information about the world outside the womb. After the child learns about the world, it becomes less necessary for him or her to respond at such a high rate.

Oral sensory processing and touch processing follow a similar developmental pattern across the birth to 36-month time period. Infants are more likely to display sensitivity to oral and touch stimuli, whereas toddlers respond less frequently to oral and touch sensory events.

Sensory Processing Features in Infants and Toddlers Who Have Disabilities

Some disability groups display significantly different patterns of sensory processing when compared to their peers without disabilities (Dunn, 2002). Children who have pervasive developmental disorders (including autism) and general developmental delays have difficulty with most areas of sensory processing when compared to peers without disabilities. Infants with reflux are significantly more sensitive when compared to infants without reflux. Preliminary evidence with children who have Down syndrome and language delays suggests that sensory processing may not be a central factor affecting their performance.

Evidence of Sensory Processing Difficulties and an Approach to Intervention

A number of authors have suggested that behaviors indicating difficulty with sensory processing are related to other developmental and behavioral problems. When caregivers come to understand the sensory processing features of these problems, they can increase their feelings of competence as they begin to have successes meeting the infants' needs. DeGangi (2000) reports on the relationship between behaviors indicative of poor sensory processing, on the one hand, and poor self-regulation, sleep disturbances, feeding difficulties, and inattention, on the other. DeGangi and Breinbauer (1997) report on the effect of hypersensitivities to touch on other developmental activities such as dressing, face washing and sitting in a car seat. For example, children 1–2 years of age with touch sensitivities are likely to have strict clothing preferences, making dressing a difficult task to master. Dunn (2002) found that infants with reflux were more likely to have sensitivities to sensory input than did their peers and hypothesizes that this might make feeding more challenging. Young children with pervasive developmental disorders, including autism, exhibit differences in their patterns of sensory processing from those of their peers without disabilities (Dunn, 2002). Although children with pervasive developmental disorders had differences in many areas of sensory processing, Ermer and Dunn (1998) identified oral sensory processing as the most distinctive feature of children with autism in a discriminant analysis comparing children with autism, those with ADHD, and those without disabilities.

There is some evidence that sensory processing approaches to intervention can be effective. Ayres and Tickle (1980) studied children with autism and found that who children who had normal responsiveness or hyperresponsiveness to sensory input responded more positively to sensory integrative interventions than those children who were underresponsive to sensory input. Other authors have reported that use of deep-pressure input is effective in reducing anxiety and arousal in persons with autism (Inamura, Wiss, & Parham, 1990a, 1990b; Creedon, 1994; Edelson, Edelson, Kerr, & Grandin, 1999; Morreau, 2000). Researchers have also studied the effects of sensory-based intervention programs on persons who have mental retardation. For example, Clark, Miller, Thomas, Kucherway, and Azin (1978) report increases in eye contact, vocalization, and postural adaptation after intervention. Younger and more involved children who have learning disabilities make significant gains in academic and motor outcomes when they receive occupational therapy using a sensory processing or a perceptual motor approach (Law, Polatajko, Schaffer, Miller, & Macnab, 1991). Kientz (1996) reports on two case studies in which a sensory processing approach of creating a sensory diet for children can be effective in helping the child develop strategies for modulating performance throughout the day. Case-Smith and Bryan (1999) studied five preschoolers, and found that a sensory-based intervention program significantly reduced nonegagement behaviors in four of five children and increased mastery play in three of five children, but peer and adult interactions did not improve during the 3 months of the study.

There continues to be a need for studies regarding the effectiveness of sensory processing approaches to intervention. There is a particular need to find ways to apply such interventions to the caregiver–infant relationship as they each experience everyday life. Currently we can only state that sensory processing challenges coexist with various disorders and difficulties with daily life function and that there is preliminary evidence to guide us regarding the way sensory processing concepts might be applied in practice.

PROVIDING SERVICES USING
A SENSORY PROCESSING APPROACH

There are many considerations that must be made in selecting any service provision approach. Professionals must understand the concepts underlying each approach so that they can make appropriate assessment choices and construct interpretations that are consistent with the approach. Interdisciplinary experts must understand who might have particular expertise so that they can harness the appropriate professional resources on a family's behalf. Those who have a particular expertise must know how to construct interventions that reflect particular approaches and how to evaluate the effectiveness of the interventions as they are occurring. Team members must also be familiar with the impact of particular approaches on the family relationships that will be needed to sustain the positive outcomes of the intervention.

A sensory processing approach is very compatible with a comprehensive service program. Sensory processing knowledge provides a framework for understanding behaviors that can augment and broaden other perspectives, thus increasing the possibilities for designing successful interventions.

ASSESSMENT OF SENSORY PROCESSING FACTORS

Target Behaviors

The most important factor to be considered when therapists are serving babies and caregivers is the impact of particular problems on the quality of interactions and life activities. Difficulties that interfere with daily life interactions can also erode the evolving relationship between the caregiver and the baby. Since sensory processing is inherent in every interaction, for example, bonding, comforting, feeding, bathing, dressing, diaper changing, sleeping, and playing, it is important to consider the contribution or interference of sensory processing patterns within all daily life interactions. It is impossible to interpret a baby's sensory processing as helpful or interfering in isolation; one must make an interpretation about the baby's and caregiver's interactions within the daily life activity to determine whether a sensory processing approach will be helpful.

Methods of Assessing Sensory Processing

Using tests, interviews, skilled observations, and questionnaires, therapists identify the caregiver's and the baby's sensory processing features (e.g., what do they like, notice, miss, become irritated by, and withdraw from), and inquire about the activities that are successful and challenging for the family. With information about the baby and caregiver and their activities, therapists consider what factors would support or create barriers to their evolving relationship and the activities of interest in their everyday lives.

Example of Sensory Processing Assessment

Karmie does not generally notice stimuli as readily as other children do. Her parents reported that Karmie has had no trouble sleeping, even in new or busy environments. However, her parents reported that her eating and playing have been frustrating times for them. Karmie wasn't responsive to their efforts to play with her and would lose interest in eating before having enough food. Lately, Dad reported that he began being more animated and physical with Karmie and that this improved her ability to respond to him. Mom wasn't having the same positive experience; she was introducing more quiet play, such as sitting and babbling and looking at books. From a sensory processing perspective, it is likely that Karmie has low registration and therefore will need additional sensory input within activities in order to interact with her parents and build their relationship. Based on this assessment, the therapist might place emphasis on the positive features of Dad's strategies, for example, adding visual, auditory, and movement characteristics to his play, to ensure that the parents have insight about the reason increasing intensity is a great choice for Karmie. Then the therapist might schedule a time to observe the family during mealtime and play, with the aim of offering some suggestions as to how to increase the intensity of stimuli during Mom's chosen activities with the baby and during mealtime.

There are also formal assessments available for documenting sensory processing patterns. DeGangi and Greenspan (1989) have provided the *Test of Sensory Functions in Infants* (TSFI), a professionally administered assessment of 4- to 18-month-old infants' responses to basic sensory input. This 24-item scale tests the infant's responses to tactile deep pressure, visual tactile integration, adaptive motor responses, oculomotor control, and vestibular stimulation. Studies have shown that the TSFI identifies sensory processing difficulties in infants with regulatory disorders and prematurity when comparing them to their peers without any diagnoses.

Questionnaires also provide a structure for eliciting sensory processing information from the family. Interdisciplinary team members may use these questionnaires in their battery of tests as a way of incorporating this perspective into their considerations. When sensory processing seems to be a challenge, the team can call upon an occupational therapist or other professional with expertise in employing a sensory processing perspective to include these ideas into intervention planning. The two questionnaires available for infants are the *Infant–Toddler*

Symptom Checklist (DeGangi, Poisson, Sickel, & Wiener, 1995) and the *Infant/Toddler Sensory Profile* (Dunn, 2002). For caregivers, the *Adolescent/Adult Sensory Profile* (Brown & Dunn, 2002) is also available.

The *Infant–Toddler Symptom Checklist* (DeGangi et al., 1995) is a screening checklist for 7- to 30-month-old children. The tool is designed to assist professionals in identifying young children who are at risk for regulatory, behavioral, sensory processing, and attentional difficulties as they grow. There is a general screening form containing 21 questions and 5 additional age-specific forms (7–9 months, 10–12 months, 13–18 months, 19–24 months and 25–30 months) that contain from 17 to 31 items each. The caregiver completes the selected form by recording how frequently the child engages in each behavior. Those children whose scores fall at or above a specified cutoff point are considered at risk, indicating further need for assessment.

The *Infant/Toddler Sensory Profile* (Dunn, 2002) is also a caregiver questionnaire. There are two forms, one for infants from birth to 6 months of age containing 36 items, the other for infants and toddlers 7–36 months of age containing 48 items. The questionnaires are organized by sensory system (i.e., auditory, visual, vestibular, tactile, oral, and general) and provides a method for calculating scores in the four quadrants from Dunn's model of sensory processing (i.e., sensation seeking, sensation avoiding, sensory sensitivity, and low registration). The caregiver completes the questionnaire by recording how frequently the child engages in each behavior (i.e., "almost never," "seldom," "occasionally," "frequently," or "almost always"). There are cut scores indicating when children are responding like age peers and when their responses are different from peers. For the youngest infants (from birth to 6 months old) cut scores indicate the need for consultation and follow-up, whereas at the older ages (7–36 months old) cut scores indicate how different the child's score is from the national sample of peers.

Sometimes it is also useful for caregivers to understand their own sensory processing patterns. The *Adolescent/Adult Sensory Profile* (Brown & Dunn, 2002) is a self-administered questionnaire containing 60 items that indicate the person's responses to sensory events in everyday life. One obtains quadrant scores for this measure as well, with indications of whether the person responds like others or more or less than others on the quadrants (sensation seeking, sensation avoiding, sensory sensitivity, or low registration). The manual provides guidance about how to make adjustments to one's daily routines to better support one's sensory processing needs.

PROVIDING INTERVENTION USING
A SENSORY PROCESSING APPROACH

The primary focus of intervention using a sensory processing perspective is creating the best match between the person's sensory processing needs and the activities and environments of interest in the person's life. We do this by providing insights as to the meaning of behaviors from a sensory processing perspective, so that families can understand the reason for selecting particular strategies along the way.

General Considerations in Implementing a Sensory Processing Approach

There are several general considerations when professionals are implementing any specialized approach to intervention. First, they must consider what expertise is needed either directly or in consultation to implement the approach effectively. Secondly, they must understand the optimal setting for implementation; sometimes approaches are harder to implement in alternative settings. Thirdly, it is helpful to know what the typical duration and pattern of services would be when one is using a particular approach. This enables the professional to gauge the appropriate selection and use of an approach with a particular family. For example, it is inappropriate to select an approach that typically requires an intensive intervention paradigm in a brief therapy environment. Dunn (1999, 2000, 2001) provides details for implementing such a sensory processing approach and includes case examples illustrating the impact on children and families.

Professional Expertise for Implementing a Sensory Processing Approach

Since sensory processing patterns are a central feature of every human experience, sensory processing knowledge can be at the root of relationship challenges. As indicated from the research completed thus far, all human experiences are rooted in sensory-based information and the same patterns of sensory processing exist across the lifespan. Therefore all professionals can enhance their ability to address relationships with infants and caregivers by understanding basic patterns of sensory processing, how people respond with each pattern, and what challenges people with each pattern have in their everyday lives.

Considering the sensory processing aspect of the relationship enables professionals to offer concrete suggestions as to the meaning of particular behaviors and possible changes that will quickly improve the baby and caregiver's ability to respond positively to each other. When caregivers are able to interpret the baby's behaviors and respond in a way that meets the baby's needs, caregivers feel more competent and receive more positive responsiveness from the baby. When caregivers understand their own sensory processing patterns, they can construct times with the baby that are mindful of their own needs as well, thus promoting positive relationship building.

Tables 7.2–7.5 provide examples of suggestions that support babies with different patterns of sensory processing during everyday life. In using these tables there are general concepts to remember for activities in each of the four quadrants. Different intervention strategies are appropriate for each of the four patterns, as follows:

1. *Low registration.* Children with this pattern can *profit from more intensity* in sensory experiences during daily life. With more intensity of sensory input, these children can continue to pay attention during daily life activities and therefore can stick with them for a longer time.

2. *Sensation seeking.* Children with this pattern can *profit from more opportunities* in sensory experiences as part of daily life, so they don't have to stop engaging in daily life activities to get the extra sensory input they desire. With more intensity of sensory input, these children can continue to pay attention during daily life activities and therefore can stick with them for a longer time.

3. *Sensory sensitivity.* Children with this pattern can profit from *more structured patterns of sensory experiences* during daily life. With more structure of sensory input, these children can continue to pay attention during daily life activities and therefore can stick with them for a longer time.

4. *Sensory avoiding.* Children with this pattern will be better able to participate in everyday life when there is *less sensory input available* in the environment. When the environment is "quiet," these children can continue daily life activities for a longer time.

Sometimes the relationship challenge is affected by sensory processing, and then suggestions such as those included in Tables 7.2 to 7.5 are insufficient to meet the baby's and caregivers needs; in these cases,

TABLE 7.2. Strategies for Supporting Babies Who Have Low Registration

Low Registration	Bathing	Dressing	General Concept: Profiting from More Intensity				
			Mealtime	Playing	Waking	Outings
Touch	Use rough and varied textures for wash cloths and towels. Use soaps with textures imbedded in them. Incorporate sprayer into bath to vary water texture.	Rub lotion on before dressing. Select highly textured socks, shirts.	Provide variety and texture in food options. Serve varied temperatures in food options.	Add texture to handles and other toy surfaces. Have child play on different surfaces (e.g., linoleum, carpet).	Move hands along the child's body while waking.	Bring textured toys along. Be sure the child is wearing textured socks, underwear.
Movement	Place bath objects and toys out of easy reach.	Place items in distant spaces so child moves around while dressing.	Have child carry utensils/items to table.	Place favorite toys in harder-to-get places.	Jostle child; pick up to vertical position.	Be extra aware of safety measures when the child is moving about (may not notice objects, stairs, changes in terrain).

(continued)

TABLE 7.2. *(continued)*

Low Registration	Bathing	Dressing	Mealtime	Playing	Waking	Outings
Visual	Incorporate soap crayons into the bath regime.	Select bright clothing.	Use contrasting plate so food shows up.	Place mirrors at floor level. Select brightly colored and contrasting toys. Add colored tape to edges of stairs.	Turn on bright lights.	Point out things you pass by. Have child look for things as you go.
Auditory	Provide lively music background. Sing during bath.	Talk about what the child/you are doing as you do it. Play the radio.	Provide lively music background.	Provide toys that make sounds while playing with them. Play TV in background.	Turn on the radio. Talk a lot, varying voice intonation.	Talk to the child. Point out sounds you hear.
Taste/smell	Use scented bath products.	Use scented lotions.	Add new aromas, tastes to foods.	Clean toys with scented cleaners.	Use spritzer scents on shoulder before picking up.	Use scented lotions on hands.
Body position	Encourage propping in tub.	Practice a routine a lot. Change the pattern each day.	Have child stand up to eat.	Select heavier objects for playing.	Vary body position frequently.	Change the child's body position frequently.

Note. Copyright by Winnie Dunn. Reprinted by permission.

TABLE 7.3. Strategies for Supporting Babies Who Have Sensation Seeking

			General Concept: Profiting from More Opportunities			
Sensation seeking	Bathing	Dressing	Mealtime	Playing	Bedtime	Outings
Touch	Provide several textures of wash cloths and let child pick one. Use exfoliating soaps. Incorporate sprayer into bath to vary water texture.	Select highly textured socks, shirts. Add accessories, such as headbands, wristbands, belts. Use body refresher spray before dressing.	Include multiple foods in one meal. Provide variety of texture and temperature in food options.	Add textures to finger paint. Add texture to toy surfaces. Encourage barefoot play on a variety of surfaces.	Create a massage ritual. Have child wear tight-fitting undergarments. Provide textured blankets/sheets of child's choice.	Bring textured toys along. Be sure the child is wearing textured socks, underwear.
Movement	Place bath objects and toys out of easy reach.	Find longer routes to clothing (e.g., put items in different places to increase opportunities for moving while dressing).	Have child help with setting the table.	Roughhouse. Place favorite toys in harder-to-get places to increase climbing crawling etc. Get a mini trampoline. Put toys away one at a time in a distant toy box.	Incorporate a rocking or swaying sequence into bedtime routine.	Select errands that require moving about (e.g., walking in aisles).
Visual	Incorporate soap crayons into the bath regime. Sort toys by color.	Select bright clothing. Put posters/other pictures up at child's eye level.	Use contrasting plate so food shows up. Provide variety of colors in one meal	Place mirrors at floor level. Select brightly colored and contrasting toys.	Leave a night-light on in the room.	Point out things as you pass by. Have child look for things as you go.

(continued)

171

TABLE 7.3. (continued)

Sensation seeking	Bathing	Dressing	Mealtime	Playing	Bedtime	Outings
Visual (cont.)		Provide extra/colored lighting in play areas.	(e.g., berries in oatmeal).			
Auditory	Provide lively music background. Sing during bath.	Talk about what the child/you are doing as you do it. Hum/sing to child, make up songs. Open windows to enable ambient sound to enter.	Provide lively music background.	Provide toys that make sounds while playing with them. Play TV in background.	Play background radio. Create bedtime voices for talking.	Talk to the child about what you see, hear, smell; ask what he or she is noticing. Get a Walkman for the child.
Taste/smell	Use scented bath products.	Use scented lotions and detergents.	Add new aromas, tastes to foods. Ask child to guess what food is by smell.	Use aroma devices in the house. Clean toys with scented cleaners.	Use a "sleep" scent on pillow.	Have scented lotions available for child to use.
Body position	Have child sit on heels or prop on knees.	Practice a routine a lot. Change the pattern each day.	Have child stand up to eat.	Select heavier objects for playing. Dance with and without music. Paint one wall with chalkboard paint.	Vary child's body position frequently.	Change child's body position frequently. Garden/dig in the dirt/sand.

Note. Copyright by Winnie Dunn. Reprinted by permission.

172

TABLE 7.4. Strategies for Supporting Babies with Sensory Sensitivity

Sensory sensitivity	Bathing	Dressing	Mealtime	Playing	Bedtime	Outings
		General Concept: Providing More Structured Patterns of Sensory Experiences				
Touch	Identify a favorite sponge/fabric for washing. Press firmly on the child's skin with whole hand. Place a mat in the bottom of the tub that is covered in a preferred texture.	Select tight clothing. Identify undergarments that are firm, without "tight" spots (e.g., elastic). Use natural fibers for clothing.	Identify favorite food flavors, textures, and temperatures and stick with them. When the child likes/dislikes a texture, name it for him or her, then continue to use these words.	Provide a buffer space for child to play without getting bumped easily. Identify preferred surface textures.	Firmly wrap the child. Use heavy blankets. Have child wear clothing that provides even pressure on skin and gives during movement. Remove blowing vents/fans from child's location.	Use firm pressure on skin to calm. Have child wear firm fitting clothing. Wrap your body around child to hold in public.
Movement	Pick one position for bathing and stick with it. Minimize bending and reaching during bath.	Place clothing at chest level in drawers/shelves. Select one position for dressing (sit, lay).	Create a seating arrangement to reduce amount of movement disruptions during meal.	Honor sedentary play. Create predictable patterns for movement play.	Use repetitive movements for calming (e.g., rocking, bouncing slowly, swaying).	Use a stroller with upright sitting position.

(continued)

173

TABLE 7.4. *(continued)*

Sensory sensitivity	Bathing	Dressing	Mealtime	Playing	Bedtime	Outings
Visual	Provide one or two selected toys for bath time.	Create a blank area for dressing (facing blank corner).	Serve foods with spaces in between them.	Provide back drops for play areas to reduce visual distractions.	Remove light sources from room.	Give child something to play with while moving in stroller to reduce strobe effect as you move.
		Have child look at you while dressing him or her.	Serve more homogeneous colors together.			
		Have child focus on one toy/poster while dressing.				
Auditory	Close the bathroom door.	Tell child what you will do; be quiet otherwise.	Use even background noise.	Allow child to move to a more remote location for play.	Turn off sound sources.	Use ear plugs/ear muffs.
	Run water before the child enters the bathroom.	Turn off radio/TV.	Talk to one person at a time.	Play even-tempo background music during playtime.	If child has preferred song or background noise, play it softly.	Select nonpeak times for outings/errands.
	Play soft background music during bath.	Turn on background sound, such as music in another room.	Use coated or plastic utensils and paper plates to reduce noise.			Limit the amount of time in loud public places.

	Tell child what you are doing, and then be quiet or hum.				
Taste/smell	Identify flavors, scents, textures child likes and incorporate them regularly.	Remove air fresheners from room. Apply own scents after dressing child.	Identify child's favorite spice and incorporate often (e.g., cinnamon). Tell child name of aromas of flavors/foods.	Be careful about cleaners for toys; use only unscented ones.	Use unscented laundry soap for bedding. Use unscented soap for hands.	Be cautious about entering stores/aisles with scented products. Reduce exposure to scents in public (e.g., food courts).
Body position	Create routines and stick with them. Have child prop up on hands/arms during bath.	Make tasks smaller in time/in parts. Have child stand to dress. Follow same sequence every day.	Create a comfortable seating structure for the child for mealtime.	Crawl in tight spaces. Carry heavy objects. Push heavy objects.	Use very heavy blankets.	Wrap child in blanket. Have child wear backpack. Place heavy toy on child's lap.

Note. Copyright by Winnie Dunn. Reprinted by permission.

175

TABLE 7.5. Strategies for Supporting Babies with Sensation Avoiding.

General Concept: Making Less Sensory Input Available

Sensation avoiding	Bathing	Dressing	Mealtime	Playing	Bedtime	Outings
Touch	Use cotton fabric pieces or T-shirt material for washcloth and toweling.	Warm wipes before using them.	Be particular about temperature of foods served (e.g., room temperature).	Identify play area with space away from other children.	Keep fans/vents from blowing on child.	Have child wear tight-fitting clothing.
	Press firmly on large surfaces of child's body when washing.	Identify undergarments without elastic (diapers, panties, socks).	Create homogeneous textures in food.		Use heavy blankets.	Keep child out of crowded spaces.
	Press soap bar directly on skin.	Have child wear firm-fitting undershirts/panties.	Try coated utensils.			Provide a heavy toy for lap.
	Do not rub on skin, only press.	Use natural fibers such as cotton for clothing; notice clothing child likes and stick with these textures.				
Movement	Pick one position for bathing and stick with it, no bending overreaching.	Gather clothing for child to dress in one place.	Select an assigned seat, with minimal passing.	Honor sedentary play; add movement from sitting in a methodical way.	Reduce movements/ rocking.	Use stroller with upright sitting position.
				Make toys/objects easily accessible.	Identify routine position.	

176

Visual	Remove toys from bath.	Keep shades drawn in rooms; add light sparsely; use pure light, like halogen.	Allow child to have one food at a time on plate. Serve plate to child.	Keep everything away in play area. Play with one toy at a time.	Remove all light sources from room. Close shades, place padding on any streams of light.	Create "blinders" on the stroller to reduce side visual input. Limit times with large unstructured time in public. Attend outings during nonpeak times.
Auditory	Close bath door. Use cloth to rinse to reduce water sounds.	Run fan (that does not blow on child) to create "white" background noise.	Create white noise to drown out unpredictable noises.	Find closed in quiet places for child to play/rest.	Turn off TV, radio, close windows.	
Taste/smell	Use unscented soaps, lotions.	Remove air fresheners from room. Use unscented products for self before dressing child. Apply own scents after dressing child.	Provide a predictable set of foods for mealtimes.	No scents. Use unscented products to clean toys.	No scents. Use unscented products on bedding, on your hands.	Name any scents so they are not unfamiliar. Do not enter stores/aisles with scented products.
Body position	Create routines and stick with them for everyday tasks that must be completed.	Use exact pattern of events every day.	Use seats/chairs, so child doesn't have to be held all the time.	Craft alone time for the child; recognize it is good.	Use very heavy blankets.	Have child carry/wear a backpack.

more specialized expertise about sensory processing will be necessary. Occupational therapists study sensory processing as part of their professional training and so are the best resource. Professionals from other disciplines may acquire this knowledge through reading the current literature, attending continuing education or graduate coursework, and/or collaborating with an occupational therapist in practice.

Settings for Services
Using a Sensory Processing Approach

The optimal setting for employing a sensory processing approach is the actual location for engaging in the daily activities of interest or concern to the family. During the assessment, the professional would seek to identify both successful and challenging times of the day for the family. It is useful to know about successful periods because these times might inform the professional about what activity and environmental and interaction characteristics are positive for this family. During the challenging life task, the therapist can observe the interactions and make hypotheses about what sensory factors might be interfering with performance. Many times, caregivers won't be aware of factors that might be creating interference, so the therapist who is observing the activity can expose factors that might not otherwise be considered. Additionally, by being right there when the activity is occurring, the therapist and caregiver can make adjustments and observe the impact of these changes on the interactions and performance. The therapist can also explain why a particular adjustment might help, thus increasing the caregivers' insights about the nature of the problem.

Duration of Services
Using a Sensory Processing Approach

Typically, the therapist meets with the family more frequently at the start of treatment (e.g., once a week for 1–1.5 hours) to find out about the relationship challenge and identify the factors that may be interfering with desired outcomes. After four or five visits, typically the therapist is available by phone and email but meets with the family only once or twice a month. Families might provide videotapes of interactions. Videotapes provide additional information and can be used to provide instruction to the caregivers about observable behaviors that might indicate sensory processing responses during these interactions. The therapist also serves as a consultant to professionals of other disciplines who are serving the baby and family, providing ways to embed the sensory processing insights into their intervention regimes. A therapist might be involved with a family for 6–12 months in this manner. With transitions to new environments and activities (e.g., from bottle feeding to self-feeding and eating, or from home-based services to center-based services), there is typically an increase in visits until new rituals have been established successfully in the new setting.

Characteristics of Intervention Using a Sensory Processing Approach

There are several tactics used when professionals are implementing a sensory processing approach to intervention. After identifying the sensory processing characteristics and the activities and settings that are likely to be challenging for the child and family, the therapist collaborates with other colleagues and the family to design an individualized intervention. Interventions include designing activities for the child and family, crafting environmental adjustments to support the child in the activities of interest, making activity adaptations to provide access to desired activities, and providing information that will enable the caregiver and infant to obtain just the right amount of just the right kind of sensory input to support their evolving relationship.

Overall Pattern of Intervention Planning

Providing intervention from a sensory processing frame of reference initially involves assessment, observation, and interviewing to obtain a substantial view of the successes and challenges, along with some data gathering about the possible interfering factors. The therapist uses this information to formulate hypotheses about what might be interfering with the relationship, particularly during desired activities, such as diapering, playing, or eating. When the therapist suspects that sensory processing is a factor that is interfering, the therapist discusses with the family and other team members the observable behaviors that might indicate sensory processing issues, the sensory processing data that supports these hypotheses, and the way sensory processing might interfere with the relationship and the desired activities. Then the therapist collaborates with other team members and the caregiver to design adjustments that will support more positive interactions between the baby and caregiver. The goal is to provide just the right amount of just the right kind of sensory information for both the baby and the caregiver so that their relationship becomes positive and generative of more interactions.

Example of Collaborative Intervention Planning
Using a Sensory Processing Approach

Gunda, the mom, was frustrated with diapering Lindsey, reporting that the infant was irritable and fussy. During skilled observation, the therapist noted that the changing table was in line with the air vent, that Lindsey winced when the powder dropped onto her skin, that Gunda was very quiet as she diapered Lindsey, and that the diaper was attached loosely. Hypothesizing that some of these sensory experiences might be overwhelming Lindsey, the therapist made a plan for introducing more calming sensory input.

First, the therapist and Gunda found a new location for the table that is not exposed to a draft. Then she showed Gunda how to press firmly on Lindsey's skin to apply the powder, providing touch pressure on the surface of the skin to provide organizing sensory input without creating arousal via the reticular formation, instructed Gunda on a firmer diaper attachment, and discussed some rhymes and chants Gunda might sing during diapering to keep Lindsey's attention. Gunda explained that she felt self-conscious about singing, so they decided to try playing a CD in the background to provide a calming auditory environment.

The therapist also discussed with Gunda that, if any of these activities made Lindsey more agitated, they would need to talk and come up with alternatives. They reviewed together what they would do and why they were making these choices, so that Gunda could begin to notice Lindsey's cues as they were in the diapering situation. The therapist videotaped Gunda changing Lindsey's diaper and talked through the ideas, so Gunda would have this to show Dad and Grandma after the therapist was gone. They agreed to talk by phone within the week to discuss how the strategies were working and what possible adjustments might need to be made.

As the reader can see, a critical feature of this intervention is that as the caregiver understands the underlying principles of the suggestions, she or he can then generate ideas for new situations as new developmental activities are encountered.

Including a Sensory Processing Approach with Other Intervention Approaches

As stated earlier, a sensory processing approach is very compatible with other approaches to intervention. In many ways, such an approach provides information about the underlying features of a child's performance and thus can be used in conjunction with most other approaches to refine the individualized nature of the intervention. For example, a sensory processing approach can be used to identify the sensitivities that the child might have to particular sensory inputs, and then this information can be integrated with a behavioral approach to design a prompting or fading sequence for learning a new skill. If we knew that a child was sensitive to touch stimuli, we could either adjust that input (e.g., by using firm touching to guide a new movement rather than light touching) or design the pattern to use an alternate input altogether (e.g., by using visual or auditory cues to guide the new movement).

Sensory processing can also be combined with psychotherapy interventions. For example, a psychotherapist might be serving a mother who has a baby that doesn't like to be nursed and cries a lot. In addition to the psychotherapy issues, the therapist might note the baby's distressed response to the sound of Mom's loud voice and suggest a softer tone to quiet the baby. The professional might also consider how the mom is holding the baby, and make suggestions for more even and firm touching while she is holding the infant, which can increase the amount of calming sensory input during feeding. Embedding these sensory-based suggestions into the psychotherapy relationship provides Mom with some immediate strategies to meet the baby's needs and increases her feelings of competence as well.

Example of an Infant and Mother Who Are Struggling to Bond with Each Other

Gretchen, the mother of 5-month-old Tobias, initially expressed concern about several daily life routines, including feeding, sleeping, dressing, and playing. She described Tobias as a fussy, demanding child. As the therapist and Gretchen talked, the mom seemed generally distressed about mothering this child. She talked about having nothing in common with Tobias and said that this made it hard for her to feel attached to him. She recalled her experience with her 3-year-old daughter, stating that her daughter was much easier to love because she knew what to do to meet her daughter's needs. Gretchen also commented on a friend's 3-year-old son who seems to her very demanding and out of control, and expresses fears that this is her son's fate.

Prior to this first visit, Gretchen had completed an *Infant/Toddler Sensory Profile*. The results verify that Tobias has very low sensory thresholds when compared to other children, with sounds, visual stimuli, and touch being particularly sensitive types of sensory input. The therapist used these data to validate Mom's experiences with Tobias and to provide guidance about which therapeutic intervention suggestions might be helpful for the family.

The therapist asked Mom to describe some of the daily life activities, that is, what happens, how things go, and what her feelings and impressions of the situations are. Mom began to describe typical days at home, and sleeping was the first topic. She described Tobias as a very light sleeper. The smallest events can wake him up such that the family only watches TV with the volume on mute, and Mom has taught her daughter how to play quietly when Tobias is sleeping so they don't disturb him. Mom has tried holding and rocking Tobias, but she said that this makes things worse. Mom felt this confirms that he doesn't like her. They have also tried to make his room completely dark, but she has been frustrated with this because if she has to enter the room to check on Tobias, the light from the hall as she opens the door seems to be enough to arouse him. During this description, Mom also told the therapist that she is exhausted from lack of sleep herself, since Tobias only sleeps for short periods at a time.

This initial description about sleeping provided a lot of information about Tobias's likely patterns of sensory processing, which the therapist verified with the *Infant/Toddler Sensory Profile*. This description also provided guidance as to suggestions that the therapist might make using a sensory processing frame of reference. However, the description also suggested that this family was living in a distressed and controlled state, that Mom felt incompetent, and that perhaps Mom considered the source of this difficult situation to be Tobias. So even though a sensory processing framework could provide guidance about some strategies for addressing the sleeping problems and their effect on the family in general, it would be of primary importance to first acknowledge both Gretchen's emotional state and her insights into her son's needs as part of comprehensive therapeutic intervention. If the therapist failed to address Mom's emotional state, mom might be unable to receive other suggestions even if they would be helpful. Sensory processing intervention ideas could help Mom feel more competent if they were framed within supporting the mother–infant bonding and as a means to build their relationship together.

The therapist commented that it sounded as if the family was living in a very controlled situation right now; Mom agreed and said, "We don't know what else we can do." The therapist then also commented about how insightful Gretchen has been to figure out all these things about Tobias and that these actions surely pointed to her ability to understand Tobias and therefore meet his needs. The mom replied that she was not feeling very successful, since Tobias was still very difficult and demanding. The therapist acknowledged that Mom was feeling frustrated about meeting Tobias's needs and said there might be some ideas that would help the situation.

The therapist then used Gretchen's own words to point out things that she had done which indicated her good insights; these insights match the findings on the *Infant/Toddler Sensory Profile*. For example, the family had taken steps to reduce the sounds in the house during rest times. The profile results verify that Tobias has low thresholds for sounds; he will notice sounds much more readily than other children his age, and this high rate of response is likely to interfere with his ability to fall asleep and stay asleep. They have also tried to reduce the intensity of the visual environment by making it dark for Tobias, another sensory area in which Tobias has sensitivity. The therapist also reassured Mom that Tobias's reactions to being held reflect his sensitivity to touch and not his response to her emotionally. The therapist also stated that she would have some suggestions to make holding Tobias more satisfying for both of them.

This pointing out of the consistencies between the scores on a standardized measure and Gretchen's own observations seemed to console her. The therapist and Gretchen then began to discuss ways to adjust the sleeping routines to both support Tobias and create a more manageable situation for the rest of the family. The therapist suggested using a dim night-light to provide a small amount of light for times when the parents need to check on Tobias; this would reduce the contrast of light coming in from the doorway. The therapist also suggested that the family keep the hall light turned off to create less contrast when they do need to enter Tobias's bedroom from the hallway. Gretchen acknowledged this was a good idea but said she had developed a habit of turning on the hall light and often didn't think of it until it woke Tobias—and then it was too late. The therapist suggested that for now they unscrew the hall light-bulb and put a night-light there as well. Finally, the therapist suggested using a baby monitor so they can check on Tobias by listening sometimes, so as not to disturb him.

The issue of the sounds was particularly important since the family's strategies for being overly quiet put a strain on everyone. They discussed the importance of finding an alternative to being quiet all the time because this builds resentment in themselves and their daughter, ultimately affecting all the family relationships. First, the therapist pointed out that it was good that the parents closed and sealed the window, including providing a heavier drapery, to reduce noise from outside. Next, the therapist suggested trying a box fan in Tobias's room, making sure that the fan did not create a breeze on him directly, but rather provided a "white noise" (i.e., continuous, even sound) in his immediate environment. The therapist explained that the proximity of this continuous sound might be able to mask sounds from the rest of the family during sleeping periods.

Then they discussed sleepware. The therapist told Gretchen about dressing Tobias in tighter-fitting sleepware, including smaller sizes and stretchy items such as tights, explaining the calming effect of firm, even pressure on the surface of the skin. The therapist also suggested using a heavy blanket to cover Tobias, explaining that the weight of the blanket would provide additional calming sensory input. Gretchen was startled and revealed that she wore tights to bed when she was a girl. This provided the therapist with an opportunity to return to the topic of her bonding and relationship building with her baby. The therapist said, "So, perhaps you do have things in common with Tobias and can use your own early experiences as a guide to understanding him a little better." They discussed how wearing tights helped her feel more secure at bedtime and how she had to fight with her parents to be allowed to wear them. Sometimes she sneaked them into her bedding so she could put them on after her parents tucked her in at night. The therapist commented that Gretchen would be able to be a much more understanding mother now that she could link her childhood sleeping experiences with those of Tobias.

Gretchen's comments about her own experiences paired with her earlier comments about fears of how Tobias would turn out prompted the therapist to continue the conversation focusing on Mom's feelings. The therapist said she had served a number of families who had babies that were sensitive like Tobias, and that although the family had been focused on the challenging aspects of his sensitivity, there were positive features of sensitivity to understand as well. She explained that people who have sensory sensitivity do notice more things than other people and that this characteristic enables them to detect small changes in circumstances, situations, or moods. This ability can contribute to their awareness of others, so that they "check in" on how others are doing. Such higher detection ability also enables people with sensitivity to express themselves creatively in various art forms because they may notice details that others miss until those details are pointed out. Gretchen began to cry and said she was an artist herself. Thus, this simple explanation of the constructive features of sensory sensitivity provided a place for Gretchen and Tobias to share common ground, with the possibility of a positive and mutually supportive outcome.

Armed with new information and insight, Gretchen went home and began to implement the strategies they discussed for bedtime. The therapist and Gretchen stayed in contact to problem solve other challenges, including the baby's eating and playing. Because Gretchen now had both a framework for understanding Tobias's behavior and a vision of the positive possibilities rather than the fear of the negative outcomes, they had more and more productive interactions and their relationship began to build. With knowledge about sensory processing, Gretchen said she was able to see Tobias as "curious" rather than "picky," and this enabled her to adjust his play and eating times to be within his tolerances, thus increasing the enjoyment for them both.

CONCLUSIONS

Sensory processing knowledge is a powerful tool to inform professionals and families about the relationships between babies and caregivers. Since every human experience contains sensory information and we use this information to understand our world and our interactions with others, it is critical to include sensory processing approaches as part of comprehensive assessment and intervention programs. Research on sensory processing indicates that there are specific patterns that we can associate with the ways in which people respond in everyday life, so this evidence can be used to guide interpretations of the interactions in the infant–caregiver relationships and to craft interventions that enable both the caregiver and the infant to get their needs met.

RESOURCES ON SENSORY PROCESSING INTERVENTIONS

Cohn, E., Miller, L., & Tickle-Degnen, L. (2000). Parental hopes for therapy outcomes: children with sensory modulation disorders. *American Journal of Occupational Therapy, 54*(1), 36–43.

Dunn, W. (1997). The impact of sensory processing abilities on the daily lives of young children and their families: A conceptual model. *Infants and Young Children, 9*(4), 23–35.

Dunn, W. (2000). *Best practice occupational therapy for serving children and families in community settings.* Thorofare, NJ: Slack.

Dunn, W., & Daniels, D. (2002). Initial development of the *Infant–Toddler Sensory Profile. Journal of Early Intervention, 25*(1), 27–41.

Williamson, G., & Anzalone, M. (2000). Sensory integration: A key component in the evaluation and treatment of young children with severe difficulties in relating and communicating. In *Assessing and treating infants and young children with severe difficulties in relating and communicating* (pp. 29–36). Washington, DC: Zero to Three.

REFERENCES

Ayres, A. J., & Tickle, L. D. (1980). Hyper-responsivity to touch and vestibular stimuli as a predictor of positive response to sensory integration procedures by autistic children. *American Journal of Occupational Therapy, 34,* 375–381.

Brown, C., Cromwell, R., Filion, D., Dunn, W., & Tollefson, N. (2002). Sensory processing in schizophrenia: Missing and avoiding information. *Schizophrenia Research, 55*(1–2), 187–195.

Brown, C., & Dunn, W. (2002). *Adolescent/Adult Sensory Profile.* San Antonio, TX: Psychological Corp.

Brown, C., Tollefson, N., Dunn, W., Cromwell, R., & Filion, D. (2001). The Adult Sensory Profile: Measuring patterns of sensory processing. *American Journal of Occupational Therapy, 55,* 75–82.

Case-Smith, J., & Bryan, T. (1999). The effects of occupational therapy with sensory integration emphasis on preschool-age children with autism. *American Journal of Occupational Therapy, 53,* 489–497.

Clark, F. A., Miller, L. R., Thomas, J. A., Kucherawy, D. S., & Azin, S. P. (1978). A comparison of operant and sensory integration methods on vocalizations and other developmental parameters in profoundly retarded adults. *American Journal of Occupational Therapy, 32,* 86–93.

Creedon, M. (1994, July). *Project SMART: Sensory modulation, assessment, research, and treatment.* Paper presented at the annual conference of the Autism Society of America, Las Vegas, NV.

Daniels, D., & Dunn, W. (2003). *The relationship between sensory processing and temperament in young children.* Manuscript in preparation.

DeGangi, G. A. (2000). *Pediatric disorders of regulation in affect and behavior.* San Diego, CA: Academic Press.

DeGangi, G. A., & Breinbauer (1997). The symptomatology of infants and toddlers with regulatory disorders. *Journal of Developmental and Learning Disorders, 1*(1), 183–215.

DeGangi, G. A., & Greenspan, S. I. (1989). *Test of Sensory Functions in Infants Manual.* Los Angeles: Western Psychological Services.

DeGangi, G. A., Poisson, S., Sickel, R. Z., & Wiener, A. S. (1995). *Infant–Toddler Symptom Checklist.* Tucson, AZ: Therapy Skill Builders.

Dunn, W. (1997). The impact of sensory processing abilities on the daily lives of young children and their families: A conceptual model. *Infants and Young Children, 9*(4), 23–35.

Dunn, W. (1999). *Sensory Profile: User's manual.* San Antonio, TX: Psychological Corp.

Dunn, W. (2000). Habit: What's the brain got to do with it? (Habits I conference.) *Occupational Therapy Journal of Research, 20*(Fall), 6S–20S.

Dunn, W. (2001). The sensations of everyday life: Empirical, theoretical, and pragmatic considerations. *American Journal of Occupational Therapy, 55,* 608–620.

Dunn, W. (2002). *The Infant/Toddler Sensory Profile manual.* San Antonio, TX: Psychological Corp.

Dunn, W., & Brown, C. (1997). Factor analysis on the Sensory Profile from a national sample of children without disabilities. *American Journal of Occupational Therapy, 51,* 490–495.

Dunn, W., & Daniels, W. (2002). Initial development of the Infant–Toddler Sensory Profile. *Journal of Early Intervention, 25*(1), 27–41.

Dunn, W., & Westman, K. (1997). The Sensory Profile: The performance of a national sample of young children without disabilities. *American Journal of Occupational Therapy, 51,* 25–34.

Edelson, S. M., Edelson, M. G., Kerr, D. C. R., & Grandin, T. (1999). Behavioral and physiological effects of deep pressure on children with autism: A pilot study evaluating the effects of Grandin's Hug Machine. *American Journal of Occupational Therapy, 53,* 145–152.

Ermer, J., & Dunn, W. (1998). The Sensory Profile: A discriminant analysis of young children with and without disabilities. *American Journal of Occupational Therapy, 52,* 283–290.

Inamura, K. N., Wiss, T., & Parham, D. (1990a). The effects of Hug Machine usage on the behavioral organization of children with autism and autistic-like characteristics: Part 1. *Sensory Integration Special Interest Section Quarterly, 18*(September), 1–5.

Inamura, K. N., Wiss, T., & Parham, D. (1990b). The effects of Hug Machine usage on the behavioral organization of children with autism and autistic-like characteristics: Part 2. *Sensory Integration Special Interest Section Quarterly, 18*(December), 1–5.

Kientz, M. A. (1996). Sensory-based needs in children with autism: Motivation for behavior and suggestions for intervention. *Developmental Disabilities Special Interest Section Newsletter, 19,* 1–3.

Kientz, M. A., & Dunn, W. (1997). A comparison of the performance of young children with and without autism on the Sensory Profile. *American Journal of Occupational Therapy, 51,* 530–537.

Law, M., Polatajko, H. J., Schaffer, R., Miller, J., & Macnab, J. (1991). The impact of heterogeneity in a clinical trial: Motor outcomes after sensory integration therapy. *Occupational Therapy Journal of Research, 11,* 177–189.

Morreau, S. (2000). *The effects of weighted vest on a preschool child with autism.* Unpublished thesis, Eastern Kentucky University, Richmond.

CHAPTER 8

A MULTIFOCAL
NEONATAL INTERVENTION

Nadia Bruschweiler-Stern

Neonatal intervention is difficult to specify because of the dynamic interplay between the intervention and the particular needs of the new family. What is done is always different because of the need to track psychic pain during a normal developmental crisis in a complex situation that evolves rapidly and usually involves three people directly: a newborn and both parents. The focus may have to be on the baby's behavior, the mother's behavior. the father's behavior, the mother's representations, the father's representations, or the couple's interactions. In addition to the dyadic, mother–baby, father–baby, and mother–father relationships, and triadic relationships between the three of them (see Fivaz-Depeursinge, Corboz-Warnery, & Keren, Chapter 6, this volume; Fivaz-Depeursinge & Corboz-Warnery, 1999), it always includes the additional relationships of the therapist to each of them as depicted in the motherhood constellation.

Interactions, representations, as well as behaviors are explored. The focus may need to shift rapidly and repeatedly. This multiple focus is specific and central to this approach. The focus is not only on the baby's behavior during a neonatal behavioral assessment (the real baby), nor on the mother's representation of her baby (the imagined baby), but also on the specific matching and dialogue between them. In terms of the model of the different possible "ports of entry" to intervene in the father–mother–infant system (see Sameroff, Chapter 1, this volume; Stern-Bruschweiler & Stern, 1989; Stern, 1995), this multifocal approach may use several ports of entry in parallel.

This shift toward multiple foci distinguishes this intervention from the traditional developmental pediatric approach of T. B. Brazelton and his colleagues, where neonatal behavioral assessments are used mostly for nonspecific education of parents about the baby's competencies, and from the original psychodynamically oriented parent–infant psychotherapy approach, where the mother's representations and their history (the origin of the imagined baby) are the central focus (see Lieberman, Chapter 5, this volume). This emphasis of the multifocal approach on the positive in the mother–baby relationship differs from that of psychoanalytic approaches which pathologize the mother by seeing her as responsible for anything that doesn't work in the relationship.

The approach has no systematic order of steps, but rather follows general guidelines for an open-ended first consultation with parents and their baby. One never knows in advance where the problem lies: it can be in the infant in terms of a hypersensitivity difficult for the parents to deal with or a physical problem like a malformation; it can be in the mother in terms of a misunderstanding of the baby's needs and signals, her wish for a girl to reproduce her ideal relationship with her mother, when she just had a boy, or in her past history of trauma or grief; it can be in the couple who discover around the crib that they have different expectations of each other as parents; it can be in the stress that can come from another domain and undermine the parents' psychological availability; or it may involve the mother's isolation from her family of origin or from her own cultural environment. Anything that prevents a smooth establishment of mutual discovery and the early attachment process that starts at birth can be the problem.

A neonatal intervention offers the opportunity to work at an early stage of perturbation (Anders, 1989; Zero to Three/National Center for Clinical Infant Programs, 1994) and less often with disturbances or disorders. The impact of this intervention has been evaluated very positively by most parents and can have effects for at least 18 months, as shown in a follow-up study (Bruschweiler-Stern, 2000).

THE SETTING FOR THIS INTERVENTION

Birth, like death, is a very special moment in life when something happens in reality that revolutionizes the habits of practical and interpersonal life (Stern & Bruschweiler-Stern, 1998), as well as the intrapsychic world. When a new life arrives, as when a life disappears, everything has to be reorganized, and this reorganization demands considerable mental and emotional energy.

The perspective on early clinical management and emotional care that underlies this multifocal neonatal intervention approach has evolved from my experience of successively wearing separate hats as a pediatrician, a child psychiatrist, and a developmentalist, and also as a parent. In these roles I learned about four different babies.

1. *The pediatric baby.* In pediatrics, we see the baby as an organism with a heart, lungs, kidneys, brain, and other organs, and the integrity and the functioning of the different systems is the focus. We see the baby as a biological organism.

More and more, the time allowed for pediatric consultations just permits technical acts—asking about symptoms, finding the diagnosis, and prescribing the treatment. The parents' anxiety or the baby's feelings get in the way of the consultation. The relationship is taken into account only if it may have an effect on the baby's health, for example, physical abuse or negligence with an impact on physical growth.

2. *The psychiatric baby.* In child psychiatry, the baby is seen linked to his or her mother, where the mother's representation of the infant is a determinant of his or her future (Lebovici, 1983). Very often, the baby is thought to be unconsciously shaped by his or her mother's unresolved conflicts. When this is so, the baby will be left lying in the crib with little attention, while the mother is asked to talk about her fantasies and her past. Child psychiatry has not yet learned to look at the infant him- or herself, because it doesn't know how to access the child's early psychological life. The baby is only the repository of the parent's plans and attributions.

3. *The competent baby of development.* From the child development point of view, one tries to demonstrate the baby's competencies, preferences, adaptation to the immediate environment, and his or her stimulus thresholds. One seeks to understand who the baby is as an individual. This is the baby as a person.

The Neonatal Behavioral Assessment Scale (NBAS; Brazelton, 1973; Brazelton & Nugent, 1995) is the tool of choice for learning about the baby's experience and way of dealing with his or her new environment. This approach has been extended for understanding early preterm newborns (Als, 1984; Als, Lester, Tronik, & Brazelton, 1982).

Who is this baby? What is this infant telling us? What is the newborn trying to do? What is his or her next developmental goal? What does the newborn need from his or her surroundings to achieve it?

4. *My baby.* The experience of different professions doesn't prepare a woman for the revolution provoked by maternity. This fourth point of view is the baby as your own child. As a mother, I had the opportunity of experiencing the intense and new emotions that emerge with this new state, facing the task of keeping the baby alive, regulating the baby's states, answering the infant's needs, and establishing a new relationship. If any of these tasks is not fulfilled, the mother's level of anxiety rises very fast. At different steps along the way, a mother will need each of the aforementioned professionals. But they will not be enough; she will also need a network of mothers and experienced women to support her in her functions.

When one considers these four babies, one realizes how partial the view of the baby is in each specialty and how far each can be removed from the parents' view and experience of their baby. This realization leads to an approach that integrates some of these four roles with the following guidelines:

- Parents always have good reasons for doing what they do.
- Parents always want the best for their baby (except in rare pathological situations).
- Parents are experts on their child.
- Health professionals are experts in techniques that may help parents and infants, but will only succeed in relieving them if they work as partners and not in a relationship of an expert with passive recipients of care.

The Psychological Setting of the Intervention

It is necessary to understand the process of becoming a mother. It is equally necessary to understand the baby's developmental process. Without both, one cannot understand particular clinical situations. The families of full-term and preterm babies undergo different experiences, but the same principles apply to both situations. The special relationship aspects of the preterm situation will be discussed below.

Fathers are in a secondary position for several reasons. Men are less likely to share their inner life, and they come less often with their baby to visit the doctor. Not experiencing the pregnancy in their own body, they have greater room to assume a wide variety of levels of involvement. But they too undergo the weight of a new responsibility; they have to ensure the security of their new family. The realization of this new responsibility hits them at various moments, and they deal with it according to their own past experience and personality. They also are in need of attention and support, and they have a full role in this multifocal approach.

Before describing the technique, it is helpful to explore further some of the elements of the psychological setting.

What the Mother Brings to the Consultation

Long before she gets pregnant, the mother has been building a representation of the child she will have—the "imagined baby." She is also constructing an "imaginary mother" that she would like to be and an "imaginary father," as well. Depending upon her personality and life experience, these representations will be more or less vague or precise.

The psychological process of preparation for a baby and a future family does not begin at the moment of conception. It has been in preparation since the mother's childhood; it evolves through various phases into adulthood until it becomes intensely active during pregnancy.

While the physical pregnancy is going on in the uterus, the mother experiences simultaneously a mental pregnancy. This mental pregnancy consists of psychological work that prepares the way for profound changes in her identity within her marriage and her family of origin, her professional and social life, and her sense of self. She works upon her image of her baby, of herself as a future mother, of her husband as a future father, of her new nuclear family, of her baby's role in this family, of the next generation of her family, and of the articulation with her husband's family. This mental work is like a "personality-o-genesis" that would be the counterpart of the organogenesis. These two simultaneous processes, physical and psychological, mutually influence one another during the entire pregnancy.

What happens to the mother's representations during the pregnancy?

The mother's representation of her baby during the pregnancy can be measured. Fava Vizziello and associates (Fava Vizziello, Antonioli,

Cocci, Invernizzi, & Cristante, F., 1993), Ammaniti (1991; see also Ammaniti & Stern, 1994), and Zeanah and associates (Zeanah, Keener, Stewart, & Anders, 1985; Zeanah, Keener, & Anders, 1986; Zeanah, 1993) have made important contributions to the assessment of these maternal representations.

Some of the results can be summarized as follow. The richness, elaboration, and specificity of the mother's representation of her baby increases slowly during the first prenatal months in parallel with her confidence in the pregnancy. The representation then makes a big leap around the fourth month (after she has the first ultrasound and first feels the baby's movements). It continues to grow progressively, reaching a high point around the seventh month. After this summit, the mother's representation of her baby loses some of its richness and specificity; the mother lets it fade and undo itself during the last weeks of pregnancy. Around that time, her concerns about the delivery take over and the baby's representation moves to the background. Generally around the birth, the mother does not remember the representations she elaborated during the previous months. The father sometimes better remembers what she was wondering about. A schematical representation of the development of a psychological pregnancy, in particular the changes in richness and specificity of the imagined baby, is shown in Figure 8.1.

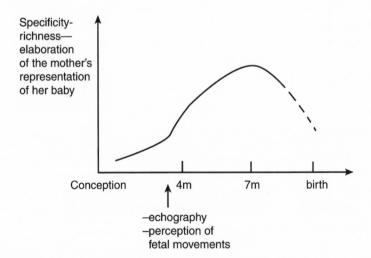

FIGURE 8.1. Psychological pregnancy: Richness of the mother's representation of her baby during the pregnancy.

The mother's representation of her baby is not a coherent and completed image of a particular personality. It is the fruit of an exploration of her wishes and fears past and present that are woven together over time and integrates real events that arose during the pregnancy.

Schematically, one could say that the mother navigates in her imagination between two groups of representations concerning her baby. One concerns the "wished-for baby": a boy or a girl, good looking, strong, athletic, charming, vivacious, smart, easy; a baby who achieves something that she had dreamed for herself, who has characteristics of her hero or heroine, as determined by the life that she has led. Simultaneously, the same imagination is working upon the feared baby: malformed, weak, with Down syndrome, ugly, myopic, who will become violent or alcoholic just like some member of her family.

During the pregnancy, she explores the field of who she will be as a mother. In the same way, thinking of her own mother, reevoking examples of mothers she admires and of others she hopes she will never be like. She does the same thing with the father, their families of origin, and the different areas of her life that are touched by the arrival of her new baby. The pregnancy is a mental laboratory where possible futures are explored, while the baby is developing in the womb (Stern & Bruschweiler-Stern, 1998).

All these representations constitute a vast repertoire of experiences in the mother's mind. Some of them will naturally or forcefully emerge when she becomes a mother, and others will be activated by people who surround her. The nature of the perinatal period is such that the social environment can have a great influence by activating representations of the mother's repertoire, which then become enacted.

Birth as a Crisis: Why Is Birth a Good Moment for Prevention and Intervention?

The birth is a moment of disequilibrium in the mother's system—a time of crisis. It is the moment when her "imagined baby" meets the "real baby." At the same time her priorities change drastically. The "motherhood constellation" (Stern, 1995) and the attachment system are activated in the following ways:

1. At the moment of birth, survival of the baby emerges as the mother's first preoccupation. When her baby is born, the mother first needs to make sure the infant is alive. She needs to make the child her

own, at a physical level: to experience the weight of the baby's body on hers; to feel the infant's texture, warmth, and animation. The moment when the baby is put on the mother's belly or chest marks this step. Mothers describe it with great emotion, and those who could not experience it often feel a strong frustration. This happens when a newborn needs resuscitation, when a preterm is taken away to the intensive care unit, or sometimes after a cesarian section. When the mother is deprived of this first physical contact, she stays in suspension until the moment when the infant is put into her arms.

The mother of a baby who died *in utero* at 37 weeks of gestation was describing her delivery and said sadly, "After the baby is out, normally, it is put here" (designating her thorax). She was expressing exactly that strong need of feeling the baby on her that set the necessary final point of the delivery and the starting point of the attachment process.

2. After the birth, she wants to know that all is going well, that her newborn son (say) is anatomically intact and in good health. She needs to see her baby naked, count his fingers, see his genitals, his front, and his back. Checking the physical status of the baby answers this question and gives a green light for the next phase.

3. When she has been reassured about the physical condition of her baby, the mother seeks to meet this new member of the family as a person. She has put out all her antennae to perceive *who* this mysterious baby boy who has been created inside her all this time really is. She is lying in wait for the slightest indication that might orient her. She will seek to appropriate him through physical resemblance, "He has his father's forehead and eyes, but he has my mouth!" and through his behavioral similarities, "When he is hungry, you've got to be there right away! He is demanding like my father," or "He sleeps a lots—in my family, we are all great sleepers."

The mother has created many different images during her imaginary voyages through her own childhood and then, more intensively, during her pregnancy, images about her baby as a person, about herself as a mother, about their very early and subsequent relationship, and about her husband in his role as a father, to name a few. All of these images are in suspension, like a cloudy emulsion in a liquid, ready to precipitate out and crystallize during the discovery process she accomplishes when she interacts with her baby. She has long imagined this baby whom she finally meets, and she latches on to each bit of information that could concern him or herself as a mother, whether it comes from her baby or from those around them.

She is particularly sensitive during this perinatal period and all input may influence her relationship with her baby.

THE INTERVENTION

Basic Guidelines

Using Positive Representations: The Good Ghosts in the Nursery

Selma Fraiberg's classic notion of "ghosts in the nursery," as revealed during consultation in child psychiatry, has taught us the potentially pathological function that representations of past relationships may have in the present (Fraiberg, Adelson, & Shapiro, 1975). As Fraiberg well knew, there are not only bad ghosts in the nursery, there are good ones too, and even good fairies, and they play an important role as inspirations and models for the mother.

Therapeutically speaking, listening very openly to the mother's representations around birth is essential. If negative representations of the past are not expressed spontaneously, they should not be looked for because the effect of this inquiry could be the activation of negative background representations that would not have come out otherwise. If aroused, these could become vivid in the mother's mind and influence her thoughts about her baby, causing her to reflect on such things as a previous baby's death and other losses or separations. If there are such events in the mother's history, she will share them easily after having built up trust in the therapeutic relationship.

Looking for the positive is accomplished by the therapist emphasizing the strengths of the baby, providing means to face any difficulties in the baby's behavior, looking for and emphasizing the mother's representations of a "good mother," those she has experienced as a support in her life and that give her confidence to offer the most secure part of her for interaction with her baby. She wants to be the good mother of her dreams or the one she didn't have. At the same time she is in a position in which she sees everything she does as wrong, and she doesn't yet realize that, guided by her emergent maternal instinct, she does exactly what fulfills her baby's needs. The therapist by revealing her positive mothering to her, emphasizing it, and eventually linking it to one of the positive representations in her repertoire, supports her in the process.

This will also contribute to providing a supportive emotional environment for the mother, who will feel cared for. This is essential to permit the building of a therapeutic alliance between mothers and care providers in the service of the family's health.

The Problem of Criticism and Negative Self-Fulfilling Prophecies

It is necessary to emphasize the very important role of the social context: the visits by friends and relatives, as well as the perinatal team. This is well represented by the fairies around the princess's crib in "Sleeping Beauty." Their comments and wishes are exclusively positive, but when the bad fairy Carabosse comes with her wish of death, it is a shock for everyone. Relief is given by the last fairy, who turns that death into a sleep 100 years long. All the wishes, good and bad, were prophecies, and they were fulfilled.

In the mother's eyes, the maternity staff has an expertise such that whatever they say during these first days may get indelibly engraved in her mind and can strongly influence her future relationship with her baby by reinforcing either a positive or negative preexisting representation.

A mother brought her 4-year-old son for a consultation because he was violent, often kicking her with his feet, and she couldn't make him obey her. Among her first words were "Already in the maternity word, a nurse said that he was bad!" That had happened 4 years ago but was still vivid in the mother's mind. Of course, the words of the nurse didn't make him bad, but they resonated with the mother's fear of having a bad baby and they left their imprint on her image of him that set her on the path of the feared baby.

One can direct a mother on the path of the wished-for baby just as easily by making positive comments. It is crucial to realize that in the neonatal period, words can have great power and a long-lasting effect.

Developmental Issues

Several developmental ideas underlie this approach and are conveyed to the parents:

1. *The newborn is a sensory being.* A newborn lives intensely at the level of senses and feelings. Research on the infant's capacity for habituation and the effect of early pain have shown that sensory functions take place first. It is only secondarily, with development, that there are responses to the sensory information, for example, the "fight-or-flight" reaction if the stimulus threshold is exceeded. In infants this reaction is

visible through the control of their states: they can escape insufficient stimulation or overstimulation by falling asleep or crying. If the overstimulation lasts, especially for a preterm infant, he or she may have autonomic nervous system reactions that can even be life threatening (e.g., bradycardia or apnea). The full-term baby will more often manifest signs of overstimulation by digestive reactions like regurgitation, hiccups, or bowel movements (Brazelton, 1992).

2. *Newborns are at the dawn of their psychological lives.* They don't yet have instrumental behaviors. They do not yet cry to get their mothers to come; they cry because they feel uncomfortable or in pain.

3. *The first weeks and months are a time of challenge and adaptation.* The time for concern with education will come later. It makes sense to keep the infants' experiences in a range of comfort and pleasure as much as possible, avoiding too much overstimulation. This helps to develop a feeling of security that will constitute a base for free exploration later on.

Research on pain has taught us that not only is the infant sensitive to pain (Anand & Hickey, 1987) but also that such early experience of pain leaves traces in the form of an increased sensitivity to later pain and more difficulty in coping with it (Taddio, Goldbach, Ipp, Stevens, & Koren, 1995). In terms of parenting, this translates as follows: instead of thinking that "because the world is a rough place, the best thing for infants is to experience it as soon as they are born," we know now that an early experience of pain makes infants more fragile to further exposures to pain, so it makes sense to protect a baby from early intense painful experiences.

Note that parallel to her infant's developing sensitivity, the mother also has a wide expansion of her own sensibility. Her sense of smell can be strongly enhanced. Her sensibility to temperature (the air, the water of the bath) is more acute. She is more responsive to the level of noise and the quality of touch (pleasure of the physical contact). Her senses and attention are directed toward her infant. She moves toward the baby to be better able to communicate and protect him or her.

She also feels a powerful need to answer her baby's distress signals, to find the reason behind them and a way to comfort the child. Motherhood includes the need to ensure her baby's survival, growth, and well-being. At this phase of life, advice like "If you pick him up every time he cries, you will make him a spoiled kid" or "he will make a slave of you" is often heard, but is inadequate. Such advice must be avoided because it puts a mother in a bind between her emergent maternal instinct and advice that does not apply to this phase of her infant's development. The mother and her infant need to be encouraged to find a way in which both of them can feel comfortable and secure.

4. *The sensorial experience of the newborn gets written in the history of his or her body and relation to the world.* The newborn's sensory processing features are identifiable: "what does he like, notice, miss, become irritated by, withdraw from" (see Dunn, Chapter 7, this volume; also Dunn, 2002; Williamson & Anzalone, 2001). Keeping the infant's sensorial system balanced is a more primitive need than the need for psychological equilibrium. Psychiatrists as well as mothers have had the tendency to ignore individual differences in sensory processing and to attribute psychological intentions to sensory reactions; an example follows.

Case 1: An Overstimulated Infant

A little boy who is very easily overloaded by stimulation and thrown into sensory processing disequilibriums, so that as he is growing up his behavior is often interpreted as impulsive and aggressive. I saw this little boy for the first time at birth when he showed a very high sensitivity to items on the Brazelton Neonatal Behavioral Assessment Scale (NBAS). His father recognized the baby's style right away, but his mother didn't at all. At 2 months of age, the mother came back with him because a little music box had fallen on his face and she noticed that he frequently startled at unexpected noises or changes in his environment. He needed a lot of support to deal with average environmental stimulation. His mother was a very intense and lively person who would dive toward his face with wonderful expressions of enthusiasm, but he didn't enjoy them at all. She was becoming discouraged and hurt by her infant's disorganization into crying and frantic motor excitement.

With the help of the intervention, she learned to protect him from overstimulation. To help him anticipate and deal with changes, she gave him support by holding and reassuring him. He constantly needed her to buffer the world around him; indeed, she became his "regulating other" (Stern, 1985). At 4½ years of age he entered kindergarten in a class of 34 kids. Because he would push, kick, and pull the other children, the teacher worried that he was too aggressive and made him sit by himself. As a result he didn't want to go to school. He was simply overwhelmed with activity and excitement—there was too much for him to deal with. When the class was split into two groups of 17, things went much better. By helping the parents and teacher understand the boy's need for a level of environmental stimulation he could deal with, the therapist prevented him from being seen as an aggressive, bad little boy and from being excluded by his group of peers.

Technique

Framework

The multifocal neonatal approach is being used in a private maternity hospital with patients of middle and high socioeconomic status. The mothers make appointments for various physical and psychological reasons: the baby may have a problem; they have a difficult personal, marital, or gynecological history; they had a difficult pregnancy or delivery; or they feel overwhelmed or isolated. Sometimes it is just to get to know their baby better.

Usually, they are seen only once or twice, but more often if needed. Some of the time the treatment lasts for months or years with decreasing frequency. It can be on a regular basis or periodically, as necessary.

Practically, the first consultation takes between 60 and 90 minutes, at the mother's bedside for inpatients or in the office for outpatients. Both parents are there most of the time. The infant has been recently fed and is usually in his or her crib.

Creating and Maintaining a Holding Environment

The very first thing is to develop a therapeutic alliance (see McDonough, Chapter 4, this volume; also McDonough, 1992, 1993). This is best accomplished by providing the mother with a holding environment from an experienced, accepting, active, and warm person. The mother must feel that the therapist is open and on her side—not on the side of a theory, the hospital, the physicians, or any other family members—and is trying to understand the way she is experiencing her path into motherhood.

Certain conditions make the creation of a holding environment possible. The therapist must—

1. Receive training that gives confidence in her ability to manipulate and evaluate the baby, deal with relational problems, and know about early development.
2. Be totally available so that she is entirely focused on the members of the family during the consultation, letting it last as long as necessary.
3. Validate the mother in her new role and avoid criticism. Be-

cause the mother is psychologically open to the negative as well as to the positive, the intervention must be constructive.

4. Be active, engaged, and curious about the mother's experience and the baby's personality and state. She should ask questions and listen, approve, express admiration, or try to find a good reason for anything that seems questionable or problematic. Feedback and guidance are given when necessary, and a model is provided for the parent's behavior when it might be helpful. There is no neutrality in this approach.

Procedure

The session starts by my asking about the parents' motive for the consultation. What will be done together is then explained.

The mother is asked how she feels about her recent experience in the form of a semistructured interview looking for the content and quality of the experience she has had. It is also important that I be alert to what, in her story, touches me, what makes me like her and want to work with her.

The interview touches on the delivery: How did it go? Is she pleased with herself? What did she feel when she saw her baby boy? Was she surprised? What did the baby look like? What did he do? When did she start to feel connected to him?

It touches on the pregnancy: Did anything particular happened? What did the baby feel like? How did he present himself? How did she imagine him then?

Then more general questions are asked including the following: Are there other babies in the family? Does she have experience with taking care of babies? How does she feel about it? How does she feel in her new role as a mother? Is she confident or worried about anything in particular? Does she have an example of a mother she admires in her life? Will her husband be at home for the first days? Does she have a support system that will be available to surround her?

Finally, I ask how she sees her baby now, both physically and in his behavior of feeding, sleeping, having a bath, awake state, and interactive moments. Is he cuddly, easy or difficult to console?

In this exchange, I would look for the quality of the experience that she had, for her sense of having the baby she expected, her self-confidence in her new role as a mother, her support network, and for the elements that will help her feel satisfied and confident.

The father's involvement is varied, so his contribution in the interview is also varied, but he is asked to express himself periodically if he doesn't do it spontaneously.

Whenever the parents go off on a question or tack of their own, I willingly interrupt the standard procedure and follow them in that direction.

This discussion of the pregnancy and delivery is often an opportunity for the parents to discover each other's experience and how each of them is dealing with the transformation into parenthood. This exchange also gives reality to their experience and reenforces their ties as a parental couple. Telling their story also can act as an initiation ritual, introducing them into parenthood. Such experiences are often missing in our culture today.

The Brazelton Neonatal Behavioral Assessment Scale

The parents are invited to step back with me and look at their baby after, but not before, a sense of mutual trust has been established and once a sense of the mother's expectations of herself and of her baby has been ascertained. This stepping back puts the parents in the perspective of discovering something new that their infant will show them about himself, as an individual with his own personality, competencies, and needs. The Brazelton NBAS is then performed with the parents close by. It should be a shared discovery of how their baby tells about how he feels, his experience.

During the NBAS the therapist makes comments and observations. Depending on the baby's state and on the mother's and father's need, the procedure can be interrupted to address their concerns or to give the mother her baby to comfort or to interact with if she shows a desire for it.

Integration of the Parent's Representations and Experience with the Baby's Behavior

When the assessment is over, the baby is usually placed in the mother's arms and comments are made about the examination. In commenting, the therapist covers the following points:

- The preoccupations the parents may have raised earlier are addressed.
- The baby's behaviors that confirm their representations or observations (the positive matches) are pointed out.
- The areas where the baby's behavior is vulnerable or may present difficulties are brought up and strategies to deal with them are devised.

- When there are negative distortions, the baby's behavior is used to correct them and to test the weight of these attributions.

During the session, the therapist aims first to promote the emerging maternal instinct and catalyze the attachment process. Promoting maternal instinct is done by exploring specific moments during the delivery, for example, after the expulsion, when her baby was put on her belly, the first time she felt connected with her baby, or what she wants to do when her baby cries. Her spontaneous actions toward her baby are validated and reinforced. It is emphasized that her own feelings are far more important than advice from others or from books. When necessary, efforts are made to ensure that the father is engaged continuously in the process.

Catalyzing the attachment process is done by aligning the mother's and father's vision of the baby and thus facilitating their encounter with respect to who the baby really is and who they really are. This promotes attachment along authentic lines during this sensitive moment in time.

At the end of the consultation, the parents are reinforced to feel more confident in their own competencies and to remember that they have an ally in their struggle as new parents; there is someone who trusts that they want the best for their baby and that they have the resources to find their way. For this reason another appointment is rarely proposed, because one wants to convey confidence (if felt). But it is made clear that the door is open, that they can reach the intervener by telephone too if they have any questions later on. They are in charge.

Of course, if there is a reason—any trouble or the mother has a high level of anxiety—a date is set for another meeting.

Clinical Vignettes

Here are a few very brief and simplified clinical vignettes to illustrate what does and can happen. Some of these seem remarkably simple but require a wide-ranging attentiveness and a positive attitude on the part of the therapist.

Case 2: A Crying Infant and Her Mother

I was called for an emergency consultation with a mother who had cried all day long beside the crib of her newborn little girl, Laura, who was also crying desperately.

In such a situation, the consultation doesn't start with an interview but with the consoling maneuvers of the Brazelton NBAS. They only succeeded when Laura had a finger or her mother's breast in her mouth. Then she would quiet down, reorganize, and become alert. With her eyes wide open, she would be ready for a conversation. She clearly showed an imperative need to suck and it was only when sucking on something that she would show interest in interacting and demonstrating her other competencies. Her mother realized it and chose to get a pacifier for Laura.

When I saw the mother 2 days later, she was radiant, the pacifier had done miracles, and she spontaneously exclaimed, "She is finally a normal baby!" This really struck me because it was as if she could recognize her baby only after the intervention. Now she knew what to do to regulate her baby's state, to be the mother she wanted to be, and to have the baby she wanted to have.

In this intervention, the point of entry was clearly the baby's behavior.

Case 3: An Infant with A Physical Anomaly

Lucas was born after an uncomplicated pregnancy and birth. After the birth, his parents discovered that their baby had a minor deformation on one foot so that it turned to the outside. This discovery was a shock and killed their joy of having a son who was otherwise in good health.

During the orientation–interaction part of the Brazelton NBAS, Lucas showed a capacity to maintain a prolonged alert state, a strong attraction to the face in front of him that he followed attentively from left to right, and an immediate and repeated orientation to his mother's voice. This response elicited intense emotion in his mother, who took him in her arms and looked at him as if, behind the screen of his deformed foot, she had never realized until that moment that there was a little guy avid for her attention and her care.

This situation illustrates the unfolding of the attachment process along the steps described earlier. The discovery of an imperfect and potentially unhealthy baby stopped the attachment process in its tracks. The parents were paralyzed. The question of the utility of such a defense in the case of a very grave pathology remains open. In this case of a very minor physical malformation, it was urgent to unblock the situation by revealing to the parents the wonderful and quiet signals of existence of their infant. In this case, the point of entry was the mother–infant interaction.

Case 4: An Introverted Baby

This example differs in the sense that it was not a consultation but a teaching session with a colleague. We borrowed a 6-day-old girl from her mother, and the observation was shared with the mother afterward.

Lea was born at term and weighed 4.2 kg. During the exam, she kept her eyes closed most of the time, concentrating on the pacifier that was indispensable to keep her from crying. Each time she was presented with a stimulus she had a tendency to seek refuge in sleep with very low muscular tone. The only way to get her into an alert state was to turn off the lights. Then she opened her eyes, ready for an interaction, but we couldn't see her anymore in the dark. Lea was a baby whose stimulation threshold was very low and who withdrew by diving into sleep very efficiently.

When the mother was asked to describe her daughter, she only said: "She is quite introverted," and then, "Her brother was much more alert and curious about what was going on around him." She went on: "During that first pregnancy, I was totally involved at each step of the process. But with her, I had to work, I was not available. . . . Maybe she felt it?" It doesn't take much to understand that this mother felt rejected by her daughter who wouldn't look at her, and she interpreted this as a punishment for her lack of interest and availability during the pregnancy. In reality, the baby only had a low tolerance for stimulation and a very good ability to protect herself by escaping into sleep instead of becoming upset and disorganized. Once it had been explained, the mother immediately could link these observations with moments when she could nicely interact with Lea during the night, when it was quiet and the light was soft. Feeling guilty, she was expecting some punishment and had interpreted her baby's neurological hypersensitivity as a negative psychological intentional act on her baby's part.

Parents need to make sense of their baby's behavior. Because the newborn's world of sensation is not yet well known, they tend to attribute psychological intentions to their sensorial baby. When a baby sleeps every time her mother tries to interact with her, the mother looks for an explanation in her repertoire of experience and representations. Having had the experience of an alert first baby boy, Lea's mother wondered what had been different that could explain this baby's behavior and found one. The very positive thing that happened is that this mother could adjust immediately to this new explanation that made sense to her. She had made a tentative attribution about her baby's behavior and not a major projection. If her attribution had persisted, that might have been the beginning of a difficult spiral of interactions and representations in a dyad where the mother who thinks that she didn't invest enough in her pregnancy feels punished by her baby from birth on.

In Lea's case the point of entry is the mother's representation.

Case 5: Stabilizing a Disorganized Baby

One Sunday morning, when I was on duty in the emergency room, I went to the maternity unit because, when we have the time, we also do physical status exams of the babies who are discharged that day.

As the consultation started, I washed my hands and talked to a new mother, while she was taking her baby girl out of her crib. She put her on the changing table, took off her clothes, and left her on her back in her diapers on the changing table. The baby started to make disorganized movements with her arms and legs and began to cry louder and louder, obviously uncomfortable. It seemed to me that she was looking for something to lean against. Her mother stepped back, saying in a tense voice, "She is nervous!"

I felt intensely that something was wrong but was unclear as to what it was. I felt I had to do something. Mother and baby were uncomfortable and tense; the baby was helpless and the mother was feeling incompetent. Without knowing exactly what to do, I looked at the mother and told her, "Let us see!" while leaning forward toward the little girl with a first goal of relieving her unhappiness.

I quietly put my hands and arms in a circle around the baby's whole body limiting the space around her. Her disorganized movements were progressively stopped by these limits, and she leaned on me with her hands and feet. Stabilized in her movements, she quieted down and opened up big wide eyes, in an alert state, ready for an interaction. Relieved and admiring of her capacity to organize herself, I turned toward the mother with a reassuring smile and said, "You see?"

She responded, "It is incredible! It is magic! How did you do it?"

"Just like this," I said. I explained to her that in the uterus, her daughter was in an enveloping limited space that provided, literally, a holding environment for her movements, that she still needed these limits and didn't like big spaces yet. I showed her how to hold the baby to help her to stabilize and quiet down and to see how then she was ready to play. The mother was relieved and enchanted.

I think that this moment provided her with a chance to reconnect with a representation of a gratifying baby that would permit her to feel like a competent mother. The threatening representation of a "nervous little girl" could fade into the background. This was a moment of meeting between the mother with a positive representation of her baby and of herself catalyzed by my intervention.

In this situation, one could observe that the mother had a distorted reading of the baby's behavioral signals and projected a nervous or irritable representation onto her daughter. This phenomenon was preparing the field for a relational mismatch. A mother–infant relationship that starts with signs of mutual misunderstanding is at risk for evolving into a negative spiral resulting in a deregulated relationship and possible problems of attachment.

In this last clinical vignette, there are several points of entry: the baby's behavior (the therapist finding the key to help her regulate her state) and the mother's behavior (by the therapist modeling behavior for her).

THE SPECIAL SITUATION OF PREMATURE BIRTH

In the development of the psychological pregnancy, a premature birth will not only produce a premature baby but also a premature mother.

As can be seen in Figure 8.1, at around 7 months of pregnancy the mother doesn't yet want to see her baby. She is at a stage of her imagination where she has a fairly well-defined image of her baby, who is closer to a vigorous, active, and gratifying 3-month-old baby than to a term neonate.

She then finds herself facing neither a gratifying 3-month-old nor even a solid and well-developed term baby, but rather a baby who is frail, not very pretty, fragile, hyperdependent, and easily overwhelmed—a baby for whom she is in no way prepared.

Moreover, this unfinished and vulnerable baby makes her feel like a mother who has not been able to fulfill her pregnancy and become a real mother, complete as a person. This incompetence is confirmed by the fact that not only are specialists and sophisticated equipment needed to care for her baby, but—even more by the fact that she cannot do much for him. This feeling of uselessness is reinforced by the physical separation from her baby, who is placed in a neonatal intensive care unit (NICU).

She is a mother who is premature, disappointed, useless, and isolated.

She experiences herself as vulnerable and having failed.

Thus, from a psychological point of view, the mother who comes to the NICU to see her premature baby is like a fragile piece of china.

One can assist a great deal by recognizing her vulnerability and helping her connect with her infant at her own pace. The mother may not be ready to be the loving mother she hoped to be. She may need time and support. For a premature mother, the holding environment must respect the timing of a woman who has been thrown into the role of mother but is not yet ready to take it on. One must gently accompany her through this accelerated metamorphosis.

Case 6: Inappropriate Diagnosis

A nurse tells the story of a preterm mother who came to the NICU for the first time to discover her newborn. She was physically hiding behind her husband, peeking over his shoulder. She was still in shock and scared. Well trained to detect early disturbed mother–infant relationships, the nurse (who had expected a mother who couldn't wait to see and be with her child) was led to write in the record "disturbed mother–infant relationship." Four years later, this was still on the list of the child's diagnoses in the medical record. The problem here is twofold: First, being a time of transition, the time of birth leaves room for evolution and change that had not been taken into account; even more, such a diagnosis may have set in concrete a behavior that might have been the expression of only transitory feelings. Second, it set forth a negative and critical prophecy that provided a specific lens for the successive members of the staff who fulfilled it.

One must be careful with diagnoses during this early period of life. They are too often to be mistrusted.

SUMMARY OF A PILOT OUTCOME STUDY

To evaluate the impact of the early intervention described above, an outcome study was conducted (Bruschweiler-Stern, 2000). The goal was to know what kind of memories remained from the intervention, whether facilitated the beginning of the infant–parent relationship, and whether the effect was transitory or lasting. Thirty-six mothers divided into three groups were interviewed by telephone up to either 6 months, 12 months, or 18 months after the intervention. An independent researcher asked the following questions:

1. *What kind of memory remains of this visit?* Ninety-five percent of the mothers had a positive memory of the consultation.

2. *Do you remember something particular?* Eighty-five percent of the mothers had a specific memory.

3. *Has this consultation helped you discover something about your baby?* Fifty-five percent of the mothers discovered something new about their baby during the consultation.

4. *Has this consultation facilitated the beginning of your relationship with your baby?* More than 55% of the mothers said yes.

5. *Have you thought about this consultation again?* Eighty-five percent of the mothers had thought about the consultation again.

6. *If the effect was positive, did it last?* Ninety-five percent of the mothers said yes during the first 6 months, and 75% said yes later.

7. *Do you think that such a consultation should be indicated for every mother?* Only 48% of the mothers thought so initially. It increased to 75% after 6 months and remained at that level through 18 months. An explanation for this may be that the intervention is so individualized that initially mothers may have the feeling that it would not apply to everyone else.

In summary, the responses were massively positive and remained so up to 18 months after the intervention.

CONCLUSION

This perspective is based on several key notions that together define the specificity of the approach:

First, we have come to recognize that moments of disequilibrium tend to open up a system for reorganization and change. Normal life crises such as birth provide such an opportunity, and in addition birth is an early point for conducting preventive or interventive acts that may have a positive effect later on.

Second, at this crisis point, one of the mother's tasks is to build a representation of her baby that integrates her "imagined baby" in her mind with the "real baby" in her arms. It is preventive and therapeutic to help her do so. This requires attention to both the baby's objective behavior and the parents' interpretation and reaction to their baby's behavior. Although the mother's imagined baby can be potentially problematic, it is far more important but less appreciated to consider her imagined baby as potentially constructive for the infant's development and to try to influence it therapeutically. Also at stake is her wondering about who she will become as a mother and her representations of herself as the "imagined mother," and more specifically her representations of a good mother.

Third, we must observe the baby's competencies and vulnerabilities, the infant's style of reacting and adapting to his or her new environment and threshold for stimulation. The Brazelton NBAS is used for that purpose. Most essential to this approach, the intervention aims to integrate representations, behaviors, and interactions. This requires a multifocal approach with equal attention to all.

Fourth, if the intervenor has been successful in providing a favorable stage for building positive experiences and representations, especially for preterm mothers and babies, she is in a privileged psychological position in the parent's mind to act as the professional coordinator of the care process and its follow-up, which is too often fragmented among several subspecialties and disciplines.

The process of facilitating the mother–newborn encounter creates very early and quickly a special therapeutic alliance that can be put to good purpose for promoting ongoing emotional and physical development.

REFERENCES

Als, H. (1984). *A manual for the naturalistic observation of the newborn (preterm and fullterm)* (rev.). Boston: Department of Psychiatry, Harvard Medical School.

Als, H., Lester, B. M., Tronik, E. Z., & Brazelton, T. B. (1982). Manual for the assessment of preterm infants' behavior (APIB). In H. E. Fitzgerald, B. M. Lester, & M. W. Yogman (Eds.), *Theory and research in behavioral pediatrics* (pp. 65–132). New York: Plenum Press.

Ammaniti, M. (1991). Maternal representations during pregnancy and early infant–mother interactions. *Infant Mental Health Journal, 12*(3), 246–255.

Ammaniti, M., & Stern, D. N. (Eds.). (1994). *Psychoanalysis and development: Representations and narrations.* New York: New York University Press.

Anand, K. J., & Hickey, P. R. (1987). Pain and its effects in the human neonate and fetus. *New England Journal of Medicine, 317,* 1321–1329.

Anders, T. F. (1989). Clinical syndromes, relationship disturbances, and their assessment. In A. J. Sameroff & R. N. Emde (Eds.), *Relationship disturbances in early childhood: A developmental approach* (pp. 124–144). New York: Basic Books.

Brazelton, T. B. (1973). Neonatal Behavioral Assessment Scale. *Clinics in Developmental Medicine, No. 50.* Philadelphia: Lippincott.

Brazelton, T. B. (1992). *Touchpoints: Your child's emotional and behavioral development.* Reading, MA: Addison-Wesley.

Brazelton, T. B., & Nugent, J. K. (1995). *Neonatal Behavioral Assessment Scale* (3rd ed.). London: Mac Keith Press.

Bruschweiler-Stern, N. (2000). Modèle d'intervention préventive au cours de la période néonatale. *Prisme, 33,* 126–139.

Dunn, W. (2002). *Infant/Toddler Sensory Profile: User's manual.* San Antonio, TX: Psychological Corp.

Fava Vizziello, G. M., Antonioli, M., Cocci, V., Invernizzi, R., & Cristante, F. (1993). From pregnancy to motherhood: The structure of representative and narrative change. *Infant Mental Health Journal, 14*(1), 4–16.

Fivaz-Depeursinge, E., & Corboz-Warnery, A. (1999). *The primary triangle: A developmental systems view of fathers, mothers and infants.* New York: Basic Books.

Fraiberg, S. H., Adelson, E., & Shapiro, U. (1975). Ghosts in the nursery: A psychoanalytic approach to the problem of impaired infant–mother relationships. *Journal of the American Academy of Child Psychiatry, 14,* 387–422.

Lebovici, S. (1983). *Le nourisson, la mère et le psychanalyste: Les interactions précoces.* Paris: Éditions du Centurion.

McDonough, S. C. (1992). Treating early relationship disturbances with interactional guidance. In G. Fava Vizziello & D. N. Stern (Eds.), *Models and techniques of psychotherapeutic intervention in the first year of life.* Milan: Rafaello Cortina Editore.

McDonough, S. C. (1993). Interaction guidance: Understanding and treating early infant–caregiver relationship disorders. In C. H. Zeanah (Ed.), *Handbook of infant mental health* (pp. 414–426). New York: Guilford Press.

Stern, D. N. (1985). *The interpersonal world of the infant.* New York: Basic Books.

Stern, D. N. (1989). The representation of the relational patterns: Some developmental considerations. In A. J. Sameroff & R. N. Emde (Eds.), *Relationship disturbances in early childhood: A developmental approach* (pp. 52–69). New York: Basic Books.

Stern, D. N. (1995). *The motherhood constellation: A unified view of parent–infant psychotherapy.* New York: Basic Books.

Stern, D. N., & Bruschweiler-Stern, N. (1998). *The birth of a mother.* New York: Basic Books.

Stern-Bruschweiler, N., & Stern, D. N. (1989). A model for conceptualizing the role of the mother's representational world in various mother–infant therapies. *Infant Mental Health Journal, 10*(3), 16–25.

Taddio, A., Goldbach, M., Ipp, M., Stevens, B., & Koren, G. (1995). Effect of neonatal circumcision on pain responses during vaccination in boys. *Lancet, 344,* 291–292.

Williamson, G. G., & Anzalone, M. E. (2001). *Sensory integration and self-regulation in infants and toddlers: Helping very young children interact with their environment.* Arlington, VA: Zero to Three.

Zeanah, C. H. (Ed.). (1993). *Handbook of infant mental health.* New York: Guilford Press.

Zeanah, C. H., Keener, M. A., & Anders, T. F. (1986). Adolescent mother's prenatal fantasies and working models of their infants. *Psychiatry, 49,* 193–203.

Zeanah, C. H., Keener, M. A., Stewart, L., & Anders, T. F. (1985). Prenatal perception of infant personality: A preliminary investigation. *Journal of the American Academy of Child Psychiatry, 24,* 204–210.

Zero to Three/National Center for Clinical Infant Programs. (1994). *Diagnostic classification 0–3: Diagnostic classification of mental health and developmental disorders of infancy and early childhood.* Arlington, VA: Author.

CHAPTER 9

LESSONS FROM STEEP™

Linking Theory, Research, and Practice for the Well-Being
of Infants and Parents

Byron Egeland
Martha Farrell Erickson

The birth of a first child is, for most people, one of life's most dramatic events. Confronted with the new realities of caring for a totally dependent infant, parents face physical and emotional demands they may never have imagined. The transition to parenthood often is a time for thinking in new ways about beliefs and values, hopes and dreams for the future, and memories of one's own childhood. Under the best of conditions, the transition to parenthood is challenging, even as it is wonderful. But for parents who have inadequate support for themselves, who struggle with the stresses of poverty, or who are haunted by memories of an abusive childhood, the birth of a child can be a time of pain and confusion for them and their infant.

For many years, we have studied the factors that support or hinder parents as they take on this new role in their lives—factors that also are critical to the long-term health and well-being of the children born to those parents. And building on findings from that research, as well as on related theory and clinical wisdom, we have developed and evaluated strategies that help parents and infants get off to a good start even in the face of high-risk circumstances.

In this chapter, we discuss that work, drawing on 16 years of experience implementing STEEP™ (Steps Toward Effective, Enjoyable Parenting), a preventive intervention program that reaches out to expectant parents and provides ongoing home visits and group support and education through the early years of the child's life. First we discuss the theory and research that guide the program, with an emphasis on attachment theory and our own longitudinal findings regarding the developmental antecedents and consequences of good parent–infant relationships. Then we describe in detail the principles, goals, and strategies that define the STEEP program. And finally, with an eye toward extending the application of this research, we discuss what we have learned about the critical ingredients and conditions for effective implementation of such a program.

HISTORY AND RATIONALE

One of the major goals of the STEEP program is to enhance the quality of the parent–child relationship in the early years. In developing the program, we were guided by theory and research on parent–child relationships, including our own research on parent–infant attachment and prospective factors associated with good and poor parenting among families in high-risk circumstances (the Minnesota Longitudinal Study of Parents and Children). Particularly important to the design of STEEP were our findings regarding the antecedents of child maltreatment (Pianta, Egeland, & Erickson, 1989) and factors (and potential mechanisms) associated with breaking the intergenerational cycle of maltreatment (Egeland, Jacobvitz, & Sroufe, 1988). Attachment theory (Bowlby, 1969, 1982; Ainsworth, Blehar, Waters, & Wall, 1978) and findings from the many studies examining the antecedents of a secure mother–infant attachment were also major influences on the development of the program.

Attachment Theory and Research

John Bowlby (1969) defines attachment as the affective bond that develops between an infant and a primary caregiver. More recently, Sroufe (1996) defined the attachment relationship as the dyadic regulation of infant emotion and arousal. Because infants are not capable of regulating their own arousal, they require the assistance of their primary caregiver in modulating arousal. Young infants are equipped to express their distress through crying and other means that require the caregiver to respond sensitively to these signals by providing contact. Caregivers who provide sensitive, emotionally responsive care during the infant's first year of life tend to have infants who are securely attached. Such infants seek comfort when distressed and easily recover from an aroused, disorganized state to a calm organized state when comforted by the caregiver. Caregivers who provide less sensitive care, who are, for example, inconsistent or less responsive, tend to have infants who are anxiously attached. They have difficulty using the caregiver effectively to regulate their arousal.

The effectiveness of the attachment relationship in regulating the infant's arousal influences the infant's willingness to use the caregiver as a "secure base" from which the infant can expand his exploration of the world. According to Sroufe (1996), infants who have learned that their caregivers will respond promptly and sensitively when they are distressed and who have learned that they will not be disorganized in the face of arousal when the caregivers are near will confidently and willingly explore the environment. As the infant becomes more mobile, regulation of arousal no longer depends solely on the caregiver's behaviors but on what the infant has come to expect about the caregiver's availability and effectiveness. The baby's regulation also is affected by his or her expectations about the potential for threat in the environment. These expectations, shaped by the baby's experience, form the basis of the child's "inner working models" of self, others, and the relationship between self and others. Such working models encompass children's learned beliefs about how they can expect their attachment figures to respond, as well as their complementary beliefs about how acceptable they are in the eyes of their attachment figures and how competent they are in eliciting responsive care when distressed (Bowlby, 1982). As infants develop and encounter the world beyond this first relationship (or relationships), the inner working models guide their behavior and expectations in subsequent relationships (Elicker, Englund, & Sroufe, 1992; Weinfield, Sroufe, Egeland, & Carlson, 1999). A major focus of the STEEP program is to assist parents in their efforts to develop effective strategies for the dyadic regulation of their infants' arousal, the ultimate goal being a secure attachment relationship.

Much is known about the factors that underlie the development of a secure or anxious attachment relationship—information that has important implications for the development of prevention and intervention programs aimed at promoting secure attachments and preventing long-term problems associated with anxious attachment (Egeland & Bosquet, 2002). Clearly, maternal sensitivity is crucial to the development of a secure attachment. However, focusing on one aspect of parenting behavior, albeit an important one, may not affect the overall parent–child relationship, particularly in high-risk families where a variety of factors likely interfere with the parent's efforts to sustain a pattern of sensitive care (Egeland, Weinfield, Bosquet, & Cheng, 2000).

Parenting and the development of the attachment relationship do not occur in isolation but within a network of influences operating on many levels. Bronfenbrenner (1977) provides a model of how personal, interpersonal, and environmental factors affect the parent–child relationship. For example, at the personal level a caregiver who suffers from depression will likely interact with her baby in a less sensitive and responsive fashion. At the interpersonal level, a supportive mate may serve as a buffer against the negative effects of maternal depression. When intervening with dyads from high-risk populations who face multiple personal and environmental challenges we believe that it is essential for the clinician to consider the many factors at different ecological levels that affect (in a positive or negative fashion) the mother–child relationship.

Antecedents of Child Maltreatment

The Minnesota Longitudinal Study of Parents and Children is a 26-year study of the development of parent–child relationships and child developmental adaptation in a poverty sample of first-time mothers enrolled in the last trimester of their pregnancy. Despite the high-risk status of the families enrolled in the project, many provided good-quality care although they lived in poverty and experienced significant life stress and adversity. Particularly enlightening for purposes of interventions are findings from parents who overcame a history of abuse in their childhood and went on to provide good care to their own children. Approximately 15% of the children in our high-risk sample experienced some form of maltreatment during the first 4 years of life. This included physical abuse, neglect, and what we have called "psychologically unavailable" parenting (Egeland & Erickson, 1987), a profound lack of emotional responsiveness to the young child. Prospective data revealed several risk factors for maltreatment. These included the parents' history of being abused (the rate of maltreatment across generations was 40%); high levels of stressful life events in the family; and a low level of psychological awareness and lack of understanding of the child's developmental needs, for example, a failure to understand that the infant's needs are independent of the parents' wishes (Pianta et al., 1989).

Even though we found that the parents' history of abuse was a major risk factor for maltreating their children in the next generation, it is important to recognize that the majority of maltreated mothers did not maltreat their children. Comparing mothers who broke the cycle of maltreatment with those who repeated the maltreatment in the next generation, we identified three critical variables (Egeland et al., 1988). Mothers who broke the cycle were (1) as children, more likely to have had foster parents or relatives who provided them with emotional support; (2) as adults, likely to be in a stable, intact, and satisfying relationship with a supportive mate; and (3) involved in long-term intensive psychotherapy. The psychotherapy appeared to enable the mothers to come to grips with and integrate the early experience of maltreatment into a coherent view of self. To test the hypothesis that mothers who broke the cycle integrated the maltreatment experience into a coherent view of self whereas those who repeated the abuse in the next generation processed information in a dissociative fashion, we compared the two groups. We found that mothers who repeated the cycle tended to dissociate (i.e., they split off the experience of childhood maltreatment and recalled childhood experience in a fragmented, disconnected, and inconsistent fashion) compared to mothers who broke the cycle (Egeland & Susman-Stillman, 1996). For the maltreated child, dissociation may be a defensive strategy for coping with pain associated with trauma and adversity. Ludwig (1983), Putnam (1993), and others note that by interfering with the normal storage and integration of thoughts, feelings, and memories, dissociation protects the individual from such traumatic experiences. However, compartmentalizing experiences and not associating thoughts, feelings, and actions make it more likely that a parent might maltreat his or her child without having empathy or feeling the pain. Mothers who broke the cycle were aware of the hurt they experienced as a child and made sure that this was not repeated with their children.

Dissociation as a coping strategy for individuals who experienced childhood adversity seems to be an important process involved in the transmission of maltreatment across generations. However, it does not account more broadly for the transmission of parenting across generations. Parenting is a complex and multifaceted activity that is the product of multiple influences. Some of the strongest and most robust influences on parenting seem to come from what individuals have experienced themselves as they were parented during infancy and childhood (Egeland et al., 2000).

Attachment theory has much to offer in terms of explaining the process by which parenting, including maltreatment, is transmitted across generations. Bowlby (1980) describes the early parent–infant attachment relationship as a prototype for later relationships. A major tenet of attachment theory (as described in the previous subsection) is that from this early relationship the infant develops a representational model of self—and of self in relationship with a significant other. At an early age, the child constructs a cognitive model that best fits the reality experienced. As the child grows older, new relationships are assimilated into existing models as long as the new experiences do not deviate greatly from the existing models. These models are maintained largely outside of awareness, and they provide the child with a set of expectations about self and relationships that in turn influence the child's behavior in relationships. Zeanah and Anders (1987) have noted that inner working models compel an individual to re-create experiences congruent with his or her relationship history. Thus, abused children expect others to be rejecting, hostile, and unavailable. Physically and emotionally neglected children expect others to be unresponsive, unavailable, and not willing to meet their needs.

From the perspective of attachment theory, it is easy to see how parenting behaviors are reenacted across generations. One of the most critical issues is how parents think about their early care—their "state of mind" with respect to attachment (Egeland, Bosquet, & Levy-Chung, 2002). Empirical data support an association between parents' inner working models and the quality of attachment they form with their infants (Benoit & Parker, 1994; Zeanah et al., 1993). This is good news for practice since we may be able to influence parents' "state of mind" through supportive intervention. In our own longitudinal study we found that the quality of mother–infant attachment, as well as parenting behavior observed at 24 and 42 months, predicted quality of attachment and parenting behavior at 24 and 42 months in the next generation (Levy, 1999).

In summary, attachment theory and research, as well as findings from studies of other aspects of parenting (particularly maltreatment), provided both the impetus and the grounding for our design of the STEEP program. With a major goal of promoting secure attachment and enhancing the parent–child relationship, we designed STEEP as a comprehensive program that addresses the many factors that influence that relationship. But at its core the program focuses on what parents learned about themselves and relationships in their own childhood, how they defend themselves against the painful parts of those lessons, and how the transition to parenthood affords a chance to move toward new models of self and other. For example, for a parent who had negative expectations about self and relationships based on representations of her childhood experiences, our goal was to provide a supportive relationship that could help modify these inner working models. For a mother who experienced trauma as a child and coped by dissociation, the goal was to assist her in integrating those experiences and enhance her understanding of how her early childhood experiences may have influenced the way she perceives and interacts with her baby.

In subsequent sections of this chapter we describe the program's format, principles, and strategies in more detail, illustrating how we have tried to achieve these goals. But first we provide a brief summary of Project STEEP, a randomized, controlled study of the effects of the program undertaken during our initial implementation of it at the University of Minnesota.

EVALUATION OF THE ORIGINAL STEEP PROGRAM

In 1987 we received funds from the National Institute of Mental Health (NIMH) to implement and evaluate the STEEP program. We enrolled 154 pregnant women through obstetric clinics in Minneapolis. Half were randomly assigned to participate in the STEEP program, and half were in a control group—all receiving assessments during pregnancy and again when the babies were 13 months, 19 months, and 2 years of age. All were first-time parents, at least 17 years of age, on welfare or poor and uninsured, and had no more than a high school education. Nearly all (92%) were single at the time of enrollment, and most reported a history of abuse in their own childhood and/or in recent relationships with partners.

The Program

Participants in the study were recruited near the end of the second trimester of their pregnancy. For those assigned to the intervention group, biweekly home visits, flexibly tailored to the unique needs, strengths, and interests of each family, began at the time of enrollment and continued until the child's first birthday. As described later, home visitors regularly videotaped parent–infant interaction in a variety of natural situations in the home, then watched the tape with the parents using the Seeing Is Believing™ approach to encourage parental understanding and sensitivity.

Around the time the babies were born, mothers in the program also began attending biweekly group sessions with others whose babies were about the same age. Reflecting the relationship-based approach that is at the heart of the program, each group was facilitated by the same person who conducted the home visits for that cohort of 8–10 families. Although group sessions were geared toward the mother and baby, fathers and other household members were engaged during home visits (including the videotaping) and periodic family events.

The Findings

To evaluate a program on its initial implementation is, in a way, setting oneself up to fail; nonetheless, Project STEEP yielded positive findings on the program's effectiveness. The areas where we failed to show positive results also taught us much, leading to hypotheses about how to refine and improve the program in subsequent implementations. As compared to the control group, mothers participating in the STEEP program demonstrated better understanding of child development, better life management skills, fewer depressive symptoms, fewer repeat pregnancies (within 2 years of the birth of their baby), and greater sensitivity to their child's cues and signals. Interestingly, life stress was associated with insensitivity in the control group; however, that was not true in the intervention group. It appeared that mothers in the intervention group learned to separate the personal effects of life stress from their interactions with their children, sustaining sensitive care even when facing difficult life circumstances. Not surprisingly, the degree of participation varied among the mothers in the program, and those who participated fully (defined as at least 60% attendance) showed the best outcomes of all.

Disappointingly, we did not demonstrate significant differences between treatment and control subjects in the quality of the mother–infant attachment when the baby was 13 or 19 months old. However, control subjects showed a tendency to move toward more anxious attachments by 19 months, while that was not true for the intervention group. Elsewhere we have discussed possible explanations for the program's lack of significant impact on quality of attachment (Egeland et al., 2000). In short, we attribute this in part to the complexity of issues the families faced and the fact that parents and facilitators were just establishing a relationship of trust and beginning to move toward deeper work at the time the program came to an end. (Note that in this initial implementation of STEEP we were funded to serve the families only for 1 year, whereas subsequent adaptations of the program have continued service at least until the child's second birthday.)

In trying to understand the limitations of the program's effectiveness, it is important to consider the cognitive and emotional status of the participants, particularly as it relates to their capacity to benefit from what is largely an insight-oriented approach. For example, seven mothers were found to have an IQ less than 70, and six of these mothers were in the treatment group. Also, a number of mothers had severe behavioral, social, and emotional problems that made it difficult for them to focus on parenting issues. This was evident when, in partnership with psychologists who were renorming the Minnesota Multiphasic Personality Inventory (MMPI), we compared the STEEP sample with a subsample of pregnant women with low educational levels selected from the larger MMPI standardization sample. The STEEP mothers scored worse on 9 of the 13 clinical and validity scales and 13 of the 15 content scales (Egeland, Erickson, Butcher, & Ben-Porath, 1991), indicating to us that we had a much more psychologically impaired group than the norm.

THE STEEP PROGRAM: FORMAT, PRINCIPLES, GOALS, AND STRATEGIES FOR CHANGE

The format of the STEEP program includes biweekly home visits beginning during the second trimester of pregnancy, as well as biweekly group sessions that include mother–infant interaction time, a shared meal, and a facilitated discussion for Moms while babies are engaged in developmentally appropriate activities with child-care providers. Periodically there also are special events for the whole family, whoever that includes according to the mother. Other than in the initial evaluation study, in which families participated until the child's first birthday, the program has served families at least until the child's second birthday. The entry into the program typically is through obstetric clinics, where STEEP facilitators personally recruit participants with assistance from clinic staff. However, in some special adaptations (mentioned below), families are referred to the program by health-care providers, child welfare workers, or the courts.

We originally developed the program to serve first-time parents whose personal history and current life circumstances present challenges to the development of good parent–child relationships. We believed that by reaching out to first-time parents before the birth of their baby (and before the parents could feel that they had failed at parenting), we would have the best chance of building a positive working alliance that would build on the parents' strengths and support them in overcoming challenges. Although we still believe first-time parents are the optimal target population, the program has been used successfully with families with multiple children. STEEP also has been adapted successfully with special populations, including families with premature, medically fragile newborns; teen parents; mothers diagnosed with postpartum depression (using a briefer, more intense version of the program); and, by far the most challenging, parents with substance abuse problems. Because of the program's emphasis on insight and self-awareness, it is not well suited to parents with a major psychiatric diagnosis or severe cognitive limitations. And when families are referred (or even court ordered) to the program because of an already-identified parenting problem, building a working alliance can be more challenging than when we reach out proactively to a pregnant first-time mother and say, "We want to share this journey with you."

A major strength of the STEEP program is the way the theoretical framework and research-based knowledge are infused into the principles, goals, and intervention strategies. As a result of findings from the evaluation of the original program and based on our experience in implementing the program in various community settings, we continue to refine our approach to meet the needs of the diverse families served (Egeland & Erickson, 1999). However, the basic structure of the program—home visits and parent–infant group sessions facilitated by the same person—has not been altered. And the program's principles, goals, and key strategies for change, which are derived from attachment theory and research on parenting in the early years, remain the same.

STEEP Principles

The purpose of STEEP is to bring support and learning to new mother–infant pairs (and the families that surround them) and to enhance the positive qualities of the parent–child relationship. STEEP is guided by the following important principles:

1. The parent–child relationship is embedded in the nuclear and extended family, the communities of which each individual or family is a part (including ethnic and cultural groups), and the larger society. Efforts focusing on the parent–child relationship must take into account the resources and challenges inherent in that larger environment.

2. The uniqueness of each baby, parent, and family served demands an individualized approach, *not* a curriculum-driven program. The focus must be specifically on this baby, not "3-month-old babies" as a group. Attention must be directed to this mother, not "mothers" in general. Also, the social context and characteristics that influence the quality of the parent–child relationship are highly varied from one dyad to the next. Finally, each family has its unique history, structure, and style— there is no stereotypical image of "family."

3. Each child, parent, and family has strengths that serve them all well; thus, the goal in working with families is to identify and build on those strengths and, in the process, to celebrate and cherish what is strong and beautiful in each individual, each family, and each culture. How we go about this is spelled out in the *STEEP Facilitator's Guide* (Erickson, Egeland, Rose, & Simon, 2002).

STEEP Goals

From among a complex array of factors contributing to what matters most for children and families in high-risk circumstances, the following eight broad goals were identified as being especially important in enhancing the quality of the parent–child relationship as well as helping parents and children move toward competence and well-being (see Table 9.1).

TABLE 9.1. STEEP Goals

1. Promote healthy, realistic attitudes, beliefs, and expectations about pregnancy, childbirth, childrearing, and the parent–child relationship.
2. Promote understanding of child development and form realistic expectations for child behavior.
3. Encourage a sensitive, predictable response to the baby's cues and signals.
4. Enhance parent's ability to see things from the child's point of view.
5. Facilitate the creation of a home environment that is safe, predictable, and conducive to optimal development.
6. Help parents identify and strengthen support networks for themselves and their child.
7. Build and support life management skills and effective use of resources.
8. Help parents recognize options, claim power, and make healthy choices.

1. *Promote healthy, realistic attitudes, beliefs, and expectations about pregnancy, childbirth, childrearing, and the parent–child relationship.* Parents who do the best with their children generally have more realistic expectations about pregnancy and parenting, recognizing both the joys and challenges that parenting brings. Parents who have difficulty with their children often have either totally positive or totally negative feelings about becoming a parent or about their children. For example, a pregnant woman might idealize the whole notion of becoming a mother, expecting that the baby will fill a gap in her life, giving her someone to love and to love her. Sometimes a mom might hope that the baby will bring the absent father of the baby back, leading to a happily-ever-after life. This is a tough role for a baby to live up to and a sure setup for disappointment.

At the other end of the continuum is the mother who thinks her life will never be her own once the baby comes. She may resent the baby for ruining her life and therefore may feel hostile and rejecting toward the child. Partnering with parents to facilitate realistic expectations about pregnancy, childbirth, and childrearing is an important first step toward healthy parent–child relationships. Helping a parent develop a balanced understanding of the daily ups and downs of parenting is a central tenet of STEEP.

2. *Promote understanding of child development and form realistic expectations for child behavior.* Underlying good care and nurture is some basic knowledge about what is normal, expectable behavior at different ages. Unrealistic expectations can lead to harsh, punitive parenting, with the parent insisting that the baby "knows better." For example, it is important for parents to know when babies might be expected to understand simple verbal directions and remember rules. Beyond just knowing what babies do and when, an understanding of the developmental meaning of certain key child behaviors is even more important. For example, parents need to understand that separation anxiety in the 8-month-old is a sign that the parent is the child's source of security at that age and that the child desperately wants to keep the parent in sight.

Likewise, parents need to understand that the toddler's negativism and noncompliance reflect his or her valiant attempts to establish a separate sense of self by moving out from the cuddly closeness of the early months of life. Saying "no" and disobeying are the only tools toddlers have for establishing their ideas and independence.

3. *Encourage a sensitive, predictable response to the baby's cues and signals.* Long before babies can speak, they have a rich repertoire of ways to tell us what they need and want. They use facial expressions,

gestures, changes in body posture, vocalizations, and varied cues to send messages to the adults around them. The parent's sensitivity to those cues and signals is an important pathway to a secure parent–child attachment and the child's subsequent competence and well-being. Sensitivity includes identifying, interpreting, and responding appropriately and consistently to the baby's cues.

When parents respond in a warm, sensitive, and consistent manner, the child learns to trust in others and to trust in her own ability to have an impact on those around her. In contrast, a child is unlikely to develop such positive expectations (and behaviors) if her parents are chronically unresponsive, highly erratic in their responses, or frequently intrusive (e.g., poking, squeezing, teasing when the child gives signals that say, "Leave me alone—I need some quiet time"). When parents' behaviors are consistently at odds with the child's desires, she learns that her actions don't count. This leaves the child feeling incompetent and increases the likelihood of later behavior problems.

4. *Enhance the parents' ability to see things from the child's point of view.* As parents increase their knowledge of child development (Goal 2) and gain in sensitivity to their infant's cues and signals (Goal 3), their ability to take the baby's perspective is enhanced. Seeing things from another person's (any person's) point of view is something that develops as people get older and become less egocentric in their thinking. People who have grown up in families with very troubled relationships may not move smoothly through that developmental change and therefore may not see things very easily from their child's perspective, or anyone else's for that matter. They may instead see most things in terms of how it impinges on them and their needs. For example, a mom with limited perspective taking may see her baby's crying as "trying to make me mad" rather than just an expression of his need for comfort or attention. Or she may see her toddler's natural exploration as "being bad" or "rebellious."

Seeing the world through the child's eyes can be an important step toward being able to meet the child's needs and gently guide the child into learning the rules of a social world. We use a variety of exercises and activities in STEEP to promote the parent's development of better perspective taking. One strategy is Seeing Is Believing (Erickson, Endersbe, & Simon, 1999), videotaping within the context of the supportive nurturing relationship between a STEEP facilitator and a family. As described later in this chapter, Seeing Is Believing focuses on the parent–child relationship, highlights the parent's expertise, and provides a new perspective from a new viewpoint (the videotape).

5. *Facilitate the creation of a home environment that is safe, predict-*

able, and conducive to optimal development. An organized and stimulating environment allows children to play and explore in ways that promote good cognitive, motor, and language development. Such an environment offers freedom for the child to explore (e.g., baby-proofing the home rather than unduly confining the child); a variety of play materials (not necessarily expensive toys, as many safe household items are great for play); organization (including a comfortable level of orderliness and a relatively predictable schedule or routine); and at least one involved, responsive adult.

6. *Help parents identify and strengthen support networks for themselves and their child.* While the STEEP facilitator is an important source of support for many program participants, it is more critical that parents make good use of natural supports that will be there long after the family's involvement in STEEP. One aim is to assist parents in learning better ways to seek and accept support from family, friends, and formal resources in the community. Sometimes parents need to work on discerning between friends or family members who truly support their efforts to be a good parent and those who undermine those efforts (e.g., the friend who begs a mom to leave her sleeping baby alone in the apartment and run out for a quick drink). When friends or family do not act in the best interest of the child, it is important to work with the parent to learn tactful but direct ways to draw boundaries and clearly let others know what she is trying to accomplish for herself and her child.

7. *Build and support life management skills and effective use of resources.* Stressful life events sometimes just happen to people and truly are beyond their control. However, many times stressful events stem from choices people make through poor planning or limited perspective taking. Through more careful planning and anticipation of possible consequences of their decisions, parents can prevent many stressful circumstances and can move toward greater stability and opportunity for themselves and their children.

To work toward this general program goal, we encourage parents to assess their current strengths and challenges and set personal objectives that will move them toward their vision for themselves and their family. This may include working toward establishing financial stability, family planning, or maintaining a "chemical-free lifestyle."

8. *Help parents recognize options, claim power, and make healthy choices.* This goal is broad and encompasses a number of issues having to do with empowerment. Many high-risk parents have a deep sense of powerlessness. They may have learned in infancy that their actions didn't count; they could not even get a response from those who were sup-

posed to care for them. They may have been stifled and slapped down when they tried to exert their independence as young children. Or perhaps they were allowed to run and explore with no limits, ultimately feeling overwhelmed by their own impulses and unable to focus on refining their skills and developing a sense of competence. For many, their sense of powerlessness was reinforced and magnified as they moved through school and into the social world of adolescence and early adulthood. Our goal is to help parents begin to recognize that they do have personal power, they do have options, and they can make wise and healthy choices for themselves and their child.

Strategies for Change

In the *STEEP Facilitator's Guide* (Erickson et al., 2002) we describe a number of techniques, strategies, and activities used as part of the intervention. While these are tailored to the specific needs of an individual or family, there are several common strategies that are used with all families in both the home and group setting. These strategies highlight how the relationship between the facilitator and the parent is used intentionally to promote change in the parent and the parent–child relationship (see Table 9.2).

Facing the Past

Perhaps the strongest influence on parenting and the developing parent–child relationship comes from what parents have experienced themselves as they were parented during infancy and childhood. As noted earlier in this chapter, infants form mental representations, or (as Bowlby [1982] called them) inner working models, of self and others and the relationship between self and others. As the infant develops and encounters the world beyond the first relationship, the inner working model guides her behavior and expectations in subsequent relationships

---

TABLE 9.2. Strategies for Change

1. Facing the past
2. Identifying coping strategies and defenses
3. Challenging all-or-nothing thinking
4. Reframing and perspective-taking
5. Problem solving
6. Guided self-observation through video feedback

as well, including parenting in the next generation. Coming from a psychoanalytic tradition, Selma Fraiberg and her colleagues (Fraiberg, Adelson, & Shapiro, 1975) believed that, in every family, influences from previous generations are evident in parental behavior and emotions. She called these unrecognized influences "ghosts in the nursery," describing them as unwelcome guests who intrude upon the parent–infant relationship. Fraiberg believed that it is necessary to recognize, remember, and contact these ghosts in order to recast and renew a troubled parent–infant relationship. Based on psychoanalytic techniques, Fraiberg developed an approach for working with parents and babies called *infant–parent psychotherapy* (see Lieberman, Chapter 5, this volume). STEEP embraces many of Fraiberg's pioneering concepts and strategies. Our approach is to develop a supportive relationship with the mother to assist her in gaining a better understanding of her childhood history and recognizing how her past experiences influence her feelings, expectations, and behavior with her own child.

As mentioned earlier, a goal of STEEP is to help the new mother look honestly at her own childhood and move toward a healthy resolution of early relationship issues in a way that frees her to respond in the best possible way to her own child. It is common for a new mother to reflect on her own childhood and the way she was parented. Using this early mothering phase as a window of opportunity, we gently explore the mom's past and reinforce her efforts to reflect on how this affects who she is today. We seek to tie a mother's current experiences with her baby to her own experiences in childhood, striving to move beyond global generalizations about the past to specific anecdotal memories of experience with caregivers. For example, we might begin by saying, "Isn't it amazing how relieved and relaxed your baby seems when you pick her up? Does holding your baby ever make you wonder about what it was like for you when you were little and needed someone to hold you?"

For many mothers, the demands of caring for a new baby may trigger their own feelings of sadness, loss, and anger because they have never really felt cared for. In our experience, some moms will (if given permission and acceptance from the facilitator and/or other group members) acknowledge feeling some resentment that they are expected to respond to their baby in a way no one ever did for them. Identifying such emotions can be an important step toward understanding how childhood history can undermine a parent's ability to respond and relate to her baby.

The STEEP group sessions provide an especially good place for some parents to examine memories of their own childhood, facilitated by the discovery that others have had similar experiences and feelings. In one activity, we put out on a table an array of messages we might have heard from our parents (in words or actions) when we were growing up. Each mother chooses the messages she remembers hearing, and blank cards are available to write her own. We then encourage mothers to remember and to talk about how it felt to experience those messages—good, bad, and everything in between. This can be a painful process but a very useful one for tapping into emotional memories. Eventually, the moms decide which messages they want to pass on to their own children and which they want to leave behind (tearing those up in a cathartic gesture!). (See the *STEEP Facilitator's Guide* [Erickson et al., 2002] for a complete description of this group exercise.)

Accessing the feelings of sadness, loss, and anger from their own childhood can help parents see things from the baby's perspective: "If I still feel sad that no one came to me when I cried, I can imagine how my baby feels when he doesn't get the attention he needs." But it seems to us the intervention process may work in a different direction as well; that is, by engaging moms in exercises that promote seeing things from the baby's view, we may help them to better understand their own emotional needs.

Also, by gradually increasing the mom's awareness and understanding of how her early experience influences her response to other life situations (e.g., relationships with partners, friends, or authority figures), we may directly or indirectly influence her relationship with her child. We have found group sessions to be an especially effective place to address these issues. A mother who has those difficulties in her own life often will seem quite skilled at seeing victimization of others and solving problems about how to change destructive patterns. It is not long before others in the group point out that she needs to look at her own life, too.

Identifying Coping Strategies and Defenses

We know from attachment theory and research that patterns of attachment and inner working models are quite stable over time (e.g., Waters, Merrick, Treboux, Crowell, & Albersheim, 2000). One reason attachment patterns persist over time is because inner working models are supported by defensive processes. Expectations about self in a relationship are, according to Bowlby (1982), built out of early emotional experiences that are intimately tied to defensive processes intended to protect individuals from the pain of difficult experiences. Defenses are adaptations in the face of difficult experiences, and change that breaks down such defenses can be detrimental if no compensatory coping strategies are available. Inner working models may be resistant to change unless alternative coping mechanisms are in place.

One aim of STEEP is to increase the mother's awareness of the strength she has shown in the face of the difficulties in her life and the way she has learned to protect herself from loss and pain. In group sessions and home visits, we talk specifically about defense mechanisms and how we use them to protect ourselves from painful feelings. We acknowledge that defense mechanisms serve an important function but point out how they also can interfere with personal well-being and relationships with children and significant others.

We also explore on an individual basis how those defenses developed in the context of early relationships. For example, for one mother it was an important discovery to see how she displaced her anger onto her son when her boyfriend treated her badly. As she talked about specific episodes from her own childhood, she could begin to understand why she learned to displace her anger in a home where it was dangerous to express it directly. This was a step toward changing this pattern in her new family.

Challenging All-or-Nothing Thinking

A tendency to look at people and situations as all good or all bad is common, especially in times of emotional stress or when we feel those around us are not being responsive to our needs. When a person has a long history of hurtful or neglectful relationships, one possible result is that this all-or-nothing thinking becomes a pattern, preventing him or her from recognizing shades of gray or understanding that people and situations are often a complex mix of qualities—good, bad, and everything in between.

While all-or-nothing thinking is typical of children and adolescents, sometimes experiences make it difficult for an individual to move beyond this type of thinking even in adulthood. This creates a problem when a mother may be unable to appreciate that the toddler who has just made her furious by breaking her favorite lamp is also the cuddly, sweet baby she loves to hug. She may swing from one extreme to the other, alternately ignoring him and smothering him with kisses, and ultimately creating confusion for the child. This same mother may react to others in her life similarly. This often happens in the case of domestic violence, when a mother, after being hurt by her boyfriend, only sees his worst qualities until he comes to her with flowers and apologizes and then she sees only the romantic guy who needs her so much.

In STEEP, we challenge all-or-nothing thinking in several ways. First of all, we look for opportunities to support the parents' own awareness of the good and bad existing together in any situation or person. We often begin by teaching the word "ambivalence," then reflect it back to parents when they seem bewildered by contradictory feelings. We are also open about our own feelings of ambivalence when it seems appropriate, modeling what we are trying to promote.

We have found the concept of a continuum to be helpful in engaging participants in a group exercise that broadens the scope of an issue and helps to heighten awareness of the area between all good and all bad. We use this concept whenever moms seem to be approaching a broad issue in a limited, dichotomous way. For example, we might draw a line on the chalkboard and label one end "sensitive" and the other "insensitive." We might ask the moms to generate a list of actions mothers do and place them on the continuum. The point is that behaviors rarely fall at the extreme end of a continuum; in fact, any judgment of a behavior depends on the context in which that behavior occurs. For example, feeding a baby may be quite sensitive if the baby is actively seeking the nipple, but it is insensitive if the baby is crying and pushing the bottle or breast away.

Reframing and Perspective Taking

Central to a good parent–child relationship is the parent's ability to see things from the child's point of view. Understanding her baby's motives and feelings can make it easier for a mother to manage even difficult behaviors. Conversely, a parent who is unable to see the baby's perspective may attribute negative qualities to the baby and misunderstand the baby's motivations and needs.

Helping the mom see behaviors of her child in light of his or her growth and development is a way to reframe the child's behavior. When we give the mom a developmental context for a particular behavior, we offer her a way to see something positive in a troublesome situation. For example, a young mother may complain that her newly mobile 8-month-old is no longer quiet and cuddly. She says he is always getting into things, and she cannot leave him for a minute. After acknowledging the frustration the mom is expressing, a facilitator can offer an alternative view of the situation such as, "Your baby is so wonderfully inquisitive and showing such growth by the way she's exploring. You must be so proud!"

Another strategy, which mothers and other family members tell us really makes them stop and think (and sometimes cry), is the writing letters to the parents from the baby's perspective. One letter from an 8-month-old who always wanted Mom in sight said, "You are the most important thing in my life right now. . . . I'd crawl for miles just to see your face. . . . Sometimes even just hearing your voice is enough to make me feel okay."

Problem Solving

Some STEEP participants have good problem-solving skills, but when faced with a crisis or major decision they struggle to work out an effective solution. Some participants, having been raised in families where crisis and chaos were everyday experiences, may never have developed the skills to go about making decisions or dealing with problems intentionally and constructively.

As outlined in the *STEEP Facilitator's Guide* (Erickson et al., 2002), a simple step-by-step framework for problem solving helps us approach decisions or difficult situations in a thoughtful, hopeful way. The steps of this generic process include (1) identifying the problem or issue; (2) brainstorming strategies to address the problem; (3) evaluating and prioritizing strategies to try; (4) implementing; and (5) evaluating success. We can talk parents through the process, naming the steps we are going through (and writing them down, if that is helpful to the parents). With repetition of this process across a variety of situations, parents discover the usefulness of such an approach for dealing with challenges in childrearing and other areas of their lives. Integrated in this process—but significant on its own merit—is the exercise of brainstorming, an effective means of involving a group in seeking new ways to handle challenges. Because brainstorming involves creative generating of ideas without judging them as good or bad, it can help a parent get "unstuck" when he or she sees no way out of a tough situation.

Guided Self-Observation through Video Feedback

A centerpiece of the STEEP program is the Seeing Is Believing strategy for videotaping parent–infant interaction and engaging parents in a process of self-observation and discovery as they watch the tape with their home visitor (Erickson et al., 1999). Mothers, fathers, and other household members participate in this activity during home visits. Through a process of open-ended questions, the STEEP facilitator encourages parents to focus on what their baby is telling them and to recognize their own skills in adapting to their baby's needs. For example, during a home visit one young mother was being rather intrusive with her new baby, getting too close to the baby's face and making clicking sounds to try to wake the baby when she dozed off. Watching the tape later, her home visitor simply asked her, "Did you notice any cues your baby was giving you here?" The new mother accurately responded, "Mom, get out of my face!" Her home visitor then was able to affirm her good observation skills and support her in letting the baby take the lead during subsequent interactions.

One new father was feeling very uncertain about how to play with his infant and, during a taping session, seemed frustrated that his baby wouldn't (couldn't!) grasp the toys he offered. But, when they watched the tape together, his home visitor asked a simple question: "What did your baby seem to like most during this session?" That prompted the young dad to discover with delight that the baby loved looking at his face and hearing him make silly sounds.

In a more dramatic example of Seeing Is Believing, one mother was clearly depressed but was not ready to admit it or seek treatment. But, with support and encouragement from her home visitor, she discovered in a video how hard her baby was working to engage her in playful interaction—to no avail. By seeing through her baby's eyes, she found the motivation to seek treatment for her depression. Videotaping helps to keep the parent–child relationship at the center of the intervention, provides a permanent record for monitoring the family's progress, and is a valuable aid when facilitators seek guidance from supervisors or consultants. Not incidentally, the tape becomes a treasured keepsake for the family—and, according to many parents, a powerful incentive for participating in the STEEP program. The major aim of Seeing Is Believing is to enhance parental sensitivity and responsiveness. But in the process of using the Seeing Is Believing strategy, we often integrate the other change strategies described in the sections above.

Relationships Change Relationships

Early in the original STEEP evaluation study, a lengthy discussion occurred at a staff meeting around the question, "What do we call ourselves?" We found many answers: *counselor, advocate, helper, worker, friend, STEEP lady, group leader, visitor,* and *big sister* were words we had heard participants use to describe us. This job does not fit neatly into any single category. We settled on the title *STEEP facilitator* because it suggests someone who supports, empowers, and encourages growth.

The relationship between the parent and the STEEP facilitator is therapeutic in that it provides a major pathway to new ways of thinking and feeling about self, others, and relationships—creating new "inner working models" in theoretical terms. The facilitator's work is to establish a supportive and sensitive relationship with the parent in order to help him or her move toward a generalized change in relationship models. This parallels in many ways what we hope for the parents' behavior with their baby: reliability, encouragement, and sensitivity.

Establishing a supportive and sensitive relationship with parents is often easier said than done. Because of their childhood history, many parents have working models of others as unavailable, unresponsive, or controlling and of self as ineffective, powerless, and unworthy of being cared for. Parents may behave in ways that set others up to perpetuate the treatment they experienced as a child. The facilitator may find herself wanting to reject or criticize a mother whose working model tends to set people up to reject and criticize her. The facilitator must understand that the individual is behaving in a way consistent with her working model and, in a patient and supportive way, proceed to contradict the mother's expectations of rejection and criticism.

In order to successfully help the parent use this new relationship as a model for other relationships, it is important for the facilitator to engage in the relationship both as a caring participant and as a benevolent observer. This requires two things. First, the facilitator engages in an honest way and communicates how she feels as an active participant in the relationship. Good communication is an essential tool in a relationship aimed at modifying working models. Listening carefully, reflecting feelings, and giving clear "I" messages can be steps toward helping a parent find new ways of interacting. It can be a major discovery for a mother to find that someone can disagree with her or dislike what she does, yet still care about her and work through the relationship. Second, facilitators gently reflect on what is happening in this relationship and relate it to other situations or relationships in the mom's life in a way that helps her see patterns or inconsistencies.

In addition, we try not to impose our own agenda on our time together, and don't expect parents to do something they do not want to do. We give parents the opportunity to identify their own needs and ask frequently how we can support and encourage them. Our agenda is flexible and responsive. There are times when we plan on one thing and end up doing something entirely different because it better suits the family's needs.

Consistent with the program principles described earlier in this chapter, we coach and support STEEP facilitators to incorporate several important attitudes into all they do with families. Discussed in more detail in the *STEEP Facilitator's Guide* (Erickson et al., 2002) we summarize a few of them here.

"I'm Not Here to Judge"

Many STEEP participants are used to being judged. They expect to be judged and even expect to be told that they're doing things all wrong. We work hard to contradict that expectation and approach parents instead with an attitude of acceptance and understanding. It is not always easy to avoid judging, especially when we see parents making choices that are not healthy for them or their children. What is critical, though, is to recognize those choices as understandable in light of the parents' own history and current life circumstances.

No matter how their actions and attitudes may be perceived by others, nearly all parents want what is best for their children. It is with this assumption that we approach STEEP participants. This allows us to feel empathy and compassion for the parents, to see their efforts as the best they have to offer at this point, and to meet them where they are in their journey to build a good life for themselves and their children.

"We're in This Together"

Accepting the role of a partner in the journey, rather than an expert, requires us to acknowledge that there are limitations to our ability to know what is best for a particular family. We define our role as collaborator, supporter, and encourager: "I can work with you to identify options and look for resources, but only you can decide what works best for you and your child."

The hope is that through the process of collaborative problem solving a parent will become more confident and better able to make healthy choices on her own when we are not there. Our own problem-solving skills are likely to improve as well. Meeting the challenges of modern life, and of parenting in particular, is difficult for all of us at times, and STEEP participants can help us and others in the program see new ways to meet those challenges. In this nonexpert, collaborative model of service delivery there is no "us" vs. "them"—only "we."

"You Can Do It!"

When we approach each family with the conscious assumption that they have strengths, we open the door to a relationship based on positive expectations and trust. For many parents, this is a new experience, having had years of hearing their own parents, teachers, and others pointing out their weaknesses and limitations, communicating to them in various ways, "You'll never make it." As described earlier, a goal of STEEP is to help parents foster their child's sense of competence and efficacy. So, an important part of our job is to engage in a parallel process with the parents, helping them become aware of their own abilities, strengths, and capacity for self-direction.

We (and the family) may at times feel overwhelmed by the challenges the family faces; at such times it is especially important to remember to focus and build on strengths. We must remember to identify, for example, parental strengths (e.g., genuine concern for the child), competence in the baby (e.g., ability to signal clearly her needs), supportive connections among family members, and resources in the larger network of which the family is a part.

As we discussed in the earlier subsection on strategies for change, sometimes identifying strengths involves reframing what the family perceives as a problem. For example, a mother's concern that her baby wants to be held all the time might be reframed as a sign that the mother is the baby's source of security and the most important thing in the baby's life at that moment—just as she should be.

Some parents have told us that STEEP was their first experience with someone who "hung in there" with them. Some even have admitted later that they "tested" their facilitator early in the program by missing appointments, acting rebellious, or trying to shock her with stories of outrageous things they had done. They also told us how their facilitator passed the test and of the powerful impact of the facilitator's acceptance and respect had on them. In one mother's words, "She was the first person who ever thought I could come through."

STEEP Facilitators

Who does this challenging work—and how they are supported in the process—are, we believe, keys to program effectiveness in any setting. In the original implementation of STEEP, the facilitators were women with a college education from a variety of backgrounds. Some, but not all, were credentialed professionals (e.g., licensed therapists, social workers, nurses, or parent educators) and all participated in STEEP's preservice orientation and training, as well as ongoing supervision and on-the-job training. Most STEEP facilitators were mothers themselves, which helped them find immediate common ground with the pregnant women recruited for the program. (It is a rare participant who doesn't want to talk about labor and delivery.) In subsequent implementations of the program, the facilitators have not necessarily had children of their own or advanced degrees.

Regardless of the facilitator's professional credentials and/or parental status, most important are attitudes and expectations. Successful facilitators need to feel and express genuine respect and compassion for the families they serve. They need to see the complexity of issues and avoid simplistic solutions for complex problems. (In hiring facilitators, we have presented candidates with a series of case vignettes and asked them to describe how they might approach such situations if they encountered them during a home visit. These vignettes have been useful in screening out applicants who oversimplified issues or responded in an overdirective way rather than trying to identify the needs and goals of the family.)

Successful facilitators also need the personal qualities of emotional maturity, stability, and clear personal boundaries. They need to be self-aware and willing to examine the way their own emotional issues come to bear on their relationships with participants. And they need to remain hopeful and see the big picture, persisting in the work without a need for immediate gratification, prompt results, or effusive gratitude. They need to recognize small signs of progress in the families they serve, and—when results are hard to see—they need to believe they may be planting a seed that can flower long after the family has left the program.

To a large extent, these are qualities that a person brings to the job. However, these qualities thrive best within a certain organizational climate and culture. We turn now to what we have learned over the years about what it takes for an organization to implement STEEP successfully.

CLIMATE FOR SUCCESSFUL IMPLEMENTATION

Because STEEP is, more than anything else, all about relationships, the program requires an organizational home that takes relationships seriously. This commitment to relationships shows up in several major ways, summarized here under three broad categories.

Program Implementation: It's in the Details

The relationship between a STEEP facilitator and the moms in her group begins at the time of recruitment. Whenever possible, facilitators go to obstetric clinics and, with the help of clinic staff, invite qualifying pregnant women to participate in the program. Facilitators tell the expectant parent (or parents, if Dad is present) they are embarking on the greatest adventure and challenge of their life. The program offers a way to help them navigate this big change in their lives and get the support and information they need to help them and their child thrive. Although using brochures to recruit would be less costly, we have found that parents are more willing to sign up when invited by the person who actually will be working with them.

Organizations implementing STEEP need to have a strong commitment to maintaining continuity of staff so that facilitators can remain with their clients throughout the duration of the program. This means offering the wages, benefits, and emotional support that will keep staff turnover to a minimum. And it means avoiding such things as arbitrary reassignment of staff to other programs within the organization or using short-term interns as primary facilitators. (Interns can fit into the program as cofacilitators or group assistants as long as a primary facilitator remains involved with families throughout their time in the program.)

This commitment to continuity also means that sometimes organizations need to stretch their geographic boundaries to follow a family when they move across town or county borders. Parents we have served typically are highly mobile, moving as many as three or four times in the first year of the baby's life. Had we not stayed with them through these moves, it is unlikely they would have found the resources and support to see them through these early days of parenthood.

In successful STEEP programs, administrators also recognize that all staff, including drivers who provide transportation to group sessions or assistants who help prepare meals, need to understand and act upon the principles of the program. Especially because so many participants have a history of rejection and failed relationships, it is critical that everyone who comes in contact with participants treat them sensitively and respectfully, reinforcing the strength-focused messages that are central to the program. When a parent's connection to a program is fragile and tenuous, as it often is in the early weeks, a thoughtless word can drive her (or him) away.

Training, Supervision, and Reflective Consultation

To do their work well, STEEP facilitators need careful preservice training and ongoing access to skilled supervisors and/or consultants to help them deal with the complexity of issues the families face. Facilitators need time to reflect on the meaning of the behaviors they see in the parents and children they serve. They need opportunities to hear and practice the words to use when they confront a difficult situation. And they need a safe and supportive environment in which to explore the ways the work with families affects them personally. Working day after day with vulnerable children and parents is difficult even for the most seasoned professional. Addressing the personal issues raised by this work is, in itself, an essential part of the work.

There are two particular aspects of the STEEP program that often seem to require special attention in supervision or reflective consultation. First is the challenge of striking an appropriate balance between being a strength-focused program, on the one hand, and, acknowledging the problems or pressing needs of the families, on the other. Although it is important to lead with the strengths of parents, children, and their networks, we do families a disservice if we slip into denial about their areas of difficulty. The second aspect of the program that challenges many facilitators is the appropriate use of self-disclosure in their relationships with families. Contrary to what mental health professionals traditionally are trained to do, STEEP facilitators are encouraged to use brief examples from their personal lives in their work with parents. For example, a facilitator might share an anecdote about a challenging time with her own child. Such self-disclosure aims to (1) give parents permission to relax their defenses and confront difficult issues; (2) cut through "all-or-nothing" thinking, which sometimes leads parents to idealize their facilitator; (3) normalize difficult emotions; and (4) model ways of acknowledging and expressing emotions without acting on hurtful impulses, such as the urge to hurt an inconsolable baby or obstinate toddler. These relaxed boundaries about self-disclosure challenge facilitators to be extra careful that their own stories don't obscure their focus on the family's feelings and experiences.

Organizational Culture

Finally, the culture of the organization needs to reflect at every level the relationship qualities that are central to the STEEP program. Administrators and supervisors need to support, encourage, and respect staff just as staff members are expected to support, encourage, and respect parents. This means identifying and building on strengths, confronting problems honestly and gently, and turning mistakes into learning opportunities. It means recognizing that, just as parents need to be healthy, well rested, and well cared for in order to care well for their children, so do staff need to be well cared for in order to serve families well. The parallel processes are striking in this kind of relationship-based work; effective practice starts at the top.

REFERENCES

Ainsworth, M. D. S., Blehar, M., Waters, E., & Wall, S. (1978). *Patterns of attachment: A psychological study of the Strange Situation.* Hillsdale, NJ: Erlbaum.

Benoit, D., & Parker, K. (1994). Stability and transmission of attachment across three generations. *Child Development, 65,* 1444–1456.

Bowlby, J. (1969). *Attachment and loss: Vol. 1. Attachment.* New York: Basic Books.

Bowlby, J. (1980). *Attachment and loss: Vol. 3. Loss.* New York: Basic Books.

Bowlby, J. (1982). *Attachment and loss: Vol. 1. Attachment* (2nd ed.). New York: Basic Books.

Bronfenbrenner, U. (1977). Toward an experimental ecology of human development. *American Psychologist, 32,* 513–531.

Egeland, B., & Bosquet, M. (2002). Emotion regulation in early childhood: The role of attachment-oriented interventions. In B. S. Zuckerman, A. F. Lieberman, & N. A. Fox (Eds.), *Socioemotional regulation: Dimensions, developmental trends, and influences* (pp. 101–124). Skillman, NJ: Johnson & Johnson Pediatric Institute.

Egeland, B., Bosquet, M., & Levy-Chung, A. (2002). Continuities and discontinuities in the intergenerational transmission of child maltreatment: Implications for breaking the cycle of abuse. In K. D. Browne, H. Hanks, P. Stratton, & C. Hamilton (Eds.), *Early prediction and prevention of child abuse: A handbook* (pp. 217–232). Sussex, UK: Wiley.

Egeland, B., & Erickson, M. F. (1987). Psychologically unavailable caregiving: The effects on development of young children and the implications for intervention. In M. Brassard, B. Germain, & S. Hart (Eds.), *Psychological maltreatment of children and youth* (pp. 110–120). New York: Pergamon Press.

Egeland, B., & Erickson, M. F. (1999). Findings from the Parent–Child Project and implications for early intervention. *Zero to Three, 20*(2), 3–10.

Egeland, B., Erickson, M. F., Butcher, J., & Ben-Porath, Y. S. (1991). MMPI-2 profiles of women at risk for child abuse. *Journal of Personality Assessment, 57,* 254–263.

Egeland, B., Jacobvitz, D., & Sroufe, L. A. (1988). Breaking the cycle of abuse. *Child Development, 59*(4), 1080–1088.

Egeland, B., & Susman-Stillman, A. (1996). Disassociation as a mediator of child abuse across generations. *Child Abuse and Neglect, 20*(11), 1123–1132.

Egeland, B., Weinfield, N. S., Bosquet, M., & Chang, V. K. (2000). Remembering, repeating and working through: Lessons from attachment-based interventions. In D. J. Osofsky & H. E. Fitzgerald (Eds.), *WAIMH handbook of infant mental health: Infant mental health in groups at high risk* (pp. 35–89). New York: Wiley.

Elicker, J., Englund, M., & Sroufe, L. A. (1992). Predicting peer competence and peer relationships in childhood from early parent–child relationships. In R. Parke & G. Ladd (Eds.), *Family-peer relationships: Modes of linkage* (pp. 77–106). Hillsdale, NJ: Erlbaum.

Erickson, M. F., & Egeland, B. (1987). A developmental view of the psychological consequences of maltreatment. *School Psychology Review, 16*(2), 156–168.

Erickson, M. F., Egeland, B., Rose, T. K., & Simon, J. (2002). *STEEP Facilitator's Guide*. Minneapolis: Regents of the University of Minnesota.

Erickson, M. F., Endersbe, J., & Simon, J. (1999). *Seeing is believing: Videotaping families and using guided self-observation to build on parenting strengths*. Minneapolis: Regents of the University of Minnesota.

Fraiberg, S., Adelson, E., & Shapiro, V. (1975). Ghosts in the nursery: A psychoanalytic approach to the problems of impaired infant-mother relationships. In S. Fraiberg (Ed.), *Clinical studies in infant mental health* (pp. 164–196). New York: Basic Books.

Levy, A. (1999). *Continuities and discontinuities in parent–child relationships across two generations: A prospective longitudinal study*. Unpublished doctoral dissertation, University of Minnesota, Minneapolis.

Ludwig, A. M. (1983). The psychological functions of dissociation. *American Journal of Clinical Hypnosis, 26*, 93–99.

Pianta, R., Egeland, B., & Erickson, M. F. (1989). The antecedents of maltreatment: Results of the Mother–Child Interaction Research Project. In D. Cicchetti & V. Carlson (Eds.), *Child maltreatment: Theory and research on the causes and consequences of child abuse and neglect* (pp. 203–253). New York: Cambridge University Press.

Putnam, F. W. (1993). Dissociative disorders in children: Behavioral profiles and problems. *Child Abuse and Neglect, 17*, 39–45.

Sroufe, L. A. (1996). *Emotional development: The organization of emotional life in the early years*. New York: Cambridge University Press.

van den Boom, D. C. (1995). Do first-year intervention effects endure?: Follow-up during toddlerhood of a sample of Dutch irritable infants. *Child Development, 66*, 1798–1816.

Waters, E., Merrick, S., Treboux, D., Crowell, J., & Albersheim, L. (2000). Attachment security in infancy and early adulthood: A 20–year longitudinal study. *Child Development, 71*(3), 543–562.

Weinfield, N. S., Sroufe, L. A., Egeland, B., & Carlson, E. (1999). The nature of individual differences in infant–caregiver attachment. In J. Cassidy & P. R. Shaver (Eds.), *Handbook of attachment: Theory, research, and clinical application* (pp. 68–99). New York: Guilford Press.

Zeanah, C. H., & Anders, T. F. (1987). Subjectivity in parent–infant relationships: A discussion of internal working models. *Infant Mental Health Journal, 8*(3), 237–250.

Zeanah, C. H., Benoit, D., Barton, M., Regan, C., Hirshberg, L., & Lipsitt, L. (1993). Representations of attachment in mothers and their one-year-old infants. *Journal of the American Academy of Child and Adolescent Psychiatry, 32,* 278–286.

CHAPTER 10

TREATING PARENT–INFANT RELATIONSHIPS IN THE CONTEXT OF MALTREATMENT

An Integrated Systems Approach

Julie A. Larrieu
Charles H. Zeanah

Multiproblem families who pose complex challenges to clinicians require comprehensive and multimodal interventions to help them. Schorr (1988, 1997) reviewed intervention programs to determine what characterized successful programs. She concluded that successful programs were (1) comprehensive, flexible, and responsive; (2) contextually organized; (3) long term rather than oriented toward a "quick fix"; (4) staffed by people who share commitment to a coherent mission; (5) linked to other "social change efforts"; and (6) characterized by staff relations built upon mutual trust and respect. Several years ago, we developed a comprehensive intervention program for abused and neglected infants and toddlers in foster care integrating the legal system, protective services, and the health system (Larrieu & Zeanah, 1998), and designed it to reflect the principles enumerated by Schorr (1988, 1997) and the relationship focus that characterizes contemporary infant mental health (Zeanah & Zeanah, 2001).

Our approach seeks to integrate several systems of care in dealing with families broken apart by abuse and neglect. Maltreatment in the earliest years of life is a serious problem for young children, who are uniquely vulnerable to the physical dangers of both abuse and neglect, as well as to the psychological effects. In fact, young children in the first 3 years of life are more likely to die from abuse and neglect than at any other 3-year period (Annie E. Casey Foundation, 2001). In addition, early childhood maltreatment increases the risk for serious problems in adolescence and adulthood, including suicide attempts (Brown, Cohen, Johnson, & Smailes, 2000), substance use disorders (Arellano, 1996), and depression (Brown et al., 2000; Heim & Nemeroff, 2001).

Maltreating parents also are known to be characterized by numerous serious risk factors for child development. Usually, the parents are poor, often unemployed or underemployed, have limited formal education, were abused themselves as children, have substance abuse and mental health disorders, have little emotional support, are involved in violent relationships, and/or live in violent neighborhoods. They often have had poor experiences with authority figures and believe that they have no one to whom they can turn for support or assistance.

Given the low expectations and poor level of trust with which these parents enter treatment, our role as sensitive and empathic guides to change becomes paramount. The characterization of successful treatment in our intervention model differs markedly from the usual presumption of facilitating personal fulfillment and structural change. Minimal competence as a parent, that is, providing "safe enough" parenting such that the children can return home, is the primary goal of the intervention. Further, the treatment has well-defined constraints. The Adoption and Safe Families Act of 1997 (ASFA) requires that a permanent plan be outlined within 12 months of the child being removed from the birth parents' home and that the permanent plan be implemented within 18 months of the child's removal.

THE POPULATION SERVED

Within a defined geographic area, every child less than 4 years of age who is validated as having been maltreated and placed in foster care is referred to us for assessment and treatment. Our referrals come exclusively from Child Protective Services, and each case that meets the geographic and age requirements is accepted. We begin work with the foster child and foster family within a week or two of the child's coming into care, but we begin to work with biological parents only after adjudication, which establishes as a legal fact that the child has been maltreated.

Over the years, we also have received referrals of children from places outside of this geographic area, generally because of a lack of availability of similar services in those locations and when there are special circumstances. On occasion, we have been asked to see maltreated young children who were not placed in foster care but are receiving interventions with their biological parents. In addition, we have at times expanded our age range to work with siblings of children less than 48 months of age; the oldest sibling with whom we have worked was a preadolescent.

Our work is intensive and typically involves several hours of weekly contact with each family. Each clinician has 5 or 6 cases for which he or she is the primary therapist. While the number of cases handled by each therapist is small, the actual workload is substantial.

THE INTERVENTION PROGRAM

Our comprehensive intervention program is known as the Infant Team. It is staffed by faculty and trainees from a medical school division of child psychiatry and includes psychiatrists, clinical and developmental psychologists, social workers, and paraprofessionals, all of whom have expertise in infant and child development and developmental psychopathology. The Infant Team is embedded administratively and physically within a public sector service delivery system that includes mental health, substance abuse, and developmental disabilities. The partnership between university faculty, trainees, and a public sector agency facilitates coordination and integration of appropriate services for families. It also makes possible one central agency that provides most of the care and assumes responsibility for coordinating all care as it relates to reunification efforts. We work in concert with a variety of systems impacting the lives of infants and toddlers, including the legal, child welfare, educational, health care, and mental health care systems, to provide assessment and treatment for these families (Larrieu & Zeanah, 1998).

MANDATE OF THE INFANT TEAM

The initial task of the Infant Team is to conduct a thorough assessment of each young child and family in order to make recommendations about what specific changes are necessary and what interventions are required to reunify these young children safely with their birth parents. These recommendations are given to Child Protective Services personnel and to the Juvenile Court. Maltreating parents are ordered to comply with assessment and treatment by the Infant Team. Once the court has ordered a case plan for the family, which is drawn largely from our assessments, our Infant Team provides the intervention. Because of the unique legal context of maltreatment, there is no confidentiality in the therapeutic relationship with both parents, as both the Juvenile Court and Child Protective Services have access to all records and require regular reporting and testimony about family progress.

If intensive multimodal intervention is not successful in making it possible for children to be reunited with their birth parents, then the children are freed for adoption. The ASFA mandates that each child who has been in care for 15 of the past 22 months must have a permanent plan, meaning return to parents, transfer of custody to a relative, or termination of parental rights. This mandate means that our interventions are necessarily time limited. Although some ASFA exceptions are possible, they are granted only when there is reason to expect that more time will allow families to progress toward reunification.

ASSESSING INFANT–CAREGIVER RELATIONSHIPS

The infant–caregiver relationship provides the primary context for therapeutic intervention and as such presents special challenges. Elsewhere, we have presented our basic model for relationship assessment (Zeanah, Larrieu, Heller, & Valliere, 2000), which we derived from Stern-Bruschweiler and Stern (1989). In this model, we assess infant–parent interaction as well as the infant's and the parent's representations of the relationship, using both structured and unstructured methods.

The representations of parents are examined by a semistructured interview, the Working Model of the Child Interview (Zeanah & Benoit, 1995), which assesses the manner in which parents discuss their relationships and the organizational quality of their discourse, particularly outlining the defensive strategies they use. We ask parents to describe their child's personality and how the child is like and unlike each parent, to give examples of the child's difficult behavior, and to describe the parent's relationship with the child. The interview assesses features of the parents' subjective representation, including its richness, flexibility, coherence, intensity of involvement, emotional integration, and affective tone. We integrate this information with our observations of the parents' overt behaviors with the infant, allowing us to interpret the goals and meanings of the parents' interactions with the child. The infant's subjective experience, of course, must be inferred. We imagine what it feels like to be that infant in that particular relationship with that specific parent at that moment in time (Larrieu & Zeanah, 1998).

Parents and infants are next observed in a standardized assessment procedure that focuses on parent–infant interaction (see Zeanah et al., 2000). This procedure involves a series of episodes, including free play, cleanup, blowing bubbles together, and teaching tasks, then a brief separation and reunion. We observe how the infant seeks out and uses support from the caregiver, whether the dyad has fun together, how comfortable they are with one another, how they share affection, the degree to which they cooperate, and how they handle disagreements. We assess the degree to which the parents can provide emotional and physical support to the child, as well as set limits, provide structure, and teach effectively. We also note the manner in which the child displays affection, complies with requests and directions, responds to learning situations, and regulates emotions and behaviors.

Other factors impacting the relationship, such as infant developmental and temperamental characteristics or maternal depression, partner violence, or history of trauma, are assessed using clinical observations, direct evaluations of behavior and skills, self-report measures, and caregiver-completed checklists.

The purpose of assessing the infant–parent relationship is to develop a treatment plan for the dyads that matches the approach to the needs of the infant and parent. Further, these needs may change over the course of the intervention, requiring use of different therapeutic modalities or approaches over time. To complicate matters further, the infant in foster care has several significant relationships, each of which must be addressed simultaneously. Thus, treatment plans for each infant must be coordinated, integrated, and individually tailored to achieve the maximum likelihood of serving the child's best interests. Accomplishing these goals in a time frame sensitive to the needs of the child requires clarity of purpose and flexibility on the part of the therapist.

UNIQUE FEATURES OF OUR INTERVENTION

With these constraints in mind, the therapist may feel some pressure to move more quickly, be more active, and confront more frequently than he or she might in a more traditional therapeutic setting. Successful in-

tervention is defined by reunification of the birth parent with the child
or freeing the child for adoption if reunification is not possible. If time
permits and the parents are able and willing, the treatment may proceed
to address more fully the myriad of difficulties with which these families
present. Reaching loftier and more ambitious goals then becomes possible.

Multiple infant–caregiver relationships are the simultaneous focus
of treatment (see Figure 10.1). The birth parent and infant typically receive intensive psychotherapy. The foster parent and infant relationship
also is a focal point, particularly to facilitate the security, stability, and responsiveness of the placement. In addition, we must maintain a focus on
the potential adoptive parent–infant relationship. Even if this "potential
parent" is the current foster parent, the nature and dynamics surrounding the adoption process elicit a variety of issues that are different when
one is fostering versus adopting. To add to the complexity, two or more
actual or potential caregivers (i.e., birth parents, foster parents, or adoptive parents) usually are identified, all of whom must be assessed and
sometimes treated with the infant.

Each caregiver or potential caregiver of the child presents with
unique concerns. Biological parents have been mandated by the Juvenile Court to participate in intervention with our Infant Team. Oversight
of the judicial system is inherent in the process, and thus the typical expectation that families are presenting "voluntarily" for intervention is
not applicable in our project. In addition to attending all evaluation and
therapy sessions, parents must show progress in meeting the ultimate
goal of being able to care for their children safely over the long term.
Thus, as clinicians, we are in the delicate position of building a working

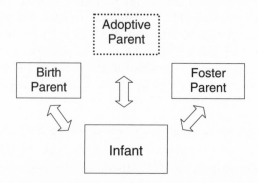

FIGURE 10.1. Multiple caregiver–child relationships in cases of maltreatment.

alliance with parents, based on trust and security, at the same time that we consult with systems who may remove the child permanently from them. To deal with this seemingly contradictory and impossible role, we explain clearly, openly, and repeatedly to biological parents the nature of our work with them and the focus of our efforts. We emphasize that it is the infant–parent relationship that is the "patient," rather than either the parent or the child alone. The task is to treat the relationship as vigorously as possible, but to evaluate its viability continuously because of the real concerns that keeping a young child in foster care and in the shadow of an unsafe relationship with a biological parent are not in the child's best interests. We emphasize that it is after the parents reveal the vulnerable and sometimes "undesirable" parts of themselves, that the work of overcoming the obstacles that brought their children into care can proceed productively.

Foster parenting presents special obstacles as well. Frequently, foster parents must care for a child without the benefit of strong preparation and education for the unique demands of the fostering role. While many foster parents have had their own biological children, they are not usually prepared for the challenges that foster children may present. They are also expected to navigate multiple systems to advocate for children about whom they frequently know little. We have found that foster parents are reluctant to ask for assistance because they fear that such requests suggest that they are incompetent at fostering. Further, foster parents are in the unique position of being asked to love a child unconditionally, even though that child may be removed from their home at a moment's notice. In the first years of our work, we found that, in spite of our early and frequent contacts with foster parents, they were not informing us about difficulties foster children were having. Sometimes, although the problems could have been treated quickly and effectively, foster parents became overwhelmed and asked for the removal of the children. Thus, we have strengthened the support and intensity of our involvement with foster parents, giving them ample room to trust us and divulge the inevitable problems encountered when a child is placed in a foster home. We have a specialized team within the larger group who provide support, education, and intervention to each foster child and parent (Heller, Smyke, & Boris, 2002).

Finally, working with adoptive parents also has challenges. Sometimes, the foster parent becomes the adoptive parent. Other times, a relative or unfamiliar nonrelative takes on that role. The task then is to build a relationship between the adoptive parent and child based on permanency and acceptance of the child for his or her lifetime. We frequently remain involved with adoptive parents and children for months following the placement to ensure its viability and stability.

TYPES OF CLINICAL INTERVENTIONS

Our therapeutic approaches are complex and multilayered. For most parents, therapeutic visitations provide the initial venue for intervention. Some parents need sessions individually with the primary clinician to prepare them before they can have productive visits with their children. Next, the core of the intervention occurs, implementing individualized plans that consist of a variety of therapies. These include (1) individual psychotherapy with the child, (2) individual psychotherapy with the biological parent, (3) infant–parent psychotherapy (see Lieberman, Chapter 5, this volume), (4) interaction guidance (see McDonough, Chapter 4, this volume), (5) couples psychotherapy, (6) family therapy, (7) group psychotherapy for the children, (8) group psychotherapy for the biological parents, (9) supportive or educational group therapy for the foster parents, (10) biological parent–infant group psychotherapy, (11) individual supportive therapy with the foster parent, and (12) psychopharmacological treatment with the biological parent. The typical therapy modalities we employ are discussed below.

THE GOALS AND PROCESS OF INTERVENTION

Because most of the biological parents with whom we work have complicated and difficult interpersonal histories, many of them have problematic perceptions of their children and themselves as parents. We believe such parents must change their distorted attributions about their children, themselves, and their relationships with their children before they can provide effective care and protection to them. Therefore, the fundamental target of our intervention is the birth parents' representations.

There are several possible transformations in a caregiver's representation that we look for to indicate progress in her ability to provide safe parenting to her children. The parent must be able to see the child as a unique individual, not as rejected parts of the self or powerful (often malevolent) figures from the parent's past. The parent also must develop an empathic appreciation of the child's experience, as well as a commitment to place the child's needs ahead of her own. She must accept responsibility for the child's maltreatment and entrance into foster care. She must be able to recognize her failure to protect the child and see herself as an effective protector. She must change her behavior as a parent to ensure the safety and protection of the infant. Understanding that help and change are possible is a basic tenet the parent must recognize, often a difficult feat for parents who themselves have had chaotic lives and been the victims of maltreatment as children.

As the Stern-Bruschweiler and Stern (1989) model illustrates (see Figure 2.1 in Chapter 2, this volume), changes in representations often change overt behaviors and conversely the route to representational changes may be behavioral. When an infant's "difficult" behaviors or symptoms are reduced, the parent may see the child as a more pleasurable companion and perceive their relationship in a more positive light. This view may bring about more satisfying interactions in the dyad, which in turn enhances the parent's positive attributions about the baby. Nevertheless, we believe it is the changes in the representation upon which enduring behavioral change is predicated.

With this framework in mind, we believe that it is crucial for parents to develop trust in authority figures, including the social services system of which we are representatives. Many have no faith that others are trustworthy or supportive, and they enter our system with the added pressure of scrutiny from Child Protection Services personnel and the Juvenile Court. Therefore, establishing trust with parents is both challenging and critical for effective treatment.

We facilitate building trust by meeting with parents regularly, in a timely fashion, and listening in a nonjudgmental way to the stories of their lives. We do so in part to communicate to them that they are worthy of help and capable of change. They must trust us as guides to change and experience us as helpful. In part to establish the parent's trust, we also coordinate our efforts with other providers, offer concrete assistance, and provide crisis intervention, as needed. We believe that by being ready to face challenges with the parents in a supportive manner, we communicate that we care about them regardless of the abusive behavior in which they have engaged with their child. This ability to accept and forgive provides a healthy model they can apply to themselves. They may be able to forgive those who violated their trust and who maltreated them and translate these changes into their relationships with their babies.

As is characteristic of our approach, the technique with which we enter a relationship to effect change is individualized for each family with whom we work. Typically, birth parents are engaged in individual, dyadic, and ancillary treatments, as we outlined above. Most caregivers are engaged in psychotherapy involving the infant, typically from the initiation of their treatment. For the birth parents, often their own experiences in childhood have been as difficult or worse than their child's experiences. Many parents report serious maltreatment, and typically are unaware of the connection between their own experiences as children and their current emotional and behavioral responses as parents. We provide intervention for at least 6–12 months, although it is not uncommon for interventions to continue for 18 months or longer, especially in cases in which the children are returned and the family requires ongoing support.

Dyadic Psychotherapies

Individual Psychotherapy with Parents

Many parents present with numerous individual difficulties that impede their ability to parent their children safely and effectively. These include psychiatric illness, particularly affective and posttraumatic stress disorders, substance use and abuse, and conflicted relationship styles. Therefore, before we begin dyadic work with the infants and parents, we require that the parents establish a commitment to treatment, as evidenced by attending individual sessions consistently. We assess whether they have an investment in remediating the circumstances in which they find themselves. Once we feel that we have established the beginnings of a collaborative therapeutic relationship and that parents have demonstrated a reasonable commitment to individual treatment, we introduce dyadic treatment. In addition, couple therapy, medication, and/or adjunctive treatments may be used concurrently with the parent(s), directed toward enhancing the infant–parent relationship.

Therapeutic Visitation

We use a variety of techniques in the treatment of infant–parent dyads. For cases in which visits between the birth parent and the infant are tumultuous or detrimental to the child, we use therapeutic visitation as a precursor to infant–parent psychotherapy. In some instances, visits between the parent and the child are compromised due to the parent's physical or emotional absence in the child's life, so that the infant does not know the parent and is frightened by being left with this "stranger."

At times, the parent is angry and unable to contain rageful feelings in the child's presence, which clearly can be traumatic for the infant. In initiating therapeutic visitation at our clinic, we hold preparatory sessions with the birth parent alone to enlist cooperation in recognizing the child's perspective in having contact with the parent. Individual sessions with the parent continue until we believe he or she can behave in a non-harmful way with the child. Then, visits occur in our clinic, where we bring the child into the session and offer support to the dyad. We assist the parent in providing structure and consistency to the visits. We also praise positive interactions and give gentle instruction when necessary. Eventually, the visitation evolves to more formal infant–parent psychotherapy.

Infant–Parent Psychotherapy

One model of dyadic psychotherapy that we use is based on the work of Alicia F. Lieberman and her colleagues (Lieberman, Silverman, & Pawl, 2000; see her Chapter 5, this volume). In this model, the parent and infant are seen together and the focus is on links between the parent's experience of her infant and her own relationship experiences, current and past. The parent's subjective experiences of herself as a mother and of herself as a child are explored. Observed interactions with the infant in the sessions are used by the clinician to discuss the mother's affective responses. A positive, trusting therapeutic relationship helps the mother to experience herself as a loving and worthy person and caregiver. We challenge negative attributions about herself and her child through sensitive support and interpretation. We believe that the mother's behaviors change as her perceptions and representations of her infant, herself, their relationship, and her prior experiences change. These representational changes are necessary for her to show meaningful modifications in her parenting behaviors.

We tend to use the Lieberman model of infant–parent psychotherapy with several types of dyads. We have found it to be very effective when the parent has the capacity for insight, curiosity about the self, and/or a pressing internal conflict about the circumstances in which she finds herself. Infant–parent psychotherapy is indicated for us when parents display intense interpersonal affect, usually toward the child. We also use this method when parents have ready access to memories for past (usually traumatic) events but have no affect associated with the memories. Therapeutic explorations may lead to new discoveries about the self as a parent and as a responsible adult, as well as discoveries about the infant. Changes in these perceptions provide the basis for constructive adaptations leading to improved interactions between the parent and the baby.

The following case illustrates the implementation of infant–parent psychotherapy with a mother who recounted, in a matter-of-fact way, her childhood experiences of horrendous physical and sexual abuse on the part of trusted family members. Her young son was active, and at times oppositional, but always filled with a zest for life and discovering what life has to offer.

Case Example: Natalie and George. Natalie, age 30, and her 3-year-old son, George, were referred to our Infant Team after she had failed to protect him from the partner violence in which she and his father were engaged. George was taken into custody and placed in a foster home. Following an extensive evaluation, we began infant–parent psychotherapy concurrently with individual psychotherapy for Natalie. Natalie presented with curiosity about the circumstances in which she found herself, but she recounted horrific memories of her past and current abuse with detachment. George presented as an active, bright boy who was inquisitive and responded well to the structure and routine maintained by his foster parents. In treatment, he became easily overstimulated by Natalie, who had problems setting limits with him. A frequent question she asked in the initial weeks of treatment was "Why can't he be good, since he knows better?"

It was only when Natalie recognized and developed empathy for the little girl inside herself, who had been ridiculed and abused, that she began to understand her behavior with George and her unrealistic expectations of him. As a child, she had been forced into a caretaking role early on, providing physical and emotional support for her siblings and her mother. When she was repeatedly sexually abused by her uncle, her mother had failed to protect her. No time had been devoted to her own emotional needs or desires, and the only playful interactions she recalled were her affectionate boxing matches with her grandfather, who had been a professional boxer.

In infant–parent psychotherapy, Natalie made connections between her own missed childhood, her anger at adults in her past, her need to be playful, and her son's desire to play as well. She wanted to provide opportunities for George to be a child, but the only play she knew was boxing. During a dyadic session, she held a boxing match with her 3-year-old, who punched her forcefully in the arm. Natalie became quite angry with him and scolded him harshly. It took some time for her to understand that in this scene she was reenacting her rage at her mother for disappointing her and at her mother's impatience and insensitivity to her experience. Gradually, she came to appreciate her difficulty in protecting George and helping him understand and express his impulses and feelings. She also came to understand that while boxing was the healthiest form of affection she had experienced as a child, she and George needed to learn other ways to demonstrate their love for one another. After more than a year of treatment, they had dealt with their issues of anger and loss, they learned healthy ways to express caring and nurturance, and Natalie consistently set appropriate limits for George. The two were then reunited.

Interaction Guidance

For cases in which the parent is young, cognitively limited, or emotionally unavailable due to chronic trauma, we often use Susan C. McDonough's psychotherapeutic approach (2000; see also Chapter 4, this volume). Interaction Guidance (IG) is a strengths-based model specifically devised for families with multiple risk factors, including poverty, substance abuse, mental illness, lack of social support, and minimal education. The parent is supported in understanding the child's development and behaviors through interactive play experiences. The clinician guides but does not undermine the parent's role as a competent caregiver. Enjoyment in the dyad's interactions is highlighted, and insensitive interactions are shaped such that they become nurturing. In IG, small samples of the videotaped session are viewed during the latter half of the therapy hour. This methodology allows for immediate feedback to the parent about her behaviors with the infant, as well as her affect during play with the baby. The clinician points out positive and satisfying interactions, and elicits comments from the parent regarding her own experience of the baby. Eventually, these strengths are used to help modify negative behaviors the parents display with their infants. The parents may at times reflect upon their own difficult experiences, either currently or in their childhood. These reflections are discussed in the context of providing relevant material for strengthening the relationship between the parent and infant. In IG, we believe that our focus on overt behaviors between the mother and infant indirectly impact caregiver and infant representations.

Case Example: Mona and Andy. The story of Mona and Andy illustrates the case of a young mother who had traumatic experiences for which she had virtually no memory, except to recall being placed in numerous foster homes due to maltreatment on the part of her mother. Andy was a quiet, affectionate toddler with his foster parents, but he expressed little affect with Mona.

Mona, age 23, and her 2-year-old son Andy were referred to our project because she had left him and his siblings alone in the home for several hours. Mona suffered from longstanding depression, and she presented to our clinic with emotional blunting and virtually no recall of her childhood. She knew she had been removed from her mother's care at 5 years of age and that she lived in an untold number of foster homes until she reached age 18. Andy presented as an adorable but reticent toddler who posed no problems for his foster parents.

Mona began with individual psychotherapy. She discussed the conditions that brought her to the attention of Child Protection Services and the unhappy relationship she had with Andy's father. She was unable to speak in any detail about current or past events and showed no discernible emotions in therapy. There were periods in which there was silence for minutes at a time. Efforts to engage her were unsuccessful.

After a few weeks, we began dyadic work with Andy using IG. During the dyadic sessions, we videotaped a few minutes of Mona and Andy playing as they typically would; in the latter half of each dyadic session, these videotaped interactions were viewed with Mona. After a few minutes of the video were reviewed, the direct interaction with Mona and Andy resumed. At first Mona was puzzled by watching the videotaped interactions, and she commented on Andy's lack of attention to her. The therapist pointed out Andy's numerous signals directed toward her, and over time she began to recognize them as well. It was easier for Mona to see Andy's bids on tape versus in the moment at which they actually occurred. However, in one instance in the clinic playroom, the therapist pointed out that when Mona looked at Andy he already was seeking her attention. This mutuality struck Mona, and she began a game with Andy by rolling the ball to him. His obvious delight and laughter elicited smiles from her. She quickly generalized these positive interactions in many more sessions with her son. However, her interactions with Andy also included passivity in response to his autonomous play and teasing in response to some of his bids to engage her in cooperative exchanges. Eventually, she was able to recognize her provocative behaviors on the videotape review, but she was unable to reflect on their meaning and on her motivations.

Meanwhile, in individual work, Mona was able to discuss her daily activities in general ways. She was unable to discuss in any detail past events, her future plans, or any feelings associated with the past, present, or future. The therapist pointed out the contrast between her warm interactions with Andy and her typical withdrawal and silence in her individual sessions. Nevertheless, we understood that in her quiet way Mona was using the therapist's presence as a secure base for her play with Andy and for reflection about herself. In both individual and dyadic work, she never missed a session and never wished to end a session prematurely. She frequently telephoned ahead to be sure the therapist would be there when she came. In individual treatment, she and the therapist sat quietly together for weeks. One day, in individual therapy, after the therapist asked her of what her current silent state reminded her, she replied, "When I laid behind the washing machine in the laundromat where my father raped me." She went on to talk about being repeatedly molested by her father since the age of 14, never having disclosed this to anyone. With this revelation, she began to address her incredible pain, her devastating losses, and her inability to hear her children's cries in the face of her own despair. She made progress in individual treatment, and her teasing and passive behavior with Andy in IG was replaced by lively and creative playful exchanges between them. After 18 months of work, they were reunified.

The foregoing two cases illustrate that both the Lieberman and the McDonough models of dyadic psychotherapy can facilitate changes resulting in a viable infant–parent relationship.

Ancillary Treatments

Adjunct therapies sometimes are necessary to remove barriers to effective functioning such that parents can begin to address issues in individual and dyadic treatment. We make referrals for these types of services to other programs inside our facility or to outside agencies. For example, substance abuse counseling, special education services, and vocational counseling for parents are referred to others. Most of the children with whom we work have both receptive and expressive language delays, and we refer them for speech and language evaluation and therapy as needed. Other services for which we make referrals include genetic and neurological evaluations and occupational and physical therapies. The Infant Team retains responsibility for coordinating and integrating treatment efforts.

SYSTEMS INTERVENTIONS

Our work is embedded within a larger social context; the families we serve are immersed in a myriad of powerful and complex systems of care. This means that our efforts are not only directed at young children and their caregivers but also at the larger systems that impact development and psychopathology. At the most proximal level, the infant is imbedded within multiple caregiving relationships overseen by a Child Protective Services caseworker (Figure 10.2). At the next level, infants and all of their caregivers are involved within the legal system (Figure 10.3). Finally, the infant and his caregivers are impacted by multiple other systems, as shown in Figure 10.4. Ports of entry for intervention are indicated by large arrows in the figures, representing the multiple avenues for connection with the families and the systems involved in our work.

Intervening at the level of the infant–caregiver relationship (Figure 10.1) includes dyadic (i.e., infant–caregiver) therapies, involving multiple relationships simultaneously, as described earlier. In addition, we must take into account the effects of various subsystems on one another. For example, at times the relationship between foster parents and birth parents is crucial, either to the child's difficulties or to amelioration of those difficulties. At other times, the relationship of the Child Protective Services caseworker to the birth or foster parents is crucial.

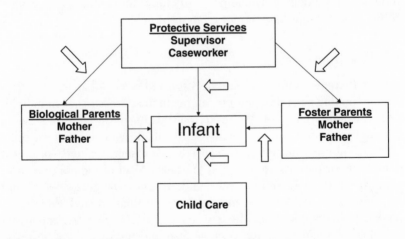

FIGURE 10.2. Ports of entry for clinical interventions in relationships impacting infants.

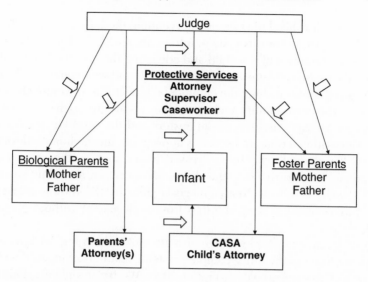

FIGURE 10.3. Ports of entry within legal systems impacting infants.

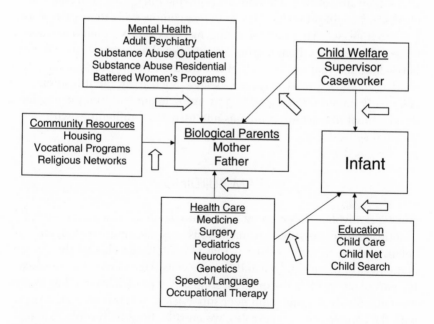

FIGURE 10.4. Ports of entry within community and service systems impacting infants.

At the next level of systems intervention, the legal system is the focus (Figure 10.3). For this system, intervention includes both advocating for the best interest of the child and educating those in the legal system about the unique and special needs of infants and very young children in foster care. These include developmental trajectories of young children, the importance of stability and consistency in caregiving, the necessity of having a primary caregiving relationship, and the need for decisions to be made within a time frame that is appropriate for the infant's development. For example, we have stressed issues such as the relationship specificity of disturbances, the distinction between attending sessions and actually achieving treatment goals, and the deleterious impact of abruptly removing young children from a placement without preparation.

At the most distal level, we also attempt to help high-risk families navigate through the other complex systems that impact infant development and psychopathology (Figure 10.4). We try to enhance families' access to services, recognizing that differing bureaucratic and administrative requirements for obtaining services are so complex and cumbersome that our families often do not avail themselves of the benefits to which they are entitled. Therefore, improving integration and coherence of services enables our families to better comply with their case plans. For example, we have helped young mothers receive child-care assistance, which allows them to pursue educational or career goals. We also have identified that virtually all of the children in our program have receptive and/or expressive speech delays. Such early identification enables early intervention aimed at preventing in our children the possible development of learning problems and associated difficulties with mastery and self-esteem.

TEAM BUILDING

Our work involves intervening with many families who are chronically chaotic and in crises, and our mandate is complex, multifaceted, and involves making recommendations that ultimately can change the course of the lives of these children and their parents. We believe that an essential part of our work is the ongoing support we provide each other in the form of individual, group, and peer supervision and consultation. To deal with the complexities of our roles, we must be flexible, receptive, and at times unflappable. We provide individual supervision at least 1 hour weekly, as well as weekly case conferences in which the details of a specific family's intervention plans and progress and the legal standing of the case are discussed with team members and Child Protective Service staff members and attorneys.

We need to support one another continually so as to be able to withstand the demands of observing repeated cases of abuse and neglect. Therefore, in addition to individual supervision and case conference consultation, we also have a dedicated time each week for talking together as a group about our individual responses to our families' strengths and weaknesses, to the frustrations and incomprehensibility of the larger systems with whom we interface, and to each other as team members. We encourage discussion of feelings, and we support one another in expressing anger, sorrow, disappointment, and aversion to the human predicaments we encounter. We process our emotions and confront our defenses in working with individuals with whom we are alike yet different, differences that potentially can set us apart. If we notice intense feelings in an Infant Team member about a child or family, we believe that it is important to point this out and begin to understand the response. Our goal is to create a working environment for the team in which it is safe to acknowledge negative feelings and reactions toward parents and children in order to identify and understand their source and enhance the therapist's sense of control.

Team members also must provide reality testing to one another at times. Because therapists must believe in their clients sometimes even more than the clients believe in themselves, the family's primary clinician generally is the most hopeful about the family's prospects for successful change. This likely is essential therapeutically, although it then becomes necessary for other team members to raise challenging questions when recommendations are made about permanency planning. The goal of these discussions is developing a more objective assessment of the situation and a recommendation that truly serves the child's best interests.

Several members of our team have worked together for more than a decade. Knowing one another professionally and personally has engendered a feeling of relationship continuity in the team itself, such that when new members enter, the transition is often facilitated by the "senior" members. This sense of family and collegiality has sustained commitment, dedication, and productivity in the face of the most challenging conditions clinicians can encounter. We believe our respect for and nurturance of our own relationships as team members enhance our abilities to provide genuine, caring intervention to families whose functioning and relationships are fragile and damaged when they enter our doors, in accord with the successful intervention principles outlined by Schorr (1997).

OUTCOMES

Recently, we examined the question of whether and how our work has effected change within larger systems. Because randomized assignment to the intervention is not possible, we examined a 4-year cohort, comparing outcomes for maltreated children in the 4 years following the intervention to the 4 years that immediately preceded the intervention. We found that intervention led to a significant change in types of outcome for young children. We demonstrated a 68% reduction in maltreatment recidivism for the same child and a 75% reduction in maltreatment recidivism for a child born subsequently to the same mother (Zeanah et al., 2001).

As with all interventions with young children, our intervention also is designed to prevent subsequent problems, thereby impacting the young child and his or her family's development long after foster care ends. The complex problems posed by young children and their families at the extremes of risk require comprehensive, integrated, and individualized treatments to enhance the relationship of these high-risk infants and parents.

CONCLUSION

Seriously disturbed parent–child relationships, as exemplified by cases of infant maltreatment, invite a relationship-based, individually tailored intervention designed to change the parent–child relationship sufficiently so that the child is at least safe (the legal mandate) and has a more adaptive developmental trajectory (the clinical mandate). We believe that fragmented interventions aimed at mental health problems of parents or children are insufficient. To be of the most benefit, they must be integrated as part of a comprehensive approach to identify and enhance strengths and to reduce or eliminate serious disturbances in parent–child relationships. The complexity, number, and magnitude of the problems experienced by young maltreated children and their families must be matched by intensive efforts to understand and address their unique challenges. A collaborative approach that incorporates clinical services into the multiple legal and social systems with which they are involved offers the optimal route to success for these families.

ACKNOWLEDGMENTS

The authors appreciate the assistance of Dr. Anna Smyke with the preparation of this chapter.

REFERENCES

Adoption and Safe Families Act of 1997, PL 105-89, 42 U.S.C. 670 *et seq.*, 111 Stat. 2115–2135.

Annie E. Casey Foundation. (2001). *Kids count data book: State profiles of child well-being.* Baltimore: Author.

Arellano, C. M. (1996). Child maltreatment and substance abuse: A review of the literature. *Substance Use and Misuse, 31,* 927–935.

Brown, J., Cohen, J., Johnson, J. G., & Smailes, E. M. (2000). Childhood abuse and neglect: Specificity of effects on adolescent and young adult depression and suicidality. *Journal of the American Academy of Child and Adolescent Psychiatry, 39,* 677–678.

Heim, C., & Nemeroff, C. B. (2001). The role of childhood trauma in the neurobiology of mood and anxiety disorders: Preclinical and clinical studies. *Biological Psychiatry, 49,* 1023–1039.

Heller, S. S., Smyke, A. T., & Boris, N. W. (2002). Very young foster children and foster families: Clinical challenges and interventions. *Infant Mental Health Journal, 23,* 555–575.

Larrieu, J. A., & Zeanah, C. H. (1998). Intensive intervention for maltreated infants and toddlers in foster care. *Child and Adolescent Psychiatric Clinics of North America, 7,* 357–371.

Lieberman, A. F., Silverman, R., & Pawl, J. H. (2000). Infant–parent psychotherapy: Core concepts and current approaches. In C. H. Zeanah (Ed.), *Handbook of infant mental health* (2nd ed., pp. 472–484). New York: Guilford Press.

McDonough, S. C. (2000). Interaction guidance: An approach for difficult-to-engage families. In C. H. Zeanah (Ed.), *Handbook of infant mental health* (2nd ed., pp. 485–493). New York: Guilford Press.

Schorr, L. B. (1988). *Within our reach: Breaking the cycle of disadvantage.* New York: Doubleday.

Schorr, L. B. (1997). *Common purpose: Strengthening families and neighborhoods to rebuild America.* New York: Doubleday.

Stern-Bruschweiler, N., & Stern, D. N. (1989). A model for conceptualizing the

role of the mother's representational world in various mother–infant therapies. *Infant Mental Health Journal, 10,* 142–156.

Zeanah, C. H., & Benoit D. (1995). Clinical applications of a parent perception
interview in infant mental health. In K. Minde (Ed.), *Child and Adolescent
Psychiatric Clinics of North America: Infant psychiatry* (Vol. 4[3], pp. 539–
554). Philadelphia: Saunders.

Zeanah, C. H., Larrieu, J. A., Heller, S. S., & Valliere, J. (2000). Infant–parent relationship assessment. In C. H. Zeanah (Ed.), *Handbook of infant mental
health* (2nd ed., pp. 222–235). New York: Guilford Press.

Zeanah, C. H., Larrieu, J. A., Heller, S. S., Valliere, J., Hinshaw-Fuselier, S.,
Aoki, Y., & Drilling, M. (2001). Evaluation of a preventive intervention for
maltreated infants and toddlers in foster care. *Journal of the American
Academy of Child and Adolescent Psychiatry, 40,* 214–221.

Zeanah, C. H., & Zeanah, P. D. (2001). Towards a definition of infant mental
health. *Zero to Three, 22,* 13–20.

PART III

CODA

CHAPTER 11

THERAPEUTIC RELATIONSHIPS IN INFANT MENTAL HEALTH AND THE CONCEPT OF LEVERAGE

Robert N. Emde
Kevin D. Everhart
Brian K. Wise

All mental health interventions involve the effects of relationships on other relationships. This is so whether we are focusing on current relationships or on future relationships, and it is so whether we are focusing on behavior or on the representational world. Traditional psychotherapy, which is not often thought about in these terms, is illustrative. It is generally referred to as a "relationship-based" form of intervention, meaning that the intervener and client establish a working relationship with a shared goal of greater understanding so that there can be less suffering and more behavior that is adaptive and satisfying. What is less often appreciated is that traditional "individual" psychotherapy involves a goal of having the working (i.e., therapeutic) relationship influence sets of other relationships. The other relationships are both represented and actual. A goal of individual psychotherapy is to influence the client's represented relationships of self in relation to other and its inner world of problematic expectations (so as to generate more reflective capacity with options and less self-defeating encumbrances). Additionally, a goal is to influence the client's current world of everyday social relationships (so as to generate interactions that are more flexible and less self defeating).

This book draws attention to the influence of the intervenor–parent (I-P) relationship on the parent–child (P-C) relationship and is thus explicit about describing how a particular relationship is intended to influence another particular relationship. The foregoing chapters, with their diversity of settings and approaches, however, compel us to extend this view to the following: another important goal of early childhood mental health interventions is to produce salutary effects on a network of relationships that surround the P-C relationship. Two of the chapters present explicit therapeutic considerations of other family relationships in their approaches (in the Lausanne Triadic Play approach of Fivaz-Depeursinge, Corboz-Warnery, and Keren [Chapter 6] and the Interaction Guidance approach of McDonough [Chapter 4]), and two of the chapters deal with multiple sets of relationships in prevention intervention settings (Egeland & Erickson in their STEEP^{TM} approach [Chapter 9] and Larrieu & Zeanah in their court-mandated approaches in maltreatment settings [Chapter 10]). Moreover, it is likely that the behavioral pediatric approach of Bruschweiler-Stern (Chapter 8) and the sensory processing approach of Dunn (Chapter 7) are both geared to influence a wider set of relationships that surround the child than the P-C relationship, and it also seems likely they aim to influence the internalized represented relationships that the child will accumulate with repeated interactions with more sensitive, available, and responsive parents. All of this extends the original multigenerational "ghosts in the nursery" model of Selma Fraiberg and her colleagues (see Fraiberg, Adelson, & Shapiro, 1975). The extension of the Fraiberg model, emphasizing psychodynamic approaches in infant parent psychotherapy, is elaborated in Chapter 2 of Stern (emphasizing therapeutic effects on internalized represented relationships) and Chapter 5 of Lieberman (emphasizing similar therapeutic effects well beyond infancy in older children).

Aside from therapeutic outcome effects, there is another reason to pay attention to a wider network of relationships than the P-C relationship as it is influenced by the I-P relationship. This concerns the process of therapeutic engagement. Prior to intervention outcomes, the network of relationships in the referral setting and in the existing family and social environment surrounding the P-C relationship can make a big difference in the levels of engagement in intervention. It is with this background that we introduce the construct of leveraging relationships. Different entry points and different action points are strategic for influencing the P-C relationship. The interventionist needs to assess the context of the intervention in terms of where there is the most opportunity, and where there is the most support for influencing a network of relationships that has prospects for initiating a cascade of positive influences for change.

RELATIONSHIPS INFLUENCING RELATIONSHIPS WITHIN A FAMILY

The approaches reviewed in this book indicate that the targeted relationships of importance for the young child are centered in the family. In thinking about opportunities for influencing family relationships, we might therefore ask about the permutations of possible influences. Mathematical considerations, surprisingly, take us beyond our usual intuitions and indicate the degree of complexity involved (Von Eye & Kreppner, 1989; Emde, 1991). Let us play out some possibilities with successive numbers. A nuclear family of 3 with a mother, a father, and a child can be seen to have 3 dyadic relationships and, correspondingly, 3 relationships where each dyad can influence the other family member. As another child is added to the family, however, the possibilities begin to expand. Now there are 15 dyadic relationships that can influence other relationships. Table 11.1 illustrates the permutations as we increase the family size to 8, with 6 children, and where there would be 28 dyadic relationships and 378 possible relationships influencing other in-

TABLE 11.1. Number of Relationships for Families with Three to Eight Members

Family size	Relationships within families (dyadic)	Relationships influencing relationships (dyadic)	Relationships within families (triadic)
Family of three (one child)	3	3	1
Family of four (two children)	6	15	4
Family of five (three children)	10	45	10
Family of six (four children)	15	105	20
Family of seven (five children)	21	210	35
Family of eight (six children)	28	378	556

dividual relationships! We could make similar calculations for the possible triadic relationships as the family grows. For our family of 8, with 6 children, there would be 56 possible triadic relationships! We invite the reader to carry on further permutations for influencing among triads, as well as even larger networks of relationships.

This complexity of influences might present a strategic nightmare for the interventionist were it not for a simple fact. For planning intervention strategies, all relationship influences within the family are not equally important. Some mean much more than others, depending on particular contexts, circumstances, and goals of the participants. In the contexts involving the care and development of the infant and young child, P-C relationships are clearly central; other relationship influences in the family may be important, but they can be considered secondary. Therefore, as in many of the intervention approaches of this book, interventions would be expected to focus on meaning and difficulties as they exist in the P-C relationship, especially as such difficulties can be influenced for the better by the I-P relationship.

Psychoanalytic and family systems theories both specify aspects of meaning that emphasize a smaller number of family relationship influences for child development. These focus on either dyadic (mother–child, M-C, or father–child, F-C) or triadic (M-F-C) configurations of influence. Based on these particular relationship experiences of early caregiving there can be maladaptive (troubled) as well as adaptive (flexible and facilitating) aspects of what the young child internalizes and brings forward to subsequent relationship experiences (see the discussions in Sameroff & Emde, 1989).

THE FRAIBERG APPROACH AND INFLUENCING
RELATIONSHIPS ACROSS GENERATIONS

Selma Fraiberg is generally celebrated as the pioneer who initiated parent–infant psychotherapy. Drawing on the work of others—especially Sigmund Freud (1920), Spitz (1961, 1965), Winnicott (1965, 1971) and Loewald (1960)—she focused on the P-C relationship within the network of family relationships as the one that carries the central responsibility for the infant's development. Beyond this, she saw the potential of parent–infant psychotherapy for favorably influencing a cascade of relationships both in mother and child. What Fraiberg and her colleagues (1975) demonstrated, using a psychoanalytic approach for understanding, was that carrying out a form of psychotherapy with a parent (typically the mother) who had her infant present during the sessions could generate insights and progress with regard to the development of the child, the development of the mother, and the development of the relationship between the two—all as a positive working alliance between the intervenor and the parent, the I-P relationship, grew over time. As Lieberman points out in Chapter 5 (this volume), Fraiberg saw it as important that this could happen before the infant developed speech and could verbally intrude; but even more important was her view that the infant's rapid development and responsiveness could be observed in therapy (with the help of the I-P relationship) and provided a huge therapeutic incentive for the mother. This led to the oft-repeated aphorism of Fraiberg: "Considering the rapid development of the infant, it's like having God on your side!" But Fraiberg's approach was also inherently three generational. As an interventionist, she could understand in a dynamic way conflicts and expectations that the parent had internalized from her previous caregiving relationship with her own parent(s), which in turn became activated with her infant and could interfere with current adaptive responses. The opportunity, with this kind of understanding, was for Fraiberg to use the infant's developmental responsiveness in a positive way to provide correction and new opportunities for the current parent to grow (and modify her internalized conflicted represented relationships for the better) as she improved her current parenting relationship. Because of the lingering unconscious aspect of such intergenerational conflicts they were captured by the metaphor of "ghosts in the nursery," that is, past conflicted relationships that haunted and needed to be put to rest. This powerful metaphor, frequently cited in the intervention work of infant mental health, was borrowed from Loewald (1960), who in turn invoked it to give an image to the uncanny aspects of Sigmund Freud's unconsciously influential repetition compulsion (1920).

The influence of internalized relationship experiences across generations has been documented most dramatically in recent attachment research. Insecure attachment patterns in a mother or father (derived from Adult Attachment Interviews done prenatally) are predictive of insecure infant attachment patterns (as observed in interactions using the Strange Situation assessment postnatally). This research can be taken to support a Fraiberg three-generation effect of relationships influencing relationships. In other words, the internalized relationships from the parent's own upbringing experiences, as manifest in the Adult Attachment Interview, in turn influence the "relationship-to-be" with the new child when that child is 1 year or 18 months of age (Fraiberg et al., 1975; Fraiberg,

1980). This is in line with other researchers' appreciation that early care-giving experiences, because of what the young child internalizes, may be influential on the later quality of the parenting relationship that results when that young child grows up to be a parent (Quinton, Rutter, & Liddle, 1984). Recently, this has been brought to bear in a parenting-to-parenting rationale for early interventions (Emde & Robinson, 2000), and it brings to mind a wise saying: "Treat your children as you would like your grandchildren to be."

The interventions discussed in this book are developmentally oriented, addressing the special considerations of early development. As in the Fraiberg approach, they also aim at enhancing the development of an adult within the parenting context. Perhaps we can elaborate on Fraiberg's simile of God as helper. There is *a strong developmental thrust* throughout life that we make use of in treatment. This thrust is especially prominent in early development. As recent research and theory indicate, it reflects basic features of human biology—what can be referred to as fundamental modes of development (Emde, 1990). But development, particularly early development, cannot be taken for granted. It requires the support of regulatory functions for survival, appreciation of times of pervasive change, and attention to directionality—all of which characterize the adaptive P-C relationship.

THREE MODELS OF EARLY DEVELOPMENT

Three models of early development represent the above principles. Based on recent research and practice, they also guide the rationale for interventions that are aimed not only at the treatment of current problems but the prevention of future developmental difficulties. The models can be presented in simplified schematics.

The first of these has to do with *regulation*. Regulation is at the core of all physiological and behavioral systems. It is a principle that involves functioning within an adaptive range of activation and is essential for life. The developmental model involves increasing self-regulation for the human infant who begins in a vulnerable condition after birth wherein much of the regulation needed for survival is supplied by the primary caregiver (Hofer, 1981). This includes much of the regulation for nourishment, warmth, safety, state maintenance, and establishment of routines, as well as for the provision of appropriate sensorimotor experiences and opportunities for learning. Self-regulation develops gradually over time within this protected regulatory relationship. So basic is this model that early development itself has been characterized as the development of self-regulation within this context (Shonkoff & Phillips, 2000). Over time, the infant–toddler–becoming young child learns to gain control not only of body temperature, fluids, and feeding but also patterns of satisfying social interaction with parents and peers. We need not dwell on this vital model but wish to refer to the simple yet poignant figure of Sameroff and Fiese (2000) showing the growth of self-regulation from the early regulation so largely dependent on the caregiving environment (see Figure 1.3 in Sameroff, Chapter 1, this volume).

A second model is equally basic and has to do with *developmental transitions*. Development does not occur in a straight line, but rather in stepwise fashion. Transitions occur when there are times of pervasive changes (e.g., in affect, attention, activity, and cognition) that are experienced as shifts not only in the child but in the child's relations with the environment. Thus when the child begins smiling socially and vocalizes to the caregiver's face at about 2 postnatal months, there are concomitant changes in sleep and wakefulness as well as in exploration and eye-to-eye contact; correspondingly, the child is typically experienced by parents as more human, responsive, and happy and is often shown more to others. Similarly when the child of 5–8 months begins crawling, he or she is likely to experience distress on the approach of strangers and separation distress when the mother or father leaves. And there are other pervasive changes. The child at this time also evidences social referencing along with the shared meaning that is expressed in peek-a-boo, ball rolling, and other games with a parent. As in the transition around 2–3 months, the child assumes a new role in the family. There is the expectation of more activity and some shared sense of rules and what is expected, as well as a clear focused sense of who is loved (i.e., a focused attachment). When one of us (RNE) began his research program, three developmental transitions were highlighted, following the pioneering observations of R. A. Spitz (1959). Now, including the postbirth transition, seven developmental transitions are included in the first 5 years and have been detailed elsewhere (Emde, 1998). The transitions are schematized in Figure 11.1. Borrowing from crisis intervention theory, Brazelton (1992) emphasizes that these times of developmental transitions are times of "dangerous opportunity" for interventions; they are both times of vulnerability and of openness for change through intervention. As such, Brazelton refers to these as "touchpoints for intervention."

DEVELOPMENTAL TRANSITIONS

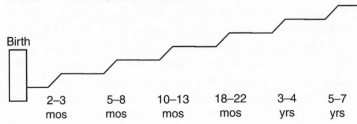

FIGURE 11.1. A schematization of seven developmental transitions. See Emde (1998).

Erikson's well-known lifespan scheme of eight stages for psychosocial development (1950) also deals with transitions. Pervasive issues or dimensions of experience are embedded in relationships and particular issues are apt to be salient at a given age although they overlap. Thus infancy has trust versus mistrust as most salient (and dependent on the caretaking environment) but also has important but less salient dimensions of experience and interactions that become more salient at later ages such as autonomy, initiative, and identity. Erikson pioneered in drawing attention to the cultural influences on the relevant issues of individual development. Less often appreciated is the fact that his scheme also draws attention to changes in the important qualities that underlie the influence of relationships on other relationships throughout life.

The third model that guides our early interventions has to do with *developmental pathways*. The image comes from Waddington (1940), who invoked pathways in his "epigenetic landscape" model for development. According to this model, the particulars of an individual's development have a cumulative tendency to proceed in a directional manner (what Waddington referred to as "canalization"). By implication, earlier deflections from an adaptive pathway have later developmental consequences with deviations that are harder to correct. John Bowlby (1988) adopted this model in discussing development and psychopathology from the perspective of his attachment theory. Two of his vivid examples of individual development with deflections and partial corrections of pathways are indicated in Figures 11.2A and 11.2B. In each, environmental events influence deflections or corrections in relation to a range of potentially healthy pathways. Thus "Mother dies" and "Unstable home" are represented as deflecting influences, while "Psychotherapy begins" and "Helpful teacher" are represented as correcting influences

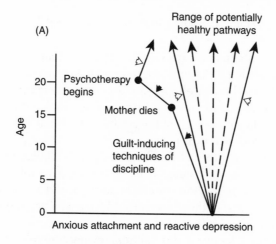

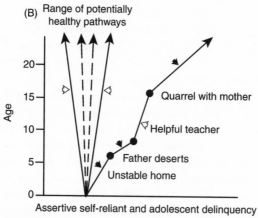

FIGURES 11.2A and 11.2B. Two examples illustrating the manner in which environmental events can influence deflections or corrections in relation to a range of potentially healthy developmental pathways. From Bowlby (1988). Copyright 1988 by the *American Journal of Psychiatry*. Reprinted by permission.

in clinical instances of reactive depression and of adolescent delinquency.

The pathways model was inherent in Anna Freud's "lines of development" (1965). It has also received considerable application in the field of development and psychopathology (Cicchetti & Toth, 1995; Cicchetti & Cannon, 1999; Rutter, 2000). The pathways model also guides thinking in the modern era of understanding gene–environment interactions across development (Rutter, 2002).

ISSUES OF DIAGNOSIS AND REFERRAL

The developmental models we have just reviewed indicate the relationship support needed for regulation, times of major change, and attention to directionality. The models provide a general background for assessment and treatment, but how children are diagnosed and referred are of practical importance for each of the settings described in this book. It is to these issues that we turn next.

Most of the chapters of this book deal with clinical problems that have been referred, and some deal with preventive intervention programs. Sources of motivation, parental concerns, and available resources are likely to vary across these domains. Moreover, what gets referred often depends on diagnosis.

Rosenblum (Chapter 3, this volume) reviews the role of diagnosis in identifying those problems in early development and infant mental health that require clinical attention. Diagnosis, which involves the classification of disorder (Axes I–III on DSM-IV [American Psychiatric Association, 1994] and DC: 0–3 [Zero to Three/National Center for Infants, Toddlers, & Families, 1994]) and the assessment of individuals (Axes IV and V on DSM-IV and DC: 0–3), is used for clinical formulation as well as linking to knowledge, communication, among professionals and connecting with services (Emde & Wise, in press). Although many would like to see diagnostic classification based more on dimensions than categories, as Rosenblum suggests, the latter are likely to remain in use since they provide "cutoffs" for clinical decisions about services as well as efficiencies in communication. She indicates that the newer classifications and assessments in DC: 0–3 appear useful for clinicians, including the innovative classifications of regulatory disorders and relationship disorders. The excellent clinical study of Keren, Feldman, and Tyano (2001) in Tel Aviv is cited, and we can now supplement their data with additional clinical trials of DC: 0–3 and additional numbers of cases that have been added to the Tel Aviv experience. Data are available from clinicians in Montreal, Paris, Lisbon, and Topeka, Kansas, as well as Tel Aviv. (The clinical data from these trials became available since the time of the workshop on which this book is based and are included in a special issue of the *Infant Mental Health Journal* (Emde & Wise, 2003; Guedeney et al., 2003; Keren, Feldman, & Tyano, 2003; Cordeiro, Caldeira da Silva, & Goldschmidt, 2003; Maldonado-Duran et al., 2003; Minde & Tidmarsh, 1997). The number of cases seen and the percentages of classifications for Axes I, II, and III across the five sites provide further documentation that DC: 0–3 is useful. The number of cases assessed at each site varied from 57 to 431. Overall, most but not all of the children referred received a Primary Diagnosis classification on Axis I (45–90% were diagnosed on this axis across sites). A substantial number received a Relationship Disorder classification on Axis II (37–62% across sites), and 19–68% received a Medical and Developmental Disorders classification on Axis III. Not only do the clinicians working at these sites appear to welcome the new system for the syndromes on Axis I, but, as important, they frequently make use of Axis II by classifying presenting problems as relationship disorders.

The settings of referral are clearly important in generating these percentages, and they cannot be considered representative of a specified population or generalizable in any way. This fact is perhaps most clearly instantiated by the different percentages on Axis III that are directly attributable to referral sources. In Tel Aviv, for example, as noted by Keren et al. (2001), there was another nearby center that provided services for disabilities resulting in a low percentage of referrals in this area (19%), whereas in Paris such referrals were expected for their setting since related services were provided (and 68% were classified on Axis III).

Table 11.2 summarizes the percentages of classifications on Axis I for DC: 0–3. Considerable variation of classification percentages by site is apparent, presumably as a reflection of referral sources. Regulatory disorders vary from 5 to 43% of diagnoses at sites; affect disorders, from

TABLE 11.2. Axis I Disorders by Percentage (from Emde & Wise, 2003)

	Montreal (N = 57)	Tel Aviv (N = 431)	Paris (N = 85)	Lisbon (N = 343)	Topeka (N = 167)
Regulatory disorder	37	5	12	7	43
Eating disorder	0	12	1	3	4
Sleep disorder	0	10	7	2	3
Affect disorder	14	9	32	26	8
Adjustment disorder	11	7	5	6	11
Traumatic stress disorder	0	1	4	2	12
Multisystem developmental disorder	5	0	13	10	10
Other disorder	12	1	0[a]	0	0
No classification	21	55	24	36[b]	10

[a]This percentage excludes 3.5% with a DSM-IV diagnosis of autism.
[b]This percentage includes 43 cases listed as "deferred" or "unknown" by the Lisbon authors.

8 to 32% of diagnoses; traumatic stress disorders, from 0 to 12% of diagnoses; and adjustment disorders, from 5 to 11%.

Settings of referral are important. To use Stern's metaphor (see Chapter 2, this volume), there can be multiple ports of entry for favorable interventions of therapeutic relationships influencing any given P-C relationship. The contributors to this book report experiences with different approaches that, by implication, yield successful outcomes in different ways. There may be some degree of equifinality across approaches, as Stern suggests, but how intervention gets started and continues, let alone moves, requires more consideration. To this consideration, we offer the concept of leverage.

THE CONCEPT OF LEVERAGE

What is leverage? We use it as a construct to indicate thinking about a maximum point of efficiency for intervention in the process of relationships influencing other relationships. Leverage has to do with perceived "best opportunities" for engaging therapeutic or preventive change in a relationship that is embedded in a network of other relationships. Thus strategic leverage has the possibility of generating positive developmental change in other relationships as well. Leverage has to do with seizing best opportunities for motivation, and it also depends upon the definitions of concern.

From where do these "best opportunities" arise? From an ecological perspective, we suggest that leverage occurs as a function of the extent to which individuals in various systems concur on the nature of a given clinical concern and the potential solutions to resolving the concern. Points of leverage must be negotiated within systems and coordinated among differing sources of motivation for change and differing concerns for the child.

Figure 11.3 illustrates a leverage point between sources of motivation and definitions of concern for the child. The arrows on either side of the leverage point reflect weights that could influence potential leverage points. Leverage is also depicted as occurring within an array of potential intervention processes, which together encompass the three R's of *redefinition, remediation*, and *reeducation* described in Sameroff, Chapter 1, this volume (also see Sameroff & Fiese, 2000). To the right of what we have depicted as the leverage point, we have arrayed potential definitions of concern for the child. Concerns related to safety from abuse or neglect are sometimes silent but have high priority. Concerns related to

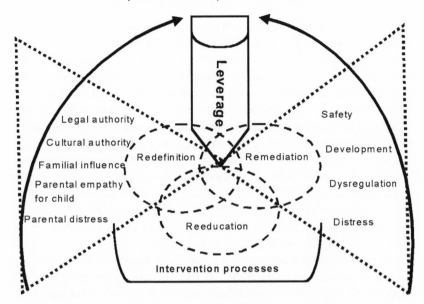

FIGURE 11.3. One view of therapeutic leverage for the P-C relationship. The figure illustrates leverage at the interface between sources of motivation, definitions of concern for the child, and the three R's of intervention.

developmental disabilities are also prominent, as are those related to dysfunctional regulatory processes and emotional distress. Note that these areas of concern, while not mutually exclusive, have the function of framing the nature of the problem to be addressed through the intervention. Also, note that clinicians often experience differences of opinion regarding which concerns deserve attention. These differences can increase in magnitude when concerns are prioritized differently by multiple individuals holding influence in the child's life.

To the left of the leverage point, we have arrayed sources of motivation. As indicated, the impetus for interventions directed toward infants and families may originate from broad systemic sources, such as legal authority (as in cases of child protection), or via referrals motivated by an observed deviance from cultural expectations (as when an infant is not "sleeping through the night"). Motivation may also originate from within a family, from a parent's empathy for the child, or even as a "cry for help" from a distressed and overwhelmed parent. These sources of motivation are not mutually exclusive. For example, cultural authority cannot easily be teased apart from legal and familial influences. Note further that any combination of sources of motivation may be paired with any combination of definitions of concern for the child. Thus, parents may be distressed by "dangerous," "impulsive," or dysregulated behaviors they have observed in their children. Similarly, a pediatrician might express concern regarding a child's attainment of developmental milestones.

As every clinician knows, motivation matters. And with different sources of motivation come different valances of authority. Aspects of authority, although not often discussed, are ubiquitous in all relationships. The parent holds authority in relation to the child. From a cultural perspective, the expert holds authority over the parent. The legal system holds authority over the expert, the parent, and the child. It is also the case that sources of authority and power may be helpful (e.g., in providing structure and resources) or not helpful (e.g., in not providing or denying access to needed structure or resources).

The motivational aspects of authority are illustrated by the work of Larrieu and Zeanah (see Chapter 10, this volume). They describe their work in attempting to reunify infants with birth parents who have been adjudicated for maltreatment. Their program reflects the structure of the Adoption and Safe Families Act of 1997 (ASFA), which mandates that a child who has been placed in out-of-home care for 15 of the past 22 months must have a permanent placement plan, meaning either return to parental custody, transfer of custody to a relative, or termination of parental rights. The program provides dyadic psychotherapy, individual therapy, and ancillary treatments, in accordance with the goal of preventing repeated victimization. According to a recent 4-year cohort study described by Larrieu and Zeanah, the program demonstrated a 68% reduction in maltreatment recidivism for the same child and a 75% reduction for maltreatment recidivism for a child born subsequently to the same mother, while simultaneously leading to more terminations [of parental rights] and fewer reunifications with birth parents. What is most germane to this discussion is that the leverage for change comes from the authority of the state—and by extension the authority of the therapist/evaluator. This leverage is applied as a means of generating change within the individual parent, out of a concern for the safety of the child (see Figure 11.3). The power differential makes use of an explicit timeline for the termination of parental rights in order to leverage parental compliance. To some this may sound harsh, but such a power differential is not new. In many ways, it merely specifies dynamics that most of us regularly encounter in our work with Child Protective Services. Through the use of a timeline, this dynamic provides focus and intensity.

Although the field of mental health in early childhood has a growing tradition of considering cultural variation and ecology (Erikson, 1950; Johnson-Powell, 1997; Garcia Coll & Magnuson, 2000; Emde & Spicer, 2000; Lewis, 2000; Christensen, Emde, & Fleming, in press), clinical theorizing sometimes tends to focus on universality in the role of maternal representations. Stern's discussion of maternal psychological reorganization, "the motherhood constellation," exemplifies this picture (see Chapter 2, this volume). Stern provides the context for a formulation of the mother–infant relationship as a new "prototypic patient," building on this formulation to suggest that there is "equifinality" with regard to the interdependence of symbolic and behavioral aspects of therapeutic strategies as they exist in different interventions. Thus, changes in maternal object relations as found in the mother's representations beget changes in caregiving behavior; similarly, changes in caregiving behavior beget changes in maternal object relations. Correspondingly, Stern suggests that ports of entry into an intervention may not make a difference. As the reader may note from the present chapter, we take issue with this suggestion. Because of different sources of motivation and parental concern, not all ports of entry are possible, and some may be more efficient than others. The interventionist needs to engage the parent and the child. For this as well as for the development of a working alliance there needs to be some agreement with regard to the nature of problems and solutions (Everhart & Wandersman, 2000). In other words, we agree that an "equifinality" can occur with outcomes from different intervention approaches, but this requires that individuals in various subsystems concur on the nature of a given clinical issue or diagnosis, goals, and potential solutions.

We would add one other point about leveraging according to individual circumstances in order to maximize the process of being helpful. This has to do with encouraging a shared narrative understanding between the interventionist and parent. A narrative can be thought of as a story—a story through which the therapist and the client may come to understand why problems develop and what can be done to remediate them. While this subjectivity may pose a challenge to clinicians who strongly identify with a particular theoretical orientation or modality of treatment, we suggest that few would disagree that successful interventions are those that are leveraged by intrinsic motivations, resources, and developmental processes within infants, parents, families, and cultures; moreover, most would agree that a coherent and shared story about what happens adds to the process.

The development of a therapeutic alliance can be thought of as a negotiation of narratives, with therapeutic leverage being derived from a shared view of the problem and the mobilization of existing resources and capacities to promote remediation. From this perspective, we can view the myriad of therapeutic approaches to working with infants and families—many of which are arrayed in this book—as examples of narratives of potential import. Indeed, it is possible to restate the concept of *redefinition* described by Sameroff in Chapter 1, this volume, as a process of narrative transformation: the story of the problem is retold, making new outcomes possible.

THERAPEUTIC LEVERAGE
BEYOND THE INFANT–PARENT RELATIONSHIP:
TWO DRAMATIC EXAMPLES

We have drawn attention to the fact that intervention involves more than the I-P relationship influencing the P-C relationship. Current applications of the Fraiberg model, as the chapters of this book illustrate, involve the influence of relationships on multiple other relationships. Moreover, the development of the P-C relationship is embedded in a network of other influential relationships. Therapeutic leverage has to do with a strategic decision about which relationships within a network provide maximum opportunities for change. Choosing which relationships to enhance (and initiating therapeutic leverage in this sense) depends upon assessments of motivation, available resources, and often political–social circumstances. These factors are particularly salient for preventive intervention programs. Two dramatic examples of such interventions, separated by 60 years, are illustrative. Each takes us well beyond leverage centered on the I-P relationship influencing the P-C relationship.

The first example of such a program, carried out in the mid-1930s, remains one of the most remarkable stories in the history of preventive intervention. We summarize this story from a 30-year follow-up of the intervention, published as a *Monograph of the Society for Research in Child Development* (Skeels, 1966). At the time the story begins, a predominant eugenics view guided practices in the United States and elsewhere. Babies who had been relinquished by their mothers were kept in orphanages for long periods of time in order to see whether they would be found suitable for adoption or, as would be expectable for a large proportion of them, instead discovered to be retarded in a way that manifested a "constitutionally inferior" state. We now know from subsequent work of Spitz (1945, 1946), Bowlby (1944, 1958, 1969), and many others that prolonged exposure to institutional environments with multiple changing caregivers largely contributed to developmental declines and "retardation"—but this was not known then. Howard M. Skeels, in the early 1930s, was a young psychologist placed in charge of a public orphanage for infants in Iowa. As was true for most such places at the time, the institution was understaffed, caregivers were multiple and changing, and there was little opportunity for play, with infant interactions typically limited to feeding, dressing, and diapering. Skeels's intervention grew out of his initial observations. When he was introduced to his orphanage, he observed a typical staffing. The discussion was designed to see if older infants brought to staffing were suitable for adoption or instead should be transferred to an institution for the mentally retarded. He took note of two girls who were frail and developmentally retarded. Those in charge of the staffing considered the girls not suitable for adoption, and they were then transferred to a nearby institution for the mentally retarded. At the time of transfer one was 15 months of age and the other 18 months of age.

Skeels's responsibilities were then increased. In addition to the orphanage, he was made responsible for two state institutions for the mentally retarded, including the locations where the two girls had been transferred. Six months after the transfer he visited the institutions and saw the two girls. They were alert, smiling, and active—looking like normal toddlers. He hardly recognized them in view of their dire prognoses. He then examined them 12 months later and found they had mental development within the normal range. What accounted for the difference? Each of the two girls had been placed on a ward with some older women, whose ages ranged from 18 to 50 years and whose mental ages ranged from 5 to 9 years, and where the girls were the only children of preschool age. Upon inquiry, he discovered that each of the girls had been "adopted" by an older inmate who became a caregiver and that others who were around served as "adoring aunts" in a way that struck Skeels as providing a rich affectionate environment that, in contrast to the orphanage, was more homelike.

At this point Skeels decided on an incredibly bold experiment. He thought of it as one to see if retardation in infancy might be reversible. From our point of view, he also seized upon an opportunity for leverage that made use of other relationships he had serendipitously discovered to be influential. He made use of limited resources and his administrative opportunity. He systematically composed an experimental (E) group of 13 children from the orphanage who were designated as unsuitable for adoption and, hence according to the rules of the time, were transferred to the institution for the mentally retarded. At the institution he made it possible for each to be a "house guest" on a ward so that a mentally retarded affectionate woman caregiver could emerge and other "aunts" could also connect to each individual infant as had happened with the two girls. He also systematically composed a contrast (C) group of 12 orphanage infants who were not considered retarded and, hence according to the rules at the time, should not be transferred to the institution for the mentally retarded. The children were then followed.

Two years later there was a developmental reversal of fortune for the two groups. The E group had an average gain of 29 IQ points, while the C group had a loss of 26 points. Five years later this trend was sustained. All in the E group were adopted by families in the community, whereas none in the C group were adopted 5 years later. On 30-year follow-up, it is difficult to imagine more dramatic results. The median grade completed for the two groups was 12.0 for the E group versus 2.75 for the C group; five had some college versus only one who went beyond eighth grade. All were self-supporting in the E group versus most who were dependent on others with five still in institutions in the C group. Finally, to put a nail in the coffin of the old eugenics idea, the 28 offspring of the children of the E group (i.e., the next generation) had a mean IQ from school records of 104.

We cannot resist a footnote to the Skeels story. The intervention period lasted only 3 years. It was ended when a change in administration of the state institutions decided it could not tolerate "such untidy procedures as having 'house guests' in an institution" (Skeels, 1966, p. 9). In Skeels's moving conclusion to his monograph, he comments on the enabling effects of the intervention relationships in allowing for regular adoptions. He then states, "It can be postulated that if the children in the contrast group had been placed in suitable adoptive homes or given some other appropriate equivalent in early infancy, most or all of them would have achieved within the normal range of development, as did the experimental subjects. . . . The unanswered questions of this study could form the basis for many lifelong research projects. If the tragic fate of the 12 contrast group children provokes even a single crucial study that will help prevent such a fate for others, their lives will not have been in vain" (pp. 56–57).

The second example is current and is a preventive intervention program that also illustrates leverage beyond the I-P relationship. Early Head Start is a national program in the United States born from a political–social awareness that many children living in circumstances of extreme poverty were unable to make gains from existing preschool opportunities; in particular, the preventive intervention activities of Head Start were often considered "too late" for such children. A 0–3 program was therefore conceptualized (U.S. Department of Health & Human Services, 1994) and, soon after the first wave of local Early Head Start programs were funded, a multisite national randomized control trial (RCT) was begun at 17 of the initial 64 sites. The idea was to determine whether new Early Head Start local programs could be successful and, if so, how they worked. The experimental trial was also bold, because usually one does not set up an RCT for evaluating first-ever new programs, let alone those that are varied due to different community needs, circumstances, and available resources. From the perspective of the present chapter, we would say that leverage points varied across programs but none centered solely or primarily on a single intervention influence on the P-C relationship. All did, however, have interventions designed to enhance child development by relationship activities of more than one staff member, and interventions were designed to enhance both parents' participation and parents' education related to their child's development. All programs also provided services to families and links to community relationships thought to be helpful. From our perspective, we could say that all programs attempted to enhance the positive development of the P-C relationship but approaches as well as the degree of specific attention to this goal varied. Some programs emphasized home visiting, others were center based, and others had elements of both approaches.

Results of the RCT involving some 3,000 families enrolled in this study were recently reported (Love et al., 2002). Significant positive impacts from Early Head Start programs were found in cognitive, language, and socioemotional development observed at both 2 and 3 years of age. There were also positive impacts at these ages in parenting, based on observations of P-C interactions and on parental self-reports. Impacts were stronger in programs independently evaluated as more fully implementing Head Start's performance standards (i.e., standards providing guidelines for quality of intervention services and continuous improvement) and in those programs that had home visiting as well as center components. Although impacts occurred across domains and demographic groups, effect sizes were modest (some 10–20%), with impacts larger in some of the subgroup analyses (e.g., 50%). The children of this study are now being evaluated at 5 years of age prior to kindergarten entry, and there is need for longitudinal study since impacting readiness to learn and socioemotional regulation for school are goals of this early intervention.

The lessons that can be learned from these two examples are many. We will mention just two.

The first is that opportunistic leverage points for successful interventions will vary, according to the parameters we mentioned. Skeels used his administrative–social opportunities, the motivational opportunities seen in the institutionalized women, and his resources at hand to generate an intervention wherein there could be salutary influences of relationships on relationships. The retarded woman–child relationship influenced the child's internalized relationships and in turn the child's developing relationships with others. Early Head Start used the national political–social opportunities, the motivations of local Head Start and other community child development leaders, as well as the resources of federal funding to generate an intervention wherein there could be multiple leverage points of relationships influencing other relationships. These included those that would influence the P-C relationship and the child's development in relation to others.

The second lesson learned concerns the importance of a longitudinal developmental perspective. The Skeels follow-up, with its dramatic results, provides value that is self-evident. The Early Head Start national program was motivated in part to improve children's readiness for school and the value of longitudinal follow up also seems self evident. Egeland and Erickson (Chapter 9, this volume) describe how the RCT of the initial STEEP program did not yield impacts on P-C attachment as assessed at 13 or 19 months, but there are strong reasons to continue follow-up of these children and their families as each child develops further. Positive effects on children may not become apparent until later. The initial positive effects Egeland and Erikson describe for parents may not yield demonstrable preventive impacts on child maltreatment (a major rationale for their program) until later. But there is now a more evidence-based reason (and we might say urgency) for longitudinal study of such early preventive interventions. Favorable longer-term effects of such programs may be pervasive and may occur in the domain of conduct. Two center-based programs originally designed with a preschool child education focus for children living in circumstances of poverty revealed such findings. As Brooks-Gunn (2003) reviewed in a recent *Social Policy Report of the Society for Research in Child Development*, both the Perry Preschool Program (see, e.g., Schweinhart, Barnes, & Weikart, 1993) and the Abecedarian Project (see Campbell & Ramey, 1994) found reductions in school dropout rates and teenage parenting rates, and the former program, in a follow-up into young adulthood, found a reduction in juvenile delinquency and crime. The results of another longitudinal study, involving a 15-year follow-up after a carefully done RCT, are even more revealing. The early intervention consisted of a program of nurse home visitation that took place during pregnancy and throughout the child's first two postnatal years (Olds et al., 1998). The reported follow-up is from the earliest RCT of three such studies of David Olds and colleagues and involves 315 children. In addition to the long-term impacts on their mothers (less welfare dependency, child maltreatment, criminality, and use of adverse substances), there were conduct effects on the children who were now adolescents. The children who had been born to unmarried mothers in low-socioeconomic-status households had fewer incidents of running away, fewer arrests, fewer convictions, fewer sex partners, and less use of cigarettes and alcohol; in addition, parents reported these children had fewer behavioral problems (Olds et al., 1998). One would have every reason to expect that more current early preventive intervention programs, giving emphasis to enhancing relationship building and socioemotional regulation such as STEEP and Early Head Start could, over time, have even more favorable influence on conduct regulation.

CONCLUSIONS

The interventions described in this book are deemed useful by those clinicians and their clients who are benefiting from them. Consistent with the goals of the book as set forth by Sameroff in Chapter 1, the other chapters have advanced a description of the "how" aspects of these interventions such that readers can understand their separate qualities, much about their workings or processes, as well as their "theories of change." We can also appreciate that, as McDonough emphasizes in Chapter 4, various approaches may supplement one another.

It seems highly unlikely, however, that all or even most approaches would be appropriate in any given circumstance. It seems equally unlikely that one could count on a "spillover effect" of relationships continuing to favorably influence other relationships, either represented or interacted. Instead, what seems likely is that successful interventions will occur when there is a matching of interests, concerns, resources and planned activities among participants. From a systems perspective, as advanced by Sameroff in Chapter 1, parts of interdependent systems can change but there needs to be openness to change in order for salutary effects to occur. We can remind ourselves that a core aspect of disorder is its resistance to change, or (to put it another way) its inflexibility or its lack of ability to make adaptive change in the midst of new circumstances. Thus from a psychodynamic point of view neuroses are understood as closed systems (Emde, 1980) and Fraiberg's ghosts in the nursery as representations that are in limbo, continuing to haunt (Fraiberg, 1980; Fraiberg et al., 1975).

It is with these considerations that we have introduced the concept of leverage—of identifying the best opportunities for engaging therapeutic or preventive change in a relationship that is embedded in a network of other relationships. In infant–parent psychotherapy (or, as we prefer to think of it, intervenor–parent influencing parent–child relationship therapy) Fraiberg was correct: the infant's rapid development, if it is appreciated, acts as an enormous incentive for development in the parent, the parenting relationship, and beyond.

This is all a background for the fascinating approaches described in this book. What we need now is more research. We need research to compare and contrast different approaches in different populations, to see what works for whom and in what circumstances, to describe and document best leverage points, and to understand outcomes not only for the child and parent but across a network of relationships. Can some approaches more than others influence salutary relationships in the family and community? Can some more than others have longer-term salutary influences on individual development and relationships? Training and research manuals for many of these approaches are becoming available, and we anticipate that additional empirical trials will take place. And, optimistically, we can anticipate longitudinal study and follow-up of these interventions. It is in the potential influences of early interventions across generations of parenting, and across a cascade of longitudinally developing relationships, that many of the interventions described in this book may have their most profound impacts.

REFERENCES

Adoption and Safe Families Act of 1997, PL 105-89, 42 U.S.C. 670 *et seq.*, 111 Stat. 2115–2135.

American Psychiatric Association. (1994). *Diagnostic and statistical manual of mental disorders* (4th ed.). Washington, DC: Author.

Bowlby, J. (1944). Forty-four juvenile thieves: Their characters and home life. *International Journal of Psycho-Analysis, 25,* 19–52, 107–127.

Bowlby, J. (1958). The nature of the child's tie to his mother. *International Journal of Psycho-Analysis, 39,* 350–373.

Bowlby, J. (1969). *Attachment and loss: Vol. 1. Attachment*. New York: Basic Books.

Bowlby, J. (1988). Developmental psychiatry comes of age. *American Journal of Psychiatry, 145*(1), 1–10.

Brazelton, T. B. (1992). *Touchpoints: Your child's emotional and behavioral development*. Reading, MA: Addison-Wesley.

Brooks-Gunn, J. (2003). Do you believe in magic?: What we can expect from early childhood intervention programs. *Social Policy Report of the Society for Research in Child Development, 17*, 1–14.

Campbell, F. A., & Ramey, C. T. (1994). Effects of early intervention on intellectual and academic achievement: A follow-up study of children from low-income families. *Child Development, 65*, 684–698.

Christensen, M., Emde R. N., & Fleming, C. (in press). Cultural perspectives for assessing infants and young children. In R. Del Carmen & A. Carter (Eds.), *Handbook of infant and toddler mental health assessment*. Oxford, UK: Oxford University Press.

Cicchetti, D., & Cannon, T. D. (1999). Neurodevelopmental processes in the ontogenesis and epigenesis of psychopathology [Special issue]. *Development and Psychopathology, 11*(3), 375–393.

Cicchetti, D., & Toth, S. L. (1995). A developmental psychopathology perspective on child abuse and neglect. *Journal of the American Academy of Child and Adolescent Psychiatry, 34*(5), 541–565.

Cordeiro, M. J., Caldeira da Silva, P., & Goldschmidt, T. (2003). Diagnostic classification: Results from a clinical experience of three years with DC: 0–3. *Infant Mental Health Journal, 24*(4), 349–364.

Emde, R. N. (1980). A developmental orientation in psychoanalysis: Ways of thinking about new knowledge and further research. *Psychoanalysis and Contemporary Thought, 3*(2), 213–235.

Emde, R. N. (1990). Mobilizing fundamental modes of development: An essay on empathic availability and therapeutic action. *Journal of the American Psychoanalytic Association, 38*(4), 881–913.

Emde, R. N. (1991). The wonder of our complex enterprise: Steps enabled by attachment and the effects of relationships on relationships. *Infant Mental Health Journal, 12*(3), 163–172.

Emde, R. N. (1998). Early emotional development: new modes of thinking for research and intervention. *Pediatrics, 102*(5, Suppl. E), 1236–1243.

Emde, R. N., & Robinson, J. L. (2000). Guiding principles for a theory of early intervention: A developmental–psychoanalytic perspective. In J. P. Shonkoff & S. J. Meisels (Eds.), *Handbook of early childhood intervention* (pp. 160–178). New York: Cambridge University Press.

Emde, R. N., & Spicer, P. (2000). Experience in the midst of variation: New horizons for development and psychopathology. *Development and Psychopathology, 12*(3), 313–331.

Emde, R. N., & Wise, B. K. (2003). The cup is half-full: Initial clinical trials of

DC: 0–3 and a recommendation for revision. *Infant Mental Health Journal,* 24(4), 437–447.

Erikson, E. (1950). *Childhood and society.* New York: Norton.

Everhart, K., & Wandersman, A. (2000). Applying comprehensive quality programming and empowerment evaluation to reduce implementation barriers. *Journal of Educational and Psychological Consultation, 11*(2), 177–191.

Fraiberg, S. (1980). *Clinical studies in infant mental health.* New York: Basic Books.

Fraiberg, S., Adelson, E., & Shapiro, V. (1975). Ghosts in the nursery: A psychoanalytic approach to the problems of impaired infant–mother relationships. *Journal of American Academy of Child Psychiatry, 14*(3), 387–421.

Freud, A. (1965). *Normality and pathology in childhood: assessments of development.* New York: International Universities Press.

Freud, S. (1920). Beyond the pleasure principle. In J. Strachey (Ed. & Trans.), *The standard edition of the complete psychological works of Sigmund Freud* (Vol. 18, pp. 7–64). London: Hogarth Press.

Garcia Coll, C., & Magnuson, K. (2000). Cultural differences as sources of developmental vulnerabilities and resources. In J. P. Shonkoff & S. J. Meisels (Eds.), *Handbook of early childhood intervention* (2nd ed., pp. 94–114). New York: Cambridge University Press.

Guedeney, N., Guedeney, A., Rabouam, C., Mintz, A. S., Danon, G., Huet, M. M., & Jacquemain, F. (2003). The zero to three diagnostic classification: A contribution to the validation of the classification from a sample of 85 under-threes. *Infant Mental Health Journal, 24*(4), 313–316.

Hofer, M. (1981). *The roots of human behavior.* San Francisco: Freeman.

Johnson-Powell, G. (1997). The culturologic interview: Cultural, social, and linguistic issues in the assessment and treatment of children. In G. Johnson-Powell & J. Yamamoto (Eds.) & G. E. Wyatt & W. Arroyo (Associated Eds.), *Transcultural child development* (pp. 349–364). New York: Wiley.

Keren, M., Feldman, R., & Tyano, S. (2001). Diagnoses and interactive patterns of infants referred to a community-based infant mental health clinic. *Journal of the American Academy of Child and Adolescent Psychiatry, 40,* 27–39.

Keren, M., Feldman, R., & Tyano, S. (2003). A five-year Israeli experience with the DC: 0–3 classification system. *Infant Mental Health Journal, 24*(4), 337–348.

Lewis, M. L. (2000). The cultural context of infant mental health: The developmental niche of infant–caregiver relationships. In C. H. Zeanah (Ed.), *Handbook of infant mental health* (2nd ed., pp. 91–107). New York: Guilford Press.

Loewald, H. W. (1960). On the therapeutic action of psycho-analysis. *International Journal of Psycho-Analysis, 41,* 16–33.

Love, J. M., Kisker, E. E., Ross, C. M., Schochet, P. Z., Brooks-Gunn, J., Paulsell, D., Boller, K., Constantine, J., Vogel, C., Fuligni, A. S., & Brady-

Smith, C. (2002). *Making a difference in the lives of infants and toddlers and their families: The impacts of Early Head Start.* Washington, DC: U.S. Department of Health & Human Services.

Maldonado-Duran, M., Helmig, L., Moody, C., Fonagy, P., Fulz, J., Lartigue, T., Sauceda-Garcia, J. M., Karacostas, V., Millhuff, C., & Glinka, J. (2003). The zero to three diagnostic classification in an infant mental health clinic: Its usefulness and challenges. *Infant Mental Health Journal, 24*(4), 378–397.

Minde, K., & Tidmarsh, L. (1997). The changing practices of an infant psychiatry program: the McGill experience. *Infant Mental Health Journal, 18*(2), 135–144.

Olds, D., Henderson, C. R.,Jr., Cole, R., Eckenrode, J., Kitzman, H., Luckey, D., Pettitt, L., Sidora, K., Morris, P., & Powers, J. (1998). Long-term effects of nurse home visitation on children's criminal and antisocial behavior: 15–year follow-up of a randomized controlled trial. *JAMA (Journal of the American Medical Association, 280*(14), 1238–1244.

Quinton, D., Rutter, M., & Liddle, C. (1984). Institutional rearing, parenting difficulties and marital support. *Psychological Medicine, 14*(1), 107–124.

Rutter, M. (2000). Resilience reconsidered: Conceptual consideration, empirical findings, and policy implications. In J. P. Shonkoff & S. J. Meisels (Eds.), *Handbook of early childhood intervention* (pp. 651–682). New York: Cambridge University Press.

Rutter, M. (2002). Nature, nurture, and development: From evangelism through science toward policy and practice. *Child Development, 73*(1), 1–21.

Sameroff, A. J., & Emde, R. N. (Eds.). (1989). *Relationship disturbances in early childhood: A developmental approach.* New York: Basic Books.

Sameroff, A. J., & Fiese, B. H. (2000). Transactional regulation: The developmental ecology of early intervention. In J. P. Shonkoff & S. J. Meisels (Eds.), *Handbook of early childhood intervention* (pp. 135–159). New York: Cambridge University Press.

Schweinhart, L. J., Barnes, H., & Weikart, D. (1993). *Significant benefits: The High/Scope Perry Preschool Study through age 27* (Monograph of the High/Scope Educational Research Foundation, No. 10). Ypsilanti, MI: High/Scope Educational Research Foundation.

Shonkoff, J. P., & Phillips, D. A. (2000). *From neurons to neighborhoods: The science of early childhood development.* Washington DC: National Academy Press.

Skeels, H. M. (1966). Adult status of children with contrasting early life experiences: A follow-up study. *Monographs of the Society for Research in Child Development, 31*(3, Serial No. 105), 1–65.

Spitz, R. A. (1945). Hospitalism: An inquiry into the genesis of psychiatric conditions in early childhood. *Psychoanalytic Study of the Child, 1*, 53–74.

Spitz, R. A. (1946). Hospitalism: A follow-up report on investigation described in Volume I, 1945. *Psychoanalytic Study of the Child, 2*, 113–117.

Spitz, R. A. (1959). *A genetic field theory of ego formation*. New York: International Universities Press.

Spitz, R. A. (1961). Some early prototypes of ego defenses. *Journal of the American Psychoanalytic Association, 9*, 626–251.

Spitz, R. A. (1965). *The first year of life*. New York: International Universities Press.

Stern, D. N. (1985). *The interpersonal world of the infant*. New York: Basic Books.

U.S. Department of Health and Human Services. (1994, September). *The statement of the Advisory Committee on Services for Families with Infants and Toddlers*. Washington, DC: Author.

Von Eye, A., & Kreppner, K. (1989). Family systems and family development: The selection of analytical units. In K. Kreppner & R. Lerner (Eds.), *Family systems and life span development* (pp. 247–269). Hillsdale, NJ: Erlbaum.

Waddington, C. H. (1940). *Organizers and genes*. Cambridge, UK: Cambridge University Press.

Winnicott, D. [O.] (1965). *The maturational processes and the facilitating environment*. New York: International Universities Press; London: Hogarth Press.

Winnicott, D. O. (1971). *Playing and reality*. New York: Basic Books.

Zero to Three/National Center for Infants, Toddlers, & Families. (1994). *DC: Zero to three (diagnostic classification of mental health and developmental disorders of infancy and early childhood)*. Washington, DC: Author.

INDEX